Lung Cancer - Modern Multidisciplinary Management

Edited by Henry S. Park

Published in London, United Kingdom

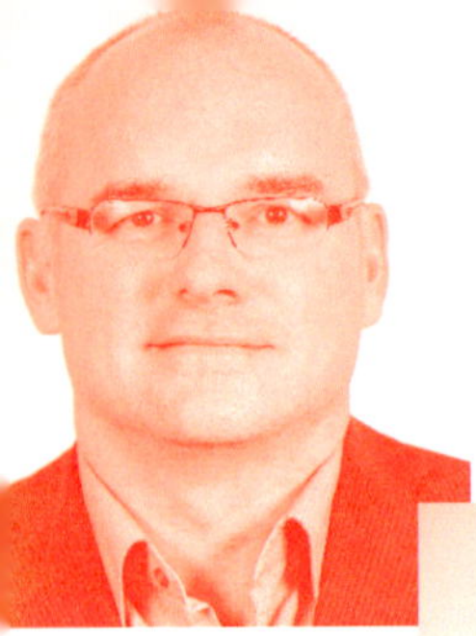
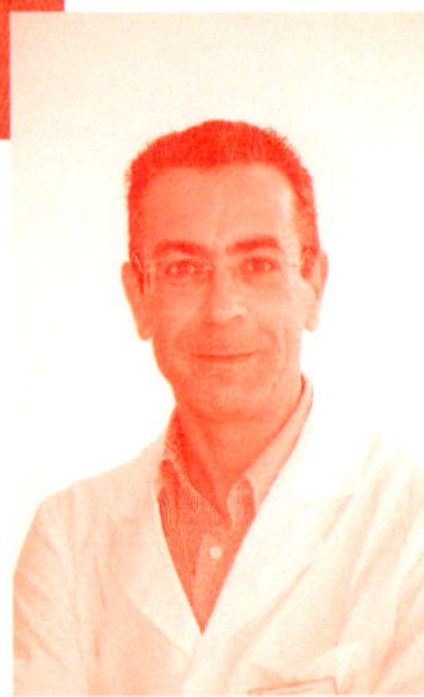
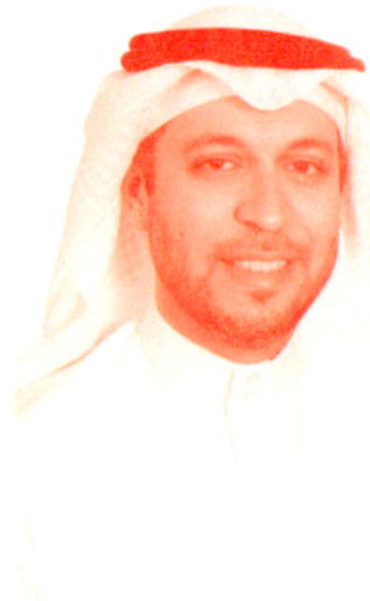
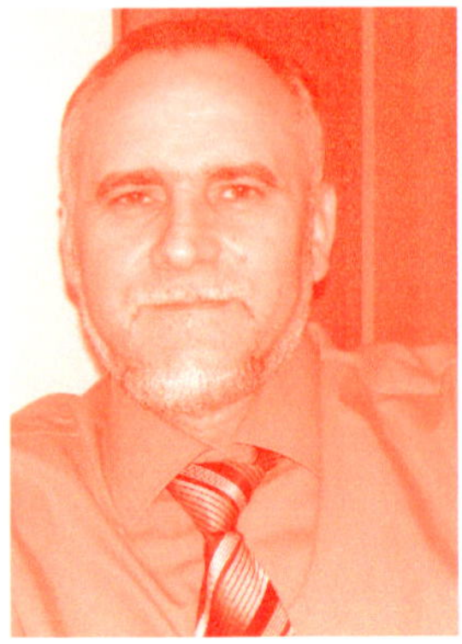
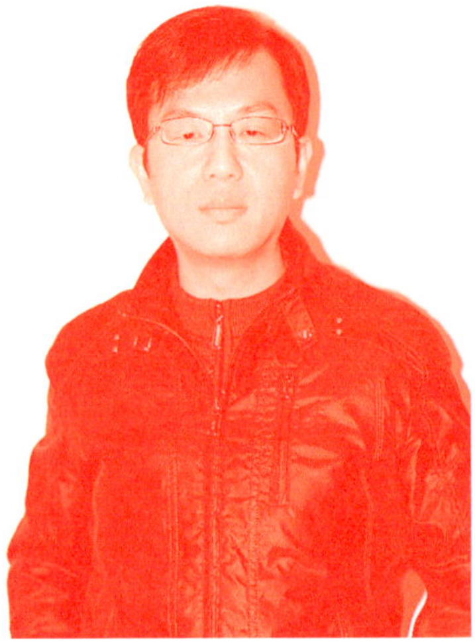
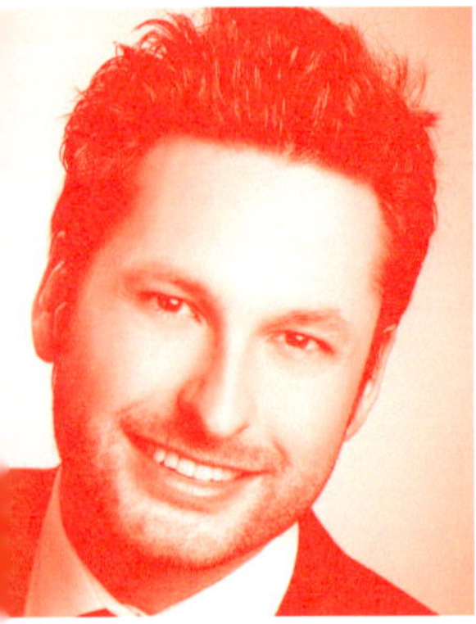
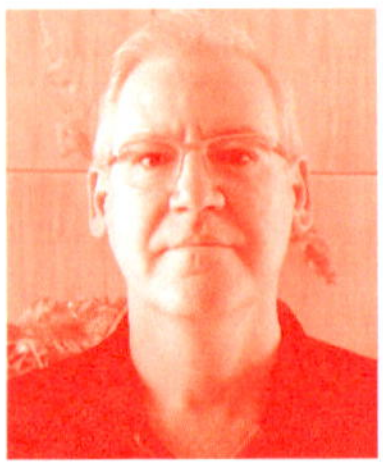

IntechOpen

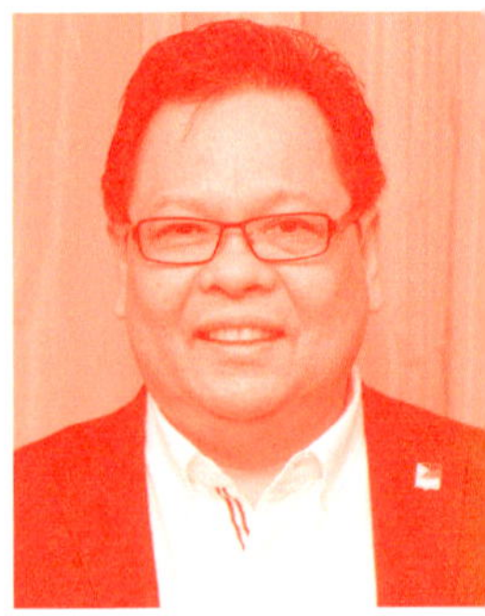
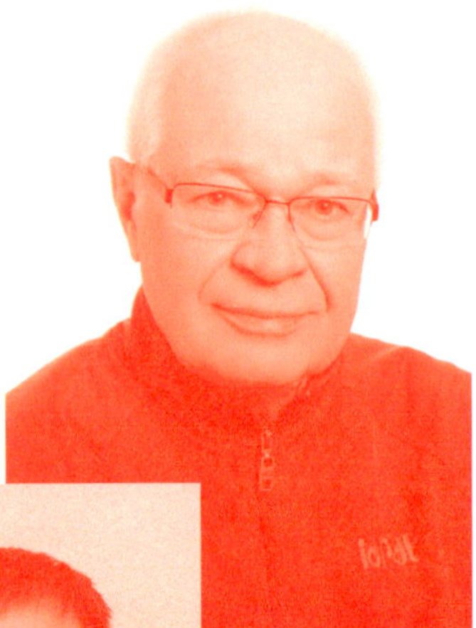
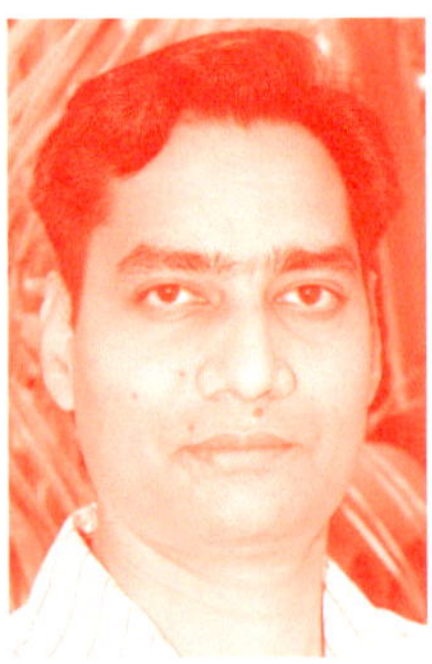
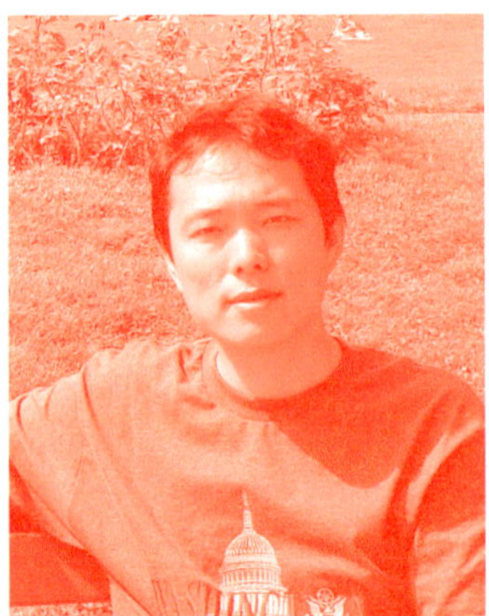
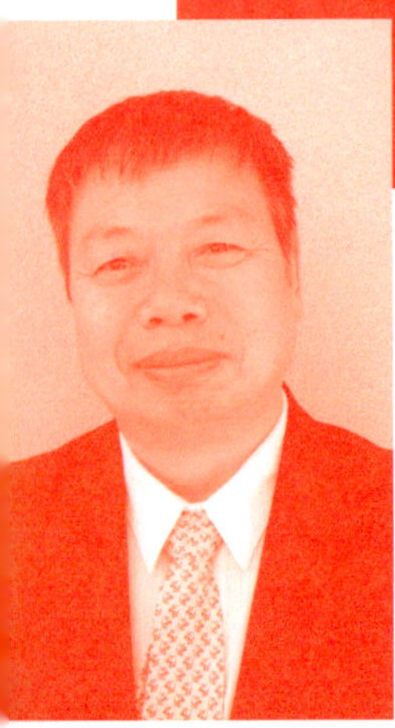
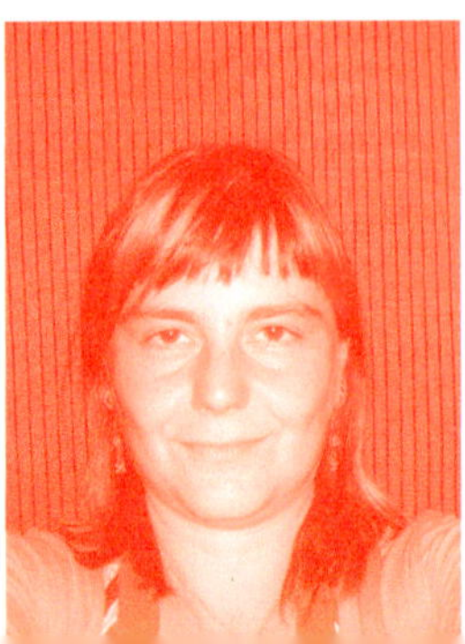

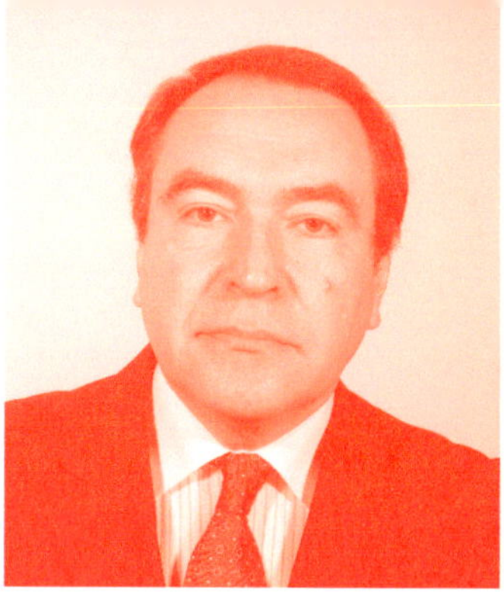
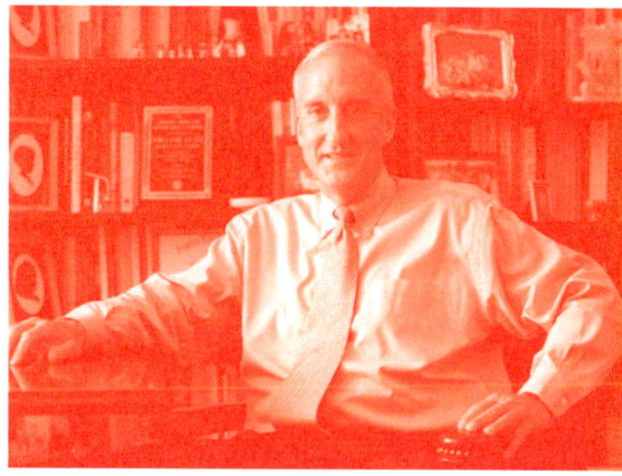
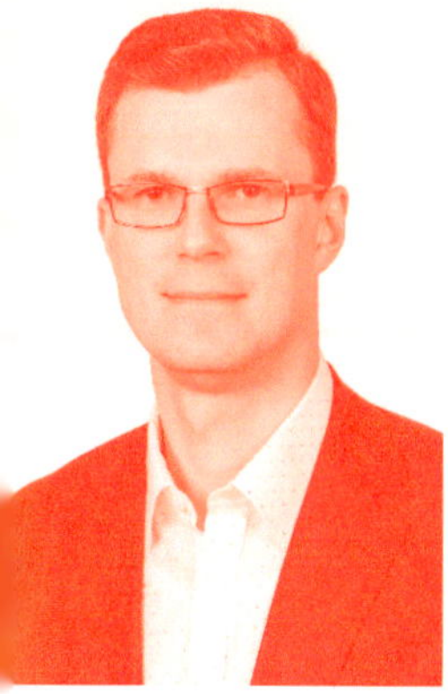
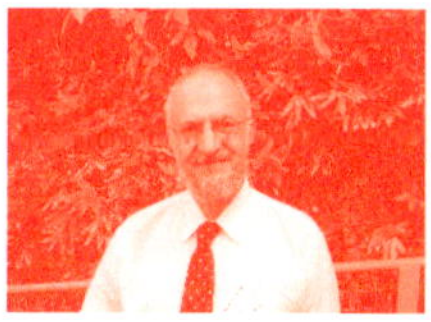
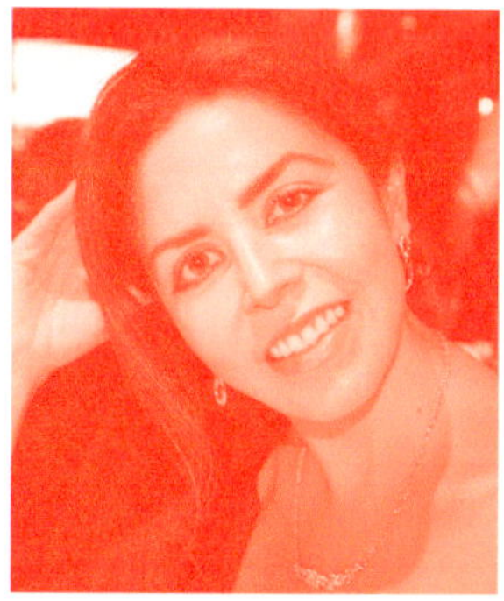

Supporting open minds since 2005

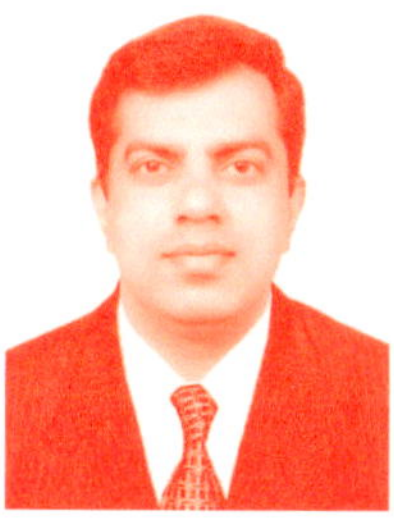
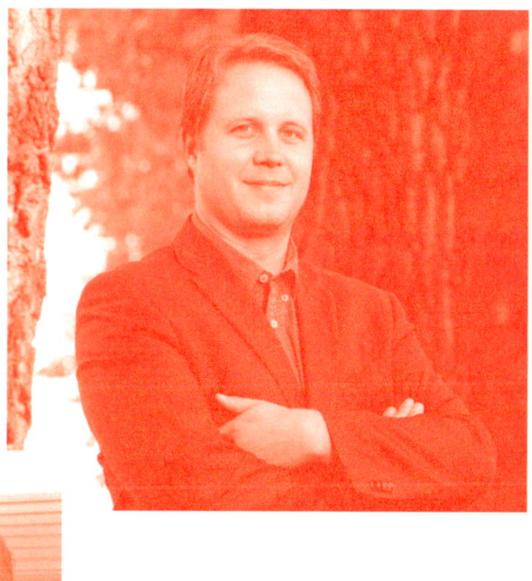
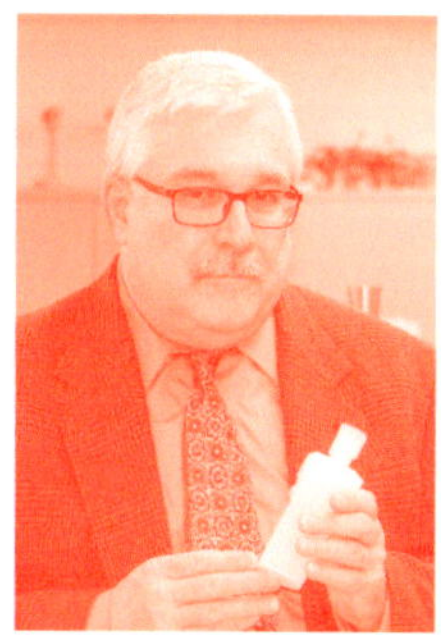
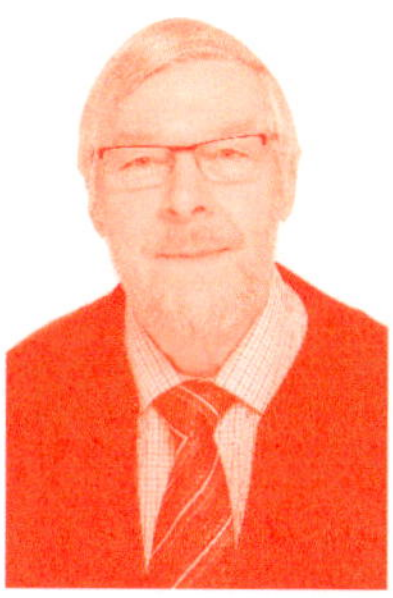
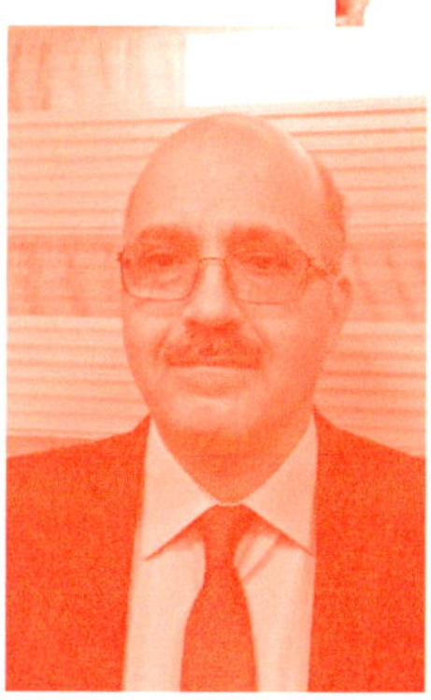
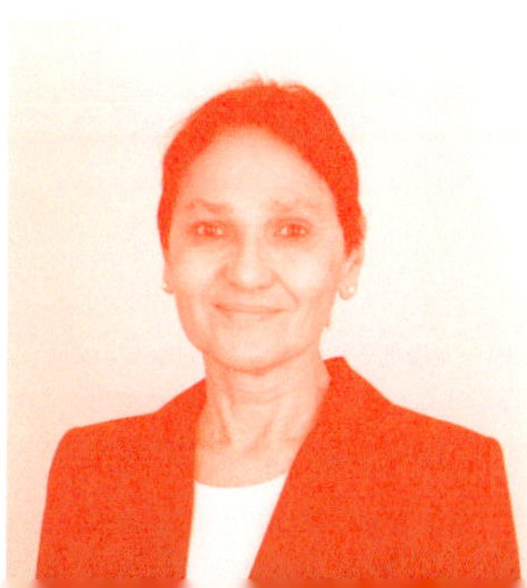
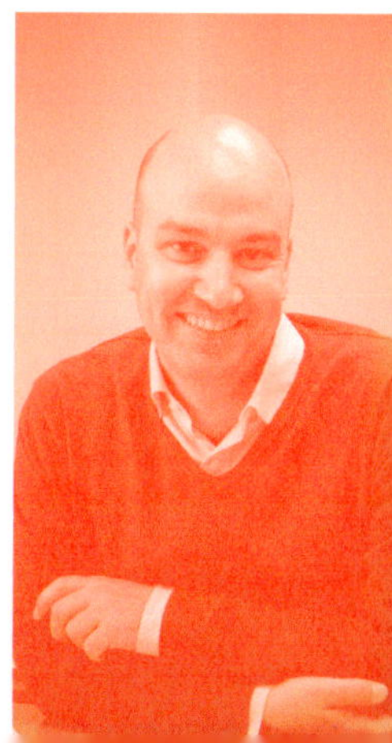

Lung Cancer - Modern Multidisciplinary Management
http://dx.doi.org/10.5772/intechopen.92053
Edited by Henry S. Park

Contributors
Joyce W.Y. Chan, Rainbow W.H. Lau, Calvin S.H. Ng, Hiroshi Doi, Kozo Kuribayashi, Beatrice Aramini, Valentina Masciale, Federico Banchelli, Roberto D'Amico, Massimo Dominici, Khawaja Husnain Haider, Paul Van Houtte, Charlier Florian, Luigi Moretti, Dirk Van Gestel, Martina Vrankar, Henry S. Park, Milad Rasouli, Nadia Fallah, Kostya (Ken) Ostrikov, Peter Ping Ping Lin, Justin Blasberg, Andrew Li, Guntug Batihan, Ana C. Belzarena, Kenan Can Ceylan

First published in London, United Kingdom, 2021 by IntechOpen
IntechOpen is the global imprint of INTECHOPEN LIMITED, registered in England and Wales, registration number: 11086078, 5 Princes Gate Court, London, SW7 2QJ, United Kingdom
Printed in Croatia

British Library Cataloguing-in-Publication Data
A catalogue record for this book is available from the British Library

Additional hard and PDF copies can be obtained from orders@intechopen.com

Lung Cancer - Modern Multidisciplinary Management
Edited by Henry S. Park
p. cm.
Print ISBN 978-1-78985-575-3
Online ISBN 978-1-78985-576-0
eBook (PDF) ISBN 978-1-78985-638-5

For EU product safety concerns:
IN TECH d.o.o., Prolaz Marije Krucifikse Kozulić 3, 51000 Rijeka, Croatia, info@intechopen.com or visit our website at intechopen.com.

Meet the editor

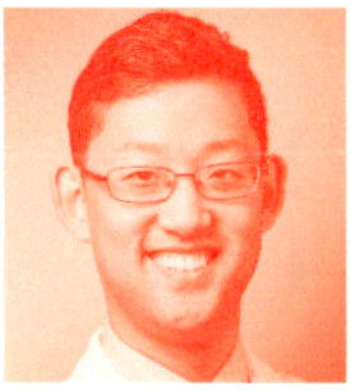

Henry Soo-Min Park, MD, MPH, is a board-certified radiation oncologist who currently serves as Assistant Professor of Therapeutic Radiology and Chief of Thoracic Radiotherapy at the Yale School of Medicine. He also serves as the department's Director of Continuing Medical Education, the Medical Student Clerkship, and the Yale Radiation Oncology Consortium e(focusing on comparative effectiveness and health services research), as well as associate director of the residency program. Dr. Park received his undergraduate degree from Yale College, master's degree from Harvard School of Public Health, and MD from Yale School of Medicine. He completed his internal medicine internship at Harvard Medical School's Beth Israel Deaconess Medical Center and returned to Yale New Haven Hospital for his residency and chief residency in radiation oncology.

Contents

Preface

Lung cancer management has undergone revolutionary changes in recent years. This book introduces the reader to some of the most relevant and exciting advances in the field. The book begins with a discussion of minimally invasive surgical techniques followed by a review of the progress in nonoperative therapies like radiotherapy and ablation. Next, the book examines systemic therapy that has moved well beyond standard cytotoxic chemotherapy and that can often be combined with local therapies even for metastatic disease. Finally, the book presents several newer diagnostic and therapeutic tools that have not yet become mainstream.

This book is dedicated to patients with lung cancer who have contributed to the acquisition and consolidation of knowledge by consenting to data collection through clinical trials or registries. By comprehensively reviewing the most impactful innovations of the modern era, we hope to inspire you to imagine what might be possible in the near future.

Henry S. Park, MD, MPH
Department of Therapeutic Radiology,
Yale School of Medicine,
New Haven, CT, USA

Section 1

Introduction

Chapter 1

Introductory Chapter: Recent Progress in Lung Cancer Treatment - The Value of Multiple Perspectives

Henry Soo-Min Park

1. Introduction

The remarkable advances in lung cancer management that we have witnessed in the past two decades did not arise in a vacuum. Surgeons, radiation oncologists, medical oncologists, pulmonologists, palliative care specialists, radiologists, pathologists, laboratory scientists, and patients have long collaborated to make the vision of improved cure rates, survival, and quality-of-life a reality.

2. Surgery

Minimally invasive surgery (MIS) has altered the landscape of thoracic surgery. Thoracotomies had been standard-of-care for lung cancer resections until the advent of video-assisted thoracoscopic surgery in the mid-1990s. While initially utilized primarily for patients with favorable anatomy and good pulmonary function, this has been increasingly adopted for use in more frail patients with more technically challenging anatomy [1]. Robotic-assisted thoracoscopic surgery was approved in the early-2000s with the help of even more sophisticated technology that imitated the manual dexterity of an open procedure.

With both approaches, there were initial concerns that there would be higher rates of complications as well as margin-positive resections that could translate into more intensive adjuvant regimens or poorer survival outcomes. Both techniques have substantial learning curves, but surgeons and centers gradually accumulated experience and increased the proportion of patients who underwent surgeries with a minimally invasive approach. Over a relatively short period of time, adoption of MIS has led to improved perioperative outcomes like pain, complications, length of hospital stay, and in-hospital costs without compromising oncologic outcomes [2, 3]. Not only has MIS allowed surgical patients to regain independence sooner than they would have otherwise, but also patients who may have not previously considered surgery due to the risk of morbidity might now be candidates for this potentially curative modality.

3. Radiotherapy and other ablative therapies

Nonsurgical local approaches have also expanded in scope due to developments in technology. Radiotherapy can now be administered with exceptional accuracy

IntechOpen

and precision despite physiologic lung motion. This is largely due to improvements in image-guidance, 4-dimensional motion management, and beam modulation approaches that allow for higher biologically effective doses to the target, less scatter doses to normal organs, and more convenient treatment schedules.

Due to these advances, more ablative doses were made possible in the form of stereotactic body radiotherapy (SBRT), also known as stereotactic ablative body radiotherapy. Since its development in the mid-2000s, SBRT has been proven to be a valid alternative to surgical resection in early-stage disease, showing local control in the 90–98% range at 3–5 years with acceptable toxicity [4, 5]. SBRT has also been increasingly utilized in oligometastatic and oligoprogressive disease, with survival benefits demonstrated when used as consolidative therapy after systemic therapy [6, 7].

For inoperable locoregionally advanced non-small cell lung cancer, fractionated radiotherapy has been traditionally combined with chemotherapy with curative intent. With improved knowledge on appropriate radiotherapy dosing and the advent of consolidative immunotherapy, we can achieve better outcomes than we have ever seen before [8, 9]. Furthermore, image-guided ablative therapies like radiofrequency ablation, microwave ablation, and cryoablation have a wide range of potential indications. They can be particularly effective in situations that are not amenable to surgical or radiotherapeutic interventions due to safety concerns.

4. Systemic therapy

For more advanced disease, precision medicine has greatly expanded in its ability to address specific mutations and biomarkers with customized combinations of chemotherapy, targeted therapy, and immunotherapy. Drugs can now specifically target mutations like EGFR and ALK, effectively controlling even the most widespread metastases. Outcomes have continued to improve with refinements in successive generations of these agents [10, 11]. In addition, immunotherapy has been successfully used as monotherapy for patients with PD-L1 expressing tumors [12], or added to chemotherapy for patients with high, low, and no PD-L1 expression [13]. This has led to standard treatment regimens for most patients with stage IV non-small cell lung cancer. These combinations have also extended to extensive-stage small cell lung cancer, with the addition of concurrent and maintenance immunotherapy representing the first major pharmacologic advance in the upfront treatment of this disease in several decades [14, 15].

Even for tumors that develop resistance to initial therapies, novel blood-based and tissue-based diagnostic testing can help clinicians formulate a truly personalized approach to oncologic management, leading to the possibility of long-term survival that was unimaginable even a decade ago. Combining these systemic therapies with local therapies in the oligometastatic and oligoprogressive setting has led to unique regimens that have dramatically altered disease trajectories.

5. Palliative care

Palliative management of bone metastases has improved due to enhanced patient selection algorithms and surgical stabilization techniques by orthopedic surgeons and neurosurgeons, in addition to the judicious use of radiotherapy. Brain metastasis management has also evolved through increased utilization of upfront stereotactic radiosurgery [16] rather than whole-brain radiotherapy, mitigating potential cognitive effects without a survival detriment [17]. Furthermore, integration of early palliative care for patients with advanced lung cancers has also contributed not only to improved quality-of-life, but also to survival [18].

6. Future directions and conclusions

Moving forward, utilization of cutting-edge technologies like circulating tumor biomarkers, machine learning, gas plasma, and nanotechnology may offer exciting new opportunities in screening, diagnosis, and therapy. While these may be in earlier stages of development than more standard modalities, they represent promising avenues for research and clinical application.

If the inspirational innovations discussed in this chapter are any indication, the future of personalized care for patients with lung cancer is exciting.

Author details

Henry Soo-Min Park
Department of Therapeutic Radiology, Yale School of Medicine,
New Haven, Connecticut, United States of America

*Address all correspondence to: henry.park@yale.edu

References

[1] McKenna RJ Jr. Lobectomy by video-assisted thoracic surgery with mediastinal node sampling for lung cancer. J Thorac Cardiovasc Surg 1994;107:879-882.

[2] Park HS, Detterbeck FC, Boffa DJ, Kim AW. Impact of hospital volume of thoracoscopic lobectomy on primary lung cancer outcomes. Ann Thorac Surg 2012;93(2):372-379.

[3] Tchouta LN, Park HS, Boffa DJ, et al. Hospital volume and outcomes of robot-assisted lobectomies. Chest 2017;151(2):329-339.

[4] Timmerman R, Paulus R, Galvin J, et al. Stereotactic body radiation therapy for inoperable early stage lung cancer. JAMA 2010;303(11):1070-1076.

[5] Timmerman RD, Hu C, Michalski JM, et al. Long-term results of stereotactic body radiation therapy in medially inoperable stage I non-small cell lung cancer. JAMA Oncol 2018;4(9):1287-1288.

[6] Gomez DR, Tang C, Zhang J, et al. Local consolidative therapy vs. maintenance therapy or observation for patients with oligometastatic non-small-cell lung cancer: long-term results of a multi-institutional, phase II, randomized study. J Clin Oncol 2019;37(18):1558-1565.

[7] Palma DA, Olson R, Harrow S, et al. Stereotactic ablative radiotherapy versus standard of care palliative treatment in patients with oligometastatic cancers (SABR-COMET): a randomized, phase 2, open-label trial. Lancet 2019;393(10185):2051-2058.

[8] Antonia SJ, Villegas A, Daniel D, et al. Overall survival with durvalumab after chemoradiotherapy in stage III NSCLC. N Engl J Med 2018;379:2342-2350.

[9] Faivre-Finn C, Vicente D, Kurata T, et al. Four-year survival with durvalumab after chemoradiotherapy in stage III NSCLC – an update from the PACIFIC trial. J Thorac Oncol 2021;Epub ahead of print.

[10] Ramalingam SS, Vansteenkiste J, Planchard D, et al. Overall survival with osimertinib in untreated, EGFR-mutated advanced NSCLC. N Engl J Med 2020;382(1):41-50.

[11] Camidge DR, Dziadziuszko R, Peters S, et al. Updated efficacy and safety data and impact of the EML4-ALK fusion variant on the efficacy of alectinib in untreated ALK-positive advanced non-small cell lung cancer in the global phase III ALEX study. J Thorac Oncol 2019;14(7):1233-1243.

[12] Mok TS, Wu YL, Kudaba I, et al. Pembrolizumab versus chemotherapy for previously untreated, PD-L1-expressing, locally advanced or metastatic non-small-cell lung cancer (KEYNOTE-042): a randomised, open-label, controlled, phase 3 trial. Lancet 2019;393(10183):1819-1830.

[13] Gandhi L, Rodriguez-Abreu D, Gadgeel S, et al. Pembrolizumab plus chemotherapy in metastatic non–small-cell lung cancer. N Engl J Med 2018;378:2078-2092.

[14] Horn L, Mansfield AS, Szczesna A, et al. First-line atezolizumab plus chemotherapy in extensive-stage small-cell lung cancer. N Engl J Med 2018;379:2220-2229.

[15] Paz-Ares L, Dvorkin M, Chen Y, et al. Durvalumab plus platinum–etoposide versus platinum–etoposide in first-line treatment of extensive-stage small-cell lung cancer (CASPIAN): a randomised, controlled, open-label, phase 3 trial. Lancet 2019;394(10212): 1929-1939.

[16] Kann BH, Park HS, Johnson SB, et al. Radiosurgery for brain metastases: changing practice patterns and disparities in the United States. J Natl Compr Canc Netw 2017;15(12): 1494-1502.

[17] Brown PD, Jaeckle K, Ballman KV, et al. Effect of radiosurgery alone vs radiosurgery with whole brain radiation therapy on cognitive function in patients with 1 to 3 brain metastases: a randomized clinical trial. JAMA 2016;316(4):401-409.

[18] Temel JS, Greer JA, Muzikansky A, et al. Early palliative care for patients with metastatic non–small-cell lung cancer. N Engl J Med 2010;363:733-742.

Section 2

Surgical Advances

Chapter 2

The Role of Minimally Invasive Surgery in the Treatment of Lung Cancer

Güntuğ Batihan and Kenan Can Ceylan

Abstract

Lobectomy plus regional lymph node dissection remains the gold standard treatment method in early-stage lung cancer. However, with the demonstration of the safety and efficacy of minimally invasive approaches, the expression of surgery in this statement, replaced by thoracoscopic anatomical lung resection. Clinical studies have demonstrated the superiority of VATS in terms of postoperative pain, drainage time, length of hospital stay, and complications, moreover, long-term oncologic results are similar or better than thoracotomy. Therefore, VATS lobectomy is the preferred surgical method in early-stage lung cancer. Different surgical techniques are available in VATS and can be modified according to the surgeon's personal experience. Uniport can be applied as well as two or three port incisions. In this book section, I plan to focus on VATS lobectomy, technique-related tricks, complication management, and long-term oncologic results in early and locally advanced lung cancer.

Keywords: Lobectomy, minimally invasive surgery, robotic surgery, video-assisted thoracic surgery

1. Introduction

Lung cancer is the most common cancer and the leading cause of cancer death in both genders [1]. Its high frequency and high mortality increase the importance of early diagnosis and treatment in this disease. Despite promising recent advances in diagnosis and treatment methods, only a minority of patients have a cure chance. Resection of the primary tumor and mediastinal lymph node dissection/sampling is the gold standard treatment method in this group of patients. However, in these patients, lung resection was performed by open thoracotomy until the end of the '90s, regardless of the size of the tumor and the extent of cancer. Severe postoperative pain and long hospitalization and drainage periods could prolong the recovery period of the patients [2].

Following the technological developments include high-definition video monitors, robot-assisted technology, specialized thoracoscopic surgical instruments, and endomechanical stapling devices, the emergence of modern imaging systems and the use of appropriate surgical equipment has created the concept of "minimally invasive surgery". In the early 2000s, patient series including Video-assisted thoracic surgery (VATS) applications began to be published. This and many subsequent studies have demonstrated the superiority of VATS over a thoracotomy in terms of less

 IntechOpen

postoperative pain and minimize complications hasten recovery and improve postoperative quality [3–6]. With the positive results of VATS, it has found a wide application area for the diagnosis and treatment of benign and malignant lung diseases.

In this section, the role and application areas of VATS in the diagnosis and treatment of lung cancer will be discussed rather than technical details.

2. Surgical technique

Although "tubeless" or "awake" VATS has been described and performed successfully by several authors, single-lung ventilation, which may be accomplished with either double-lumen endobronchial tubes or with single-lumen tubes and bronchial blockers, is often required for thoracoscopic lobectomy [7, 8].

The patient is positioned in full lateral decubitus position with slight flexion of the table at the level of the mid-chest, which allows slight splaying of the ribs to improve exposure in the absence of rib spreading.

The instruments and surgical technique used vary according to the number, location, and width of the port incisions. Although the number of port incisions and locations are the surgeon's preference, different applications and techniques have emerged over time.

2.1 Posterior approach

The posterior approach was first described by Walker WS in 1992. The main components of this approach include [6, 9]:

- The surgeon stands posterior to the patient.
- The utility incision is made at the 6th or 7th intercostal space anterior to latissimus dorsi muscle.
- The camera port is made through the auscultatory triangle, instead of the lower anterior axillary line;
- The aim is to dissect the hilar structures from the posterior to the anterior. For this purpose, the interlobar fissure must be opened first to identify and isolate pulmonary arterial branches.

The main advantages of the posterior approach include:

- Easy access to the posterior hilum.
- Easy access to subcarinal lymph nodes.
- A clear view of the posterior hilum allows safe dissection of the segmental artery and bronchial branches.

However, the interlobar fissure is incomplete in a considerable number of patients, and fissure dissection may cause parenchymal damage and prolonged air leak in the postoperative period. If the posterior approach is preferred, the interlobar fissure should be carefully dissected. Tissue glues, absorbable patches, or fibrin sealants can be used in the repair of injuries and air leaks that may occur in the parenchyma.

2.2 Anterior approach

The anterior approach, also known as the fissureless technique, was applied firstly in open thoracotomy in 1999. The application of this technique to VATS has been described recently [10–12]. In this technique, the surgeon stands anterior to the patient, and the camera port is placed at the anterior axillary line. The hilar structures are dissected from the anterior to the posterior. After the dissection of the bronchovascular structures is completed, the interlobar fissure is divided with endoscopic staplers and the lobe is removed from the thorax.

This approach aims to prevent postoperative air leaks due to fissure dissection.

2.3 3-port VATS

In this technique, the camera port-anterior port is located in the 7th or 8th intercostal space in the anterior axillary line, and the posterior port is located in the posterior axillary line in the same intercostal space. The utility port was usually placed in the anterior axillary line 4th intercostal space for an upper lobectomy or 5th intercostal space for a lower lobectomy (**Figure 1**). While the posterior port was

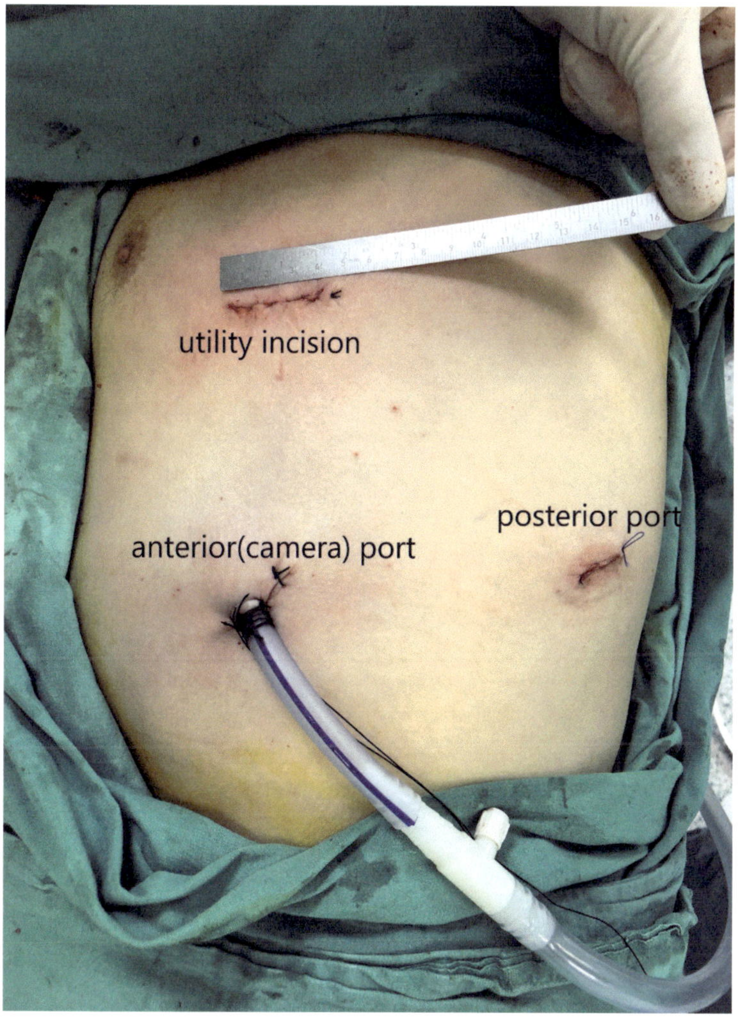

Figure 1.
Port incisions in the 3-port VATS technique.

previously placed from the upper and rear levels, it was modified over time, and the localization we described became more frequently applied [13].

2.4 2-port VATS

Since the additional contribution of the posterior port is not essential, VATS has become applied with two ports in some centers. The need for surgical retraction and manipulation can be provided by using another instrument via the utility port (**Figure 2**). However, apart from providing retraction, another feature of the posterior port that makes it useful is the introduction of the endoscopic stapling devices. Therefore, the absence of the posterior port should be compensated by appropriate maneuver and retraction of the lung.

2.5 Uniportal VATS

Uniportal VATS is firstly described by Dr. Gaetano Rocco for minor thoracic procedures include lung biopsies and pneumothorax operations [14]. Dr. Diego

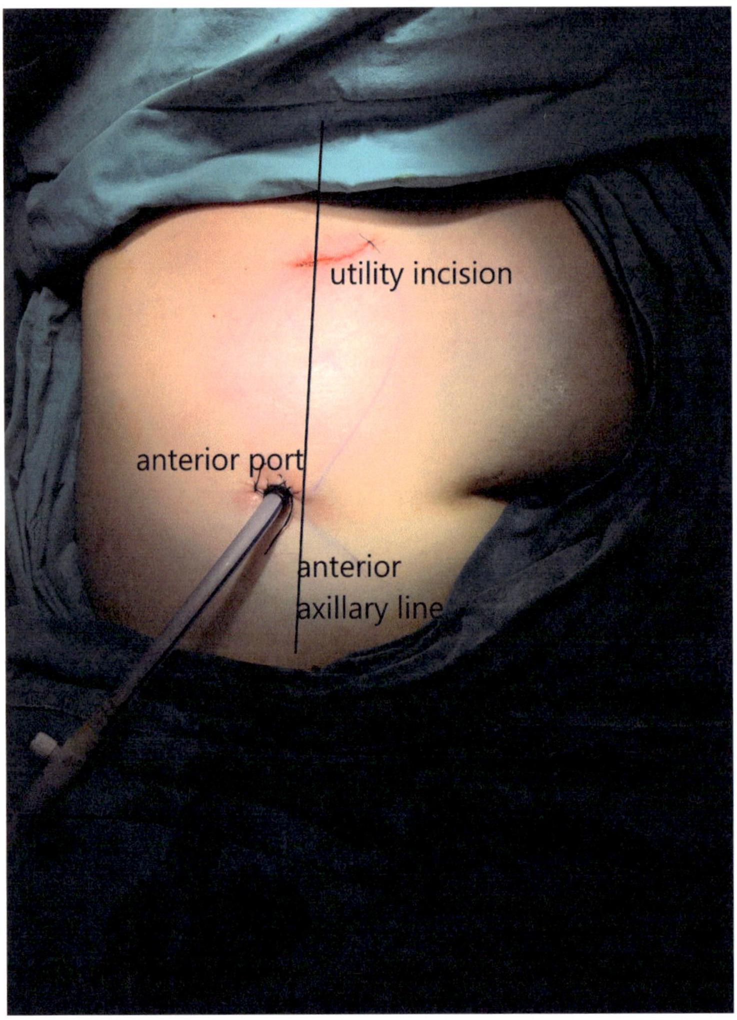

Figure 2.
Port incisions in the 2-port VATS technique.

Gonzalez Rivas shared his single port VATS lobectomy experience and became a pioneer in this regard [15, 16]. It has become preferred by many surgeons due to its advantages, such as causing less tissue damage and providing direct vision.

3–5 cm uniport incision is placed in the 5th intercostal in the anterior axillary line. A 5 mm diameter 30° video-thoracoscope is inserted through the same incision. Thus, the assistant and the surgeon share the same vision of direction. Although this is beneficial in terms of team cooperation, the working environment of the surgeon is somewhat limited.

Moreover, Gonzales Rivas successfully performed extended lung resections include bronchial, arterial, and double sleeve resections and raised the bar in uniportal VATS lobectomy [17]. Despite favorable surgical results, whether uniportal VATS has an additional benefit over traditional VATS is still controversial.

2.6 Needlescopic VATS

The main goal of this technique is to reduce the size of the incisions rather than the number of ports. It was aimed to minimize intercostal nerve damage and achieve better cosmetic results with the use of instruments and ports with a diameter of 3–5 mm instead of 10 mm ones used in conventional VATS [18].

The placement of the ports and the direction of the vision are the same as the 3-port VATS technique, and the utility port has to remain at 3–5 cm to extract the resection material. Surgeons who have appropriate instruments include 3 mm trocar, 3 mm 30° video-thoracoscope, and needlescopic grasper and do not prefer the uniportal VATS may prefer this technique.

2.7 Robot-assisted thoracic surgery

Advances in technology have enabled robots to be used in surgical procedures, and some authors started to share their first experiences in robotic thoracic surgery in the early 2000s [19].

It is thought that robotic surgery, which provides 3-dimensional vision and has articulated modern instruments, may allow the surgeon a safer dissection. With increasing experience, many thoracic surgery procedures are successfully performed with robotic surgery [20].

However, its use has not become widespread worldwide due to the system's higher cost, the time-consuming installation, and the lack of tactile feedback during surgery. It is possible to achieve similar surgical results with much less expense without sacrificing minimal invasiveness.

3. Diagnostic performance of VATS in patients with lung cancer

Despite advances in imaging technology techniques, including positron emission tomography (PET), integrated PET/computed tomography (CT) scans, PET/magnetic resonance imaging (MRI), multi-slice computed tomography, invasive diagnostic procedures continue to play an essential role in the management of the patient with lung cancer.

VATS provides the opportunity to evaluate for solitary pulmonary nodules, mediastinal or chest wall invasion by the primary tumor, pleural effusions/nodules, and mediastinal lymph nodes. Especially in the recent period, the use of targeted treatment methods has increased the need for tissue for mutation analysis. This situation has increased the diagnostic value of VATS and has widened its usage area.

3.1 Mediastinal staging

Evaluate the mediastinal and hilar lymph node status is essential for accurate staging of the lung cancer and to choose the appropriate treatment modality.

Noninvasive mediastinal staging methods include CT and PET/CT provide valuable clinical information however sensitivity, specificity, and negative predictive values insufficient to guide treatment decisions [21–23].

Abnormal lymph node (LN) is described as an LN with a short-axis diameter $\geq$ 1 cm). The median sensitivity and specificity of CT for identifying mediastinal lymph node metastasis are 55% and 81% [21].

PET can provide more accurate information about the differentiation of malignant and benign lymph nodes than CT. The median sensitivity and specificity of PET/CT for detecting lymph node metastases is ranges 80%- 88%, PET is successfully used in clinical staging and monitoring response to treatment in patients with lung cancer. However, the risk of false negativity is relatively high in lesions smaller than 1 cm and tumors with low metabolic activity (e.g. well-differentiated adenocarcinoma) [22, 23].

Cervical mediastinoscopy is the gold standard method for preoperative mediastinal lymph node staging in patients with lung cancer. The 2nd, 4th, and 7th station lymph nodes can be sampled by mediastinoscopy [24, 25]. Nowadays, cervical mediastinoscopy is performed with the help of a videomediastinoscope and it is named "video-assisted mediastinoscopy (VAM)" or "video-assisted mediastinal lymphadenectomy (VAMLA)" depending on the application technique [26].

Endobronchial ultrasound (EBUS) and endoscopic ultrasound (EUS), which are parts of minimally invasive procedures, are successfully applied with high sensitivity and specificity for mediastinal staging. Combined application of EBUS and EUS allows sampling of lymph node stations numbered 2R, 2 L, 4R, 4 L, 7, 8, and 9 with the sensitivity of 86% (95% CI, 82–90%) [21, 24, 27].

VATS is very useful in the evaluation of lymph nodes as well as the evaluation of the T factor of the tumor. It allows for access to almost every mediastinal lymph node station and total mediastinal lymphadenectomy can be applied [28]. With the right-sided VATS, lymph node stations numbered 2,4,7,8 and 9 can be sampled (**Figures 3** and **4**). Left-sided VATS is an ideal approach for sampling the 5th and 6th lymph node stations that cannot be reached by EBUS and mediastinoscopy.

Although the awake/tubeless VATS procedure has been described, general anesthesia and intubation with a double-lumen tube are usually required and it can only evaluate one side of the mediastinum. In conclusion, it is an approach that offers

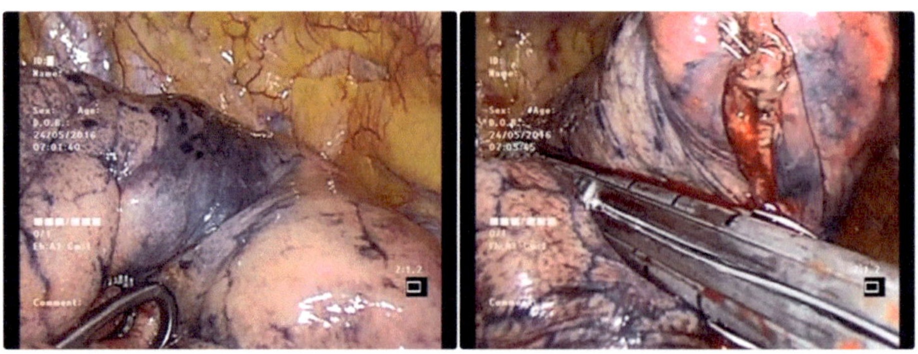

Figure 3.
Intraoperative image of the lung parenchyma after the CT-guided methylene blue labeling.

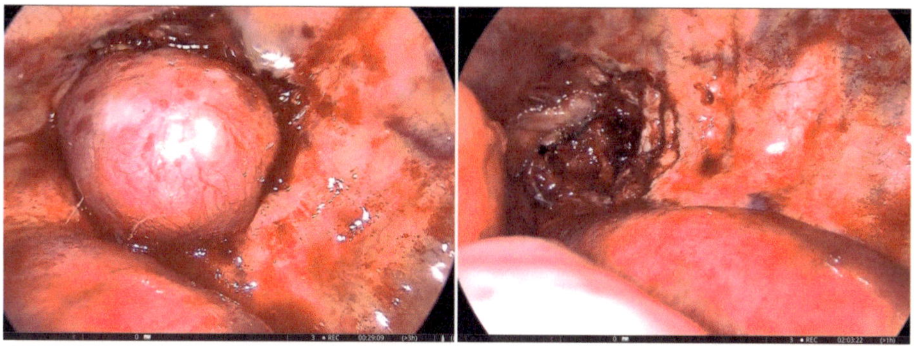

Figure 4.
VATS is also an effective method in the diagnosis and treatment of undiagnosed lesions located in the mediastinum. Para-aortic large mass resected and diagnosed as ectopic mediastinal thyroid.

high specificity and sensitivity values, especially in patients who require sampling of 5th and 6th lymph node stations or in whom complete lymph node dissection is planned.

3.2 Investigation of the pulmonary nodules

With the widespread use of radiological imaging methods, patients with newly detected pulmonary nodules constitute an important part of daily practice.

According to the recommendations of the Fleischner Society, solitary pulmonary nodules larger than 8 mm are recommended for further examination include tissue sampling regardless of cancer risk status [29]. CT-guided percutaneous transthoracic needle aspiration or transbronchial biopsy can be applied to pulmonary nodules with appropriate location and size. However, regardless of the location or size of the pulmonary nodule, sufficient material cannot always be obtained for cytopathological examination by transthoracic and transbronchial biopsy.

VATS is a useful approach for pulmonary nodules that cannot be sampled with minor diagnostic procedures. However, probe or digital palpation is very difficult for ground-glass opacity (GGO) lesions and nodules smaller than 1 cm. To solve this problem several pre-operative and perioperative marking techniques were described in the literature:

- Preoperative CT-guided injection of methylene blue [30].
- CT-guided positioning of a metal wire [31].
- CT-guided placement of a micro coil [32].
- Pleural dye marking using electromagnetic navigation bronchoscopy with or without radial endobronchial ultrasound [33].
- Gamma probe assessment after marking with Technetium-99 [34].
- The intrathoracic stamping method [35].

Each of the methods listed above has advantages and disadvantages and it is controversial which is the best method for marking the pulmonary nodules. We use the "CT-guided injection of methylene blue" method for marking the pulmonary nodules in our clinic (**Figure 5**). It is a simple, safe and effective procedure.

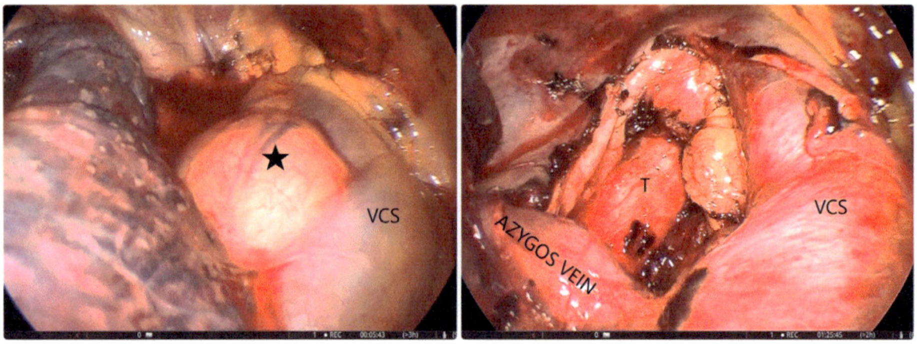

Figure 5.
The paratracheal lymph node, which could not be diagnosed by EBUS, was totally excised with VATS (VCS: Superior vena cava, T: Trachea, asterisk indicates paratracheal lymph node).

However, in order to ensure optimal labeling, the radiologist and the surgeon must be in good collaboration and the time between labeling and operation must be kept as short as possible.

4. The role of VATS in the surgical treatment of the lung cancer

Surgical resection in lung cancer has a relatively long history. First successful en bloc pneumonectomy reported by Graham and Singer in 1933 for the treatment of lung cancer. Lobectomies and segmentectomies were reported in the 1940s and 1950s and the first successful sleeve resection with right upper lobectomy for carcinoma in 1952 by Allison [36–38].

Today, anatomic pulmonary resection remains the best curative option in patients with early-stage lung cancer. The first VATS lobectomy series was reported in 1992 by Lewis [39].

In the following years, different surgeons defined unique techniques and pioneered the development of VATS however, the variability in the technique and the skeptical approach to published results prevented VATS from being widely accepted until the 2000s [40–42].

In addition to being technically feasible, superior postoperative results compared to thoracotomy have been effective in the general acceptance of VATS (**Figure 5**).

Long et al. conducted a prospective randomized trial comparing the quality of life after VATS vs. open lobectomy for clinically early-stage NSCLC [42]. It was stated that a month after operation both dyspnea and pain score were significantly lower in the VATS group.

In another study, Andretti et al. documented the results of 145 patients and compared the postoperative pain of patients who underwent VATS and mini thoracotomy. It was stated that significantly less pain was observed in the VATS group at the 1st, 12th, 24th and 48th postoperative hours [43].

The advantages of VATS over thoracotomy have also been revealed in other studies conducted with large patient groups:

McKenna Jr. et al. published experiences of 1,100 cases and reported 0.8% mortality and 15.3% morbidity [4].

In another study, Boffa et al. analyzed data of 9033 pulmonary resections for primary lung cancer by using the database of the Society of Thoracic Surgeons. In this study, VATS resection was performed in 2429 of 9033 patients. In the VATS group, the mortality rate was 2% and the overall morbidity was 32% [44].

Laursen et al. analyzed the results of 1379 patients who underwent lobectomy. In this study minor and major complications were found significantly lower in the VATS group [45].

Compared to the mortality (%1–2) and morbidity (%32–37) of open lobectomies from large series in the literature, the results are highly satisfactory [46].

The risk of compromising the oncological principles in VATS has been a matter of debate for a long time. However, in the retrospective large-scale studies, no significant difference was found between VATS and thoracotomy in terms of oncological results. Watanabe et al. reported no differences in the total number of lymph nodes, nodal stations, mediastinal nodes, and stations sampled during systematic lymph node dissection between VATS and thoracotomy groups [47].

Moreover, Yang et al. reported the long-term results of VATS and open lobectomy based on the National Cancer Data Base of the U.S. About three thousand patients with stage I NSCLC was matched with propensity score from >7,000 patients; the 5-year OS rates of the two groups were similar [48].

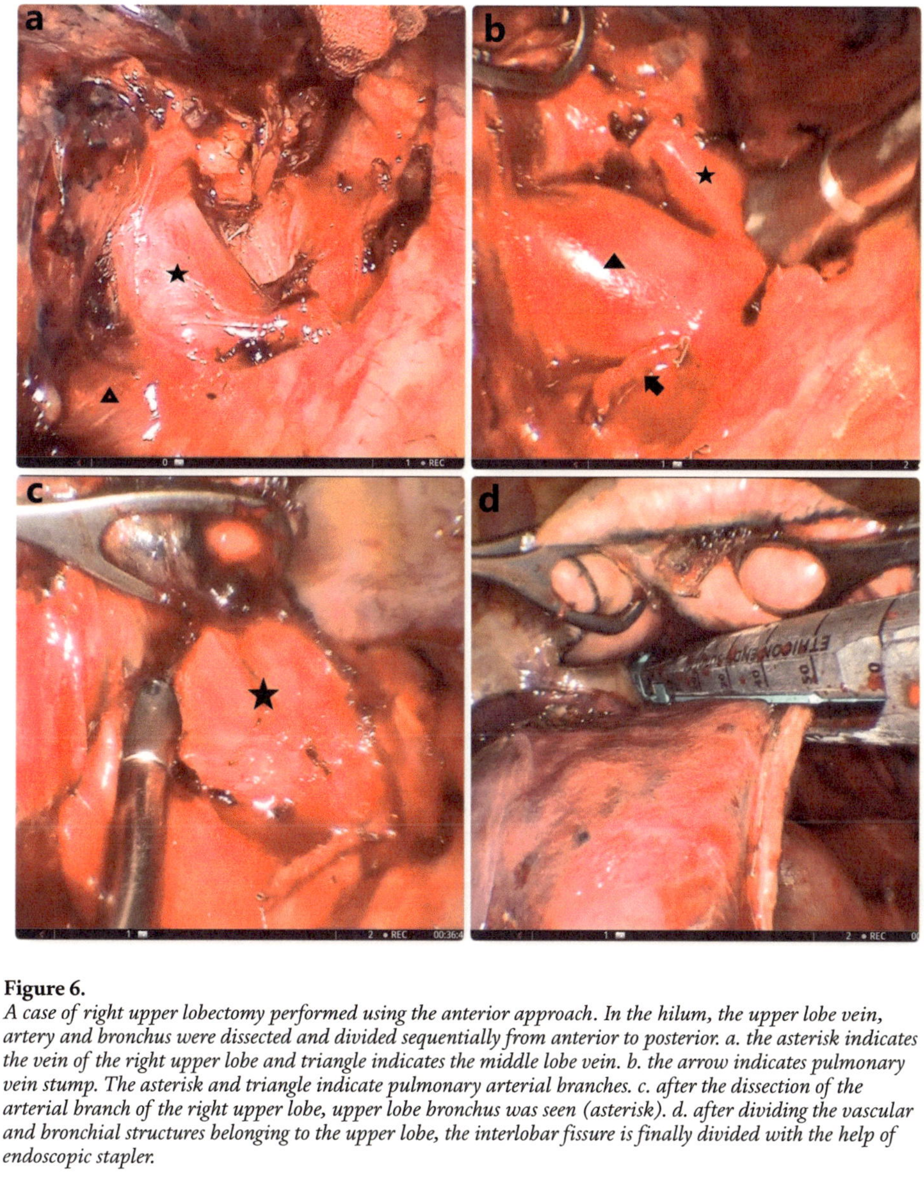

Figure 6.
A case of right upper lobectomy performed using the anterior approach. In the hilum, the upper lobe vein, artery and bronchus were dissected and divided sequentially from anterior to posterior. a. the asterisk indicates the vein of the right upper lobe and triangle indicates the middle lobe vein. b. the arrow indicates pulmonary vein stump. The asterisk and triangle indicate pulmonary arterial branches. c. after the dissection of the arterial branch of the right upper lobe, upper lobe bronchus was seen (asterisk). d. after dividing the vascular and bronchial structures belonging to the upper lobe, the interlobar fissure is finally divided with the help of endoscopic stapler.

Nowadays, the indications of VATS have expanded with the increasing experience. It can be successfully applied in cases with neoadjuvant therapy, tumor larger than 5 cm, chest wall invasion, need of sleeve resection, which was previously considered as a relative or absolute contraindication.

Park BJ et al. analyzed 428 patients who underwent induction chemotherapy for lung cancer and compared thoracotomy and minimally invasive surgical approaches in this patient group. There were not seen any differences in disease-free and overall survival between minimally invasive surgery and thoracotomy groups [49].

Huang et al. presented the results of 118 patients who underwent VATS bronchial sleeve lobectomy and postoperative complications were reported in only 2 patients.

In a study, we conducted in our clinic, which included 60 patients with tumors larger than 5 cm, mean drainage time and postoperative length of hospital stay were significantly shorter [50] (**Figure 6**).

5. Contraindications for VATS anatomic lung resection

With the widespread use of the VATS technique, many contraindications related to the procedure have been described [51]. However, these contraindications have changed over time, thanks to the increasing experience in VATS and the need-oriented developments and diversity of thoracoscopic instruments.

Many conditions such as the presence of endobronchial lesions, history of neoadjuvant treatment, pleural adhesions, and tumor larger than 3 cm, which were previously contraindicated for VATS, are not considered as contraindications by many surgeons today.

Sleeve resections with VATS can be successfully applied in patients with endobronchial lesions.

Moreover, many studies have demonstrated that VATS can be applied with low complication rates after neoadjuvant therapy or in cases with large tumors [49–52].

Large mediastinal vessel, pericardium, carina, and chest wall invasions can be considered relatively contraindicated for VATS. These kinds of major resections must be performed in high-volume institutions and by experienced surgeons.

6. Learning curve for VATS

Mc Kenna has been suggested that the length of the VATS lobectomy learning curve should consist of 50 lobectomies however, there are several personal and environmental factors that affect the learning curve associated with VATS lobectomy [53]. If we put aside personal factors such as instrument use, anatomy mastery and 3-dimensional thinking ability, there are 2 main factors affecting the learning curve: The size of the center and the presence of experienced surgeons who can supervise [51, 53, 54].

The prolongation of the time between the two cases will adversely affect the learning process. In centers where there are not many cases, this deficiency can be partially eliminated with VATS videos or simulators.

7. Conclusions

Minimally invasive thoracic surgery has made great progress in the past 20 years and today it has an important role in both diagnosis and treatment of lung cancer. However, VATS lobectomy is a relatively young technique and is still evolving.

The search for a less invasive technique is not specific to thoracic surgery and is a process that occurs in all surgical specialties. Fortunately, advancing technology supports this search in the best possible way.

Conflict of interest

The author declares no conflict of interest.

Acronyms and abbreviations

CT	Computed tomography
EBUS	Endobronchial ultrasound
EUS	Endoscopic ultrasound
MRI	Magnetic resonance imaging
NSCLC	Non-small cell lung cancer
PET	Positron emission tomography
VATS	Video-assisted thoracic surgery
VCS	Superior vena cav

Author details

Güntuğ Batihan* and Kenan Can Ceylan
University of Health Sciences Turkey, Dr. Suat Seren Chest Diseases and Chest Surgery Training and Research Center, İzmir, Turkey

*Address all correspondence to: gbatihan@hotmail.com

References

[1] Ferlay J, et al. GLOBOCAN 2012v1.0, Cancer Incidence and Mortality Worldwide. IARC Cancer Base No. 11. Lyon, France: International Agency for Research on Cancer (2013).

[2] Lazdunski LL. Surgery for nonsmall cell lung cancer. Eur Respir Rev 2013; 22: 382-404

[3] Roviaro G, Rebuffat C, Varoli F, et al. Videoendoscopic pulmonary lobectomy for cancer. Surg Laparosc Endosc 1992;2:244-7

[4] McKenna RJ, Jr, Houck W, Fuller CB. Video-assisted thoracic surgery lobectomy: experience with 1,100 cases. Ann Thorac Surg 2006;81:421-5; discussion 425-6

[5] Onaitis MW, Petersen RP, Balderson SS, et al. Thoracoscopic lobectomy is a safe and versatile procedure: experience with 500 consecutive patients. Ann Surg 2006;244:420-5

[6] Walker WS, Codispoti M, Soon SY, et al. Long-term outcomes following VATS lobectomy for non-small cell bronchogenic carcinoma. Eur J Cardiothorac Surg 2003;23:397-402

[7] Gonzalez-Rivas D, Bonome C, Fieira E, et al. Non-intubated video-assisted thoracoscopic lung resections: the future of thoracic surgery? Eur J Cardiothorac Surg 2016;49:721-31.

[8] Cui F, Liu J, Li S, et al. Tubeless video-assisted thoracoscopic surgery (VATS) under non-intubated, intravenous anesthesia with spontaneous ventilation and no placement of chest tube postoperatively. J Thorac Dis 2016;8:2226-32.

[9] Yan TD. Surgical atlas of thoracoscopic lobectomy and segmentectomy. Ann Cardiothorac Surg. 2014;3(2):183-191. doi:10.3978/j.issn.2225-319X.2014.03.11

[10] Temes RT, Willms CD, Endara SA, et al. Fissureless lobectomy. Ann Thorac Surg 1998;65:282-4.

[11] Cerfolio RJ, Bryant AS, Singh S, Bass CS, Bartolucci AA. The management of chest tubes in patients with a pneumothorax and an air leak after pulmonary resection. Chest 2005; 128:816-20.

[12] Stamenovic D, Bostanci K, Messerschmidt A, Jahn T, Schneider T. Fissureless fissure-last video-assisted thoracoscopic lobectomy for all lung lobes: a better alternative to decrease the incidence of prolonged air leak? Eur J Cardiothorac Surg. 2016 Jul;50(1):118-23.

[13] Sihoe AD. The evolution of minimally invasive thoracic surgery: implications for the practice of uniportal thoracoscopic surgery. J Thorac Dis. 2014;6(Suppl 6):S604-S617.

[14] Rocco G, Khalil M, Jutley R. Uniportal video-assisted thoracoscopic surgery wedge lung biopsy in the diagnosis of interstitial lung diseases. J Thorac Cardiovasc Surg 2005;129: 947-8.

[15] Gonzalez-Rivas D, Paradela M, Fernandez R, et al. Uniportal video-assisted thoracoscopic lobectomy: two years of experience. Ann Thorac Surg 2013;95:426-32.

[16] Gonzalez D, Paradela M, Garcia J, et al. Single-port video-assisted thoracoscopic lobectomy. Interact Cardiovasc Thorac Surg 2011;12:514-5.

[17] Gonzalez-Rivas D, Fieira E, Delgado M, de la Torre M, Mendez L, Fernandez R. Uniportal video-assisted thoracoscopic sleeve lobectomy and

other complex resections. J Thorac Dis. 2014;6(Suppl 6):S674-S681.

[18] Chou SH, Li HP, Lee JY, et al. Needlescopic video-assisted thoracic surgery for primary spontaneous pneumothorax. Minim Invasive Ther Allied Technol 2009;18:221-4.

[19] Melfi FM, Menconi GF, Mariani AM, et al. Early experience with robotic technology for thoracoscopic surgery. Eur J Cardiothorac Surg 2002;21:864-8.

[20] Veronesi G, Galetta D, Maisonneuve P, et al. Four-arm robotic lobectomy for the treatment of early-stage lung cancer. J Thorac Cardiovasc Surg 2010;140:19-25.

[21] Detterbeck FC, Jantz MA, Wallace M, Vansteenkiste J, Silvestri GA; American College of Chest Physicians. Invasive mediastinal staging of lung cancer: ACCP evidence-based clinical practice guidelines (2nd edition). Chest. 2007 Sep;132(3 Suppl):202S–220S.

[22] van Tinteren H, Hoekstra OS, Smit EF, et al. Effectiveness of positron emission tomography in preoperative assessment of patients with suspected non-small cell lung cancer: The PLUS multicentre randomized trial. Lancet. 2002;359:1388-93.

[23] Gelberg J, Grondin S, Tremblay A. Mediastinal staging for lung cancer. Can Respir J. 2014;21(3):159-161.

[24] Block MI, Tarrazzi FA. Invasive mediastinal staging: Endobronchial ultrasound, endoscopic ultrasound, and mediastinoscopy. Semin Thorac Surg. 2013;25:218-27.

[25] Lemaire A, Nikolic I, Petersen T, et al. Nine-year single center experience with cervical mediastinoscopy: Complications and false negative rate. Ann Thorac Surg. 2006;82:1185-90.

[26] Leschber G, Holinka G, Linder A. Video-assisted mediastinoscopic lymphadenectomy (VAMLA)--a method for systematic mediastinal lymphnode dissection. Eur J Cardiothorac Surg. 2003 Aug;24(2):192-5

[27] Dong X, Qiu X, Liu Q, et al. Endobronchial ultrasound-guided transbronchial needle aspiration in the mediastinal staging of non-small cell lung cancer: A meta-analysis. Ann Thorac Surg.

[28] Hiebinger A, and Velano D, Bodner. VATS-lymph node dissection, staging and restaging in advanced malignancy/ the Munich experience. Video-assist Thorac Surg 2018;3:29.

[29] MacMahon H, Naidich DP, Goo JM et al. "Guidelines for management of incidental pulmonary nodules detected on CT images: from the Fleischner Society 2017," Radiology, vol. 284, no. 1, pp. 228-243, 2017.

[30] Wang YZ, Boudreaux JP, Dowling A, Woltering EA. Percutaneous localisation of pulmonary nodules prior to video-assisted thoracoscopic surgery using methylene blue and TC-99. Eur J Cardiothorac Surg. 2010 Jan;37(1):237-8.

[31] Wang T, Ma S, Yan T, Song J, Wang K, He W, Bai J. [Computed Tomography Guided Hook-wire Precise Localization and Minimally Invasive Resection of Pulmonary Nodules]. Zhongguo Fei Ai Za Zhi. 2015 Nov;18(11):680-5. Chinese.

[32] Alharbi SR. Computed Tomography-guided Pulmonary Nodule Microcoil Localization Technique, Misplacement Errors, and Complications: A Pictorial Essay. J Clin Imaging Sci. 2018 Mar 9;8:8.

[33] Ozgul G, Cetinkaya E, Ozgul MA, et al. Efficacy and safety of electromagnetic navigation bronchoscopy with or without radial

endobronchial ultrasound for peripheral lung lesions. Endosc Ultrasound. 2016;5(3):189-195.

[34] Sugi K, Kaneda Y, Hirasawa K, Kunitani N. Radioisotope marking under CT guidance and localization using a handheld gamma probe for small or indistinct pulmonary lesions. Chest. 2003 Jul;124(1):155-8.

[35] Kawada M, Okubo T, Poudel S, et al. A new marking technique for peripheral lung nodules avoiding pleural puncture: the intrathoracic stamping method. Interact Cardiovasc Thorac Surg. 2013;16(3):381-383.

[36] Kittle CF. The history of lobectomy and segmentectomy including sleeve resection. Chest Surg Clin N Am 2000;10:105-130.

[37] Evarts A, Graham MD, Singer JJ. Successful removal of an entire lung for carcinoma of the bronchus. JAMA 1984; 251: 257-260.

[38] Allison PR. Meeting of the Association of Thoracic Surgeons; quoted by Jones PH. Ann R Coll Surg Engl25:20, 1959

[39] Lewis RJ, Sisler GE, Caccavale RJ. Imaged thoracic lobectomy: should it be done? Ann Thorac Surg 1992; 54:80-83

[40] Lewis RJ, Caccavale RJ, Bocage JP, Widmann MD. Video-assisted thoracic surgical non-rib spreading simultaneously stapled lobectomy: a more patient-friendly oncologic resection. Chest. 1999 Oct;116(4):1119-24.

[41] Walker W. VATS lobectomy: the Edinburgh experience. Semin Thorac Cardiovasc Surg 1998; 10:291-299

[42] Roviaro G. VATS major pulmonary resections: the Italian experience. Semin Thorac Cardiovasc Surg 1998; 10:313-320

[43] Andreetti C, Menna C, Ibrahim M, et al. Postoperative pain control: videothoracoscopic versus conservative mini-thoracotomic approach. Eur J Cardiothorac Surg 2014;46:907-12. 10.1093/ejcts/ezu092

[44] Boffa DJ, Allen MS, Grab JD, Gaissert HA, Harpole DH, Wright CD. Data from The Society of Thoracic Surgeons General Thoracic Surgery database: the surgical management of primary lung tumors. J Thorac Cardiovasc Surg. 2008 Feb;135(2):247-54.

[45] Laursen LØ, Petersen RH, Hansen HJ, Jensen TK, Ravn J, Konge L. Video-assisted thoracoscopic surgery lobectomy for lung cancer is associated with a lower 30-day morbidity compared with lobectomy by thoracotomy. Eur J Cardiothorac Surg. 2016 Mar;49(3):870-5.

[46] Watanabe S, Asamura H, Suzuki K, Tsuchiya R. Recent results of postoperative mortality for surgical resections in lung cancer. Ann Thorac Surg. 2004;78(3):999-1002.

[47] Watanabe A, Koyanagi T, Ohsawa H, et al. Systematic node dissection by VATS is not inferior to that through an open thoracotomy: A comparative clinicopathologic retrospective study. Surgery 2005;138:510-7.

[48] Yang CJ, Kumar A, Klapper JA, et al. A National Analysis of Long-term Survival Following Thoracoscopic Versus Open Lobectomy for Stage I Non-small-cell Lung Cancer. Ann Surg 2019;269:163-71.

[49] Park BJ, Yang HX, Woo KM, et al. Minimally invasive (robotic assisted thoracic surgery and video-assisted thoracic surgery) lobectomy for the treatment of locally advanced non-small cell lung cancer. J Thorac Dis 2016;8: S406-13.

[50] Batihan G, Ceylan KC, Usluer O, et al. Video-Assisted Thoracoscopic Surgery vs Thoracotomy for Non-Small Cell Lung Cancer Greater Than 5 cm: Is VATS a feasible approach for large tumors?. J Cardiothorac Surg 2020;15: 261.

[51] Hanna JM, Berry MF, D'Amico TA. Contraindications of video-assisted thoracoscopic surgical lobectomy and determinants of conversion to open. J Thorac Dis. 2013 Aug;5 Suppl 3 (Suppl 3):S182-9.

[52] Huang J, Li S, Hao Z, et al. Complete video-assisted thoracoscopic surgery (VATS) bronchial sleeve lobectomy. J Thorac Dis 2016;8:553-74.

[53] McKenna RJ., Jr. Complications and learning curves for video-assisted thoracic surgery lobectomy. Thorac Surg Clin 2008;18:275-80.

[54] Long H, Lin ZC, Lin YB, Situ DR, Wang YN, Rong TH. [Quality of life after lobectomy for early stage non-small cell lung cancer--video-assisted thoracoscopic surgery versus minimal incision thoracotomy]. Ai Zheng. 2007 Jun;26(6):624-8.

Chapter 3

Robotic Surgery for Non-Small Cell Lung Cancer

Andrew X. Li and Justin D. Blasberg

Abstract

Pulmonary resection has been a cornerstone in the management of patients with non-small cell lung cancer (NSCLC) for decades. In recent years, the popularity of minimally-invasive techniques as the primary method to manage NSCLC has grown significantly. With smaller incisions and a lower incidence of peri-operative complications, minimally-invasive lung resection, accomplished through keyhole incisions with miniaturized cameras and similarly small instruments that work through surgical ports, has been shown to retain equivalent oncologic outcomes to the traditional gold standard open thoracotomy. This technique allows for the safe performance of anatomic lung resection with complete lymphadenectomy and has been a part of thoracic surgery practice for three decades. Robotic-assisted thoracoscopic surgery (RATS) represents another major advancement for lung resection, broadening the opportunity for patients to undergo minimally invasive surgery for NSCLC, and therefore allowing a greater percentage of the lung cancer population to benefit from many of the advantages previously demonstrated from video assisted thoracoscopic surgery (VATS) techniques. RATS surgery is also associated with several technical advantages to the surgeon. For a surgeon who performs open procedures and is looking to adopt a minimally invasive approach, RATS ergonomics are a natural transition compared to VATS, particularly given the multiple degrees of freedom associated with robotic articulating instruments. As a result, this platform has been adopted as a primary approach in numerous institutions across the United States. In this chapter, we will explore the advantages and disadvantages of robotic-assisted surgery for NSCLC and discuss the implications for increased adoption of minimally invasive surgery in the future of lung cancer treatment.

Keywords: non-small cell lung cancer, pulmonary resection, minimally invasive surgery, robotic surgery, robotic-assisted thoracoscopic surgery

1. Introduction

Surgical resection for early stage non-small cell lung cancer (NSCLC) (Stage I and II) is associated with the lowest risk for local and distant recurrence and the best 5-year survival compared to other available treatment options [1]. The preferred approach for the surgical management of resectable, early-stage NSCLC has shifted in recent years from open thoracotomy to minimally-invasive surgery (MIS). Although thoracotomy has evolved over several decades to utilize muscle sparing incisions and improved postoperative pain control using epidural and para-vertebral catheter systems, this technique is associated with more significant muscle dissection, rib spreading, and increased risk for morbidity and mortality after surgery. This includes a protracted period of recovery following hospital discharge, a slower return to baseline quality of life, and the potential for chronic pain associated with a larger thoracotomy incision.

With fewer perioperative complications and quicker recovery, minimally invasive surgery offers expanded opportunities for surgical resection in patients who otherwise would not tolerate the morbidity of thoracotomy. There are additional benefits to minimally invasive resection, including significantly improved postoperative pain control, shorter hospital length of stay, quicker return to baseline quality of life, and earlier return to work that enhance and support the utilization of this platform for NSCLC [2–4]. These advantages have resulted in a significant shift in the surgical management of NSCLC patients, where formerly open resection and up to a week-long hospitalization were standard even without significant postoperative complications, current expectations for VATS lung resection include discharge to home in the majority of cases within 4–5 days or less [5]. Additionally, in cases where there may be a recommendation for adjuvant therapy, MIS patients are more likely to have recovered and be ready to receive such therapy earlier in their treatment course. Therefore, minimally invasive resection has significant advantages, especially when considering some percentage of thoracotomy patients might not receive adjuvant therapy given a challenging recovery from their index lung resection.

Video-assisted thoracoscopic surgery (VATS) for lung resection has been a part of the thoracic surgeon's toolbox for the past three decades. Lewis et al. first described the use of VATS in 1992 [6]. The technique was quickly adapted to lobectomy in elderly patients with early-stage NSCLC, where some of the first cases were completed with similar or better results to historical controls [7]. Since these initial reports, VATS surgery has become increasingly common, with expanded use in complex lung resections, pneumonectomy, bronchovascular sleeve resections, and tumors that include the chest wall [8–10]. While only 8% of lobectomies in the United States were performed thoracoscopically in 2003, this figure has increased significantly over time, up to 54% as reported in 2014, especially among high-volume surgeons [11–13]. Trends that favor VATS adoption include being a dedicated thoracic surgeon in a high-volume center, performance of lung resection in a larger hospital, and lung resections performed in the Northeast. In one multi-variate analysis, there was a significant association between VATS adoption and surgeon volume (>15 lobectomies performed per year), which is not unexpected given the technical challenges associated with becoming proficient with this technique [11]. Although VATS adoption has significantly improved, there remains a large number of both general, dedicated thoracic, and cardiothoracic surgeons who continue to perform a thoracotomy for NSCLC, limited by both volume challenges and the learning curve associated with VATS lobectomy. Although the percentage of open lung resection has declined over time, this technique still represents a large proportion of early stage NSCLC surgery performed in the United States. As a result, there is an opportunity to expand on the availability of minimally invasive lung resection to patients, and to do so using technology that favors a natural transition for otherwise traditional open surgeons.

This need has led to another major technical innovation in thoracic surgery over the last two decades with the adoption of the Da Vinci robotic system (Intuitive Surgical Inc., Sunnyvale, CA, USA), a platform that is at the forefront of minimally-invasive lung, esophageal, and mediastinal tumor resection. In robotic-assisted thoracoscopic surgery (RATS), the surgeon is seated at a console adjacent to the sterile field which operates a bedside patient cart with several robotic arms (**Figure 1**). Attached to these arms are robotic instruments that enter the pleural space via keyhole incisions and robotic ports. At the console, the surgeon manipulates the robotic

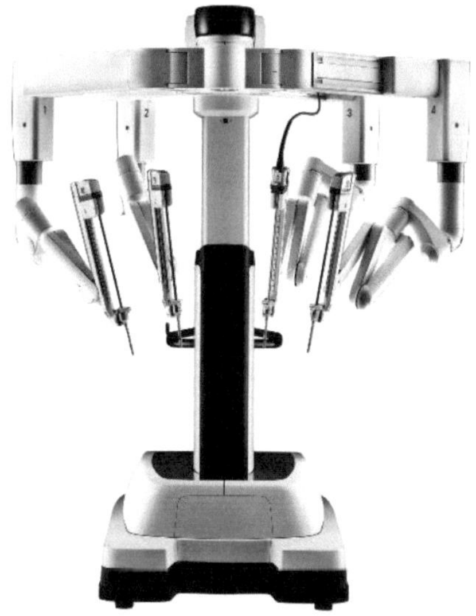

Figure 1.
Da Vinci XI patient cart with four robotic arms. Image courtesy of © [2020] Intuitive Surgical, Inc.

arms with three-dimensional controls which translate the surgeon's hand movements to the wristed instruments on each of the robotic arms. A RATS platform aids the surgeon by enhancing visualization with a three-dimensional high-definition view, minimizing hand tremors, and improving dexterity of the instruments by functioning with multiple degrees of freedom. Wristed instruments mimic the surgeon's actual hand movements, simulating open surgery, allowing for the precise dissection of vascular structures and a thorough lymphadenectomy, key steps to success when performing minimally invasive lung resection. While this technique is a dramatic change from either open or VATS procedures as the surgeon is not at the patient's bedside, repetition and the frequency of performing robotic cases helps one's personal comfort as they transition to RATS.

Although the technical advantages of RATS make the platform desirable, the adoption of minimally-invasive robotic surgery is associated with some challenges. While benefits such as reduced postoperative pain, decreased peri-operative morbidity, reduce risk for postoperative air leak, and shorter hospital length of stay have been described, concern over upfront investment and increased cost per operation may be considered a barrier to access. Additional training for operating room staff is required, capital investment into larger operating rooms and to modernize traditional open surgery rooms that might like technological infrastructure, as well as increased operating times impact the opportunity cost of performing other operations and can contribute to some level of adoption apprehension for hospitals that have no robotic experience. Despite any misgivings, there is clear evidence that the adoption of robotic surgery for lung resection is on the rise. In just two years, from 2010 to 2012, robotic surgery increased in popularity by 3-fold, accounting for 9.1% of lung resections annually in 2012 [14]. More recently, an estimated 17.5% of lobectomies were performed robotically in 2017 [15]. Trends in robotic adoption seem to suggest that the technical advantages associated with robotic lung resection outweigh the capital and educational investment needed to make such a program successful. What specific metrics drive robotic adoption and improve outcomes in thoracic surgery are defined in the literature. This chapter will address the advantages and disadvantages of MIS for NSCLC, including the role of robotic surgery, and discuss its future directions in this field.

2. Advantages of robotic-assisted and video-assisted thoracoscopic surgery

Minimally-invasive thorascopic surgery, and in turn RATS, have several advantages over traditional open surgery. Compared to thoracotomy, VATS and RATS utilize small incisions to access the chest cavity, reducing peri-operative morbidity and enhancing recovery. This allows the surgeon to select a larger range of patients who may otherwise be unable to tolerate open resection. Avoiding the muscle dissection/division and rib spreading associated with thoracotomy, while not compromising on the oncologic efficacy of the procedure, are the key advantages to both VATS and RATS procedures. For the facile VATS surgeon, lung resection and complete lymphadenectomy can be accomplished with a high rate of success, low risk of complication, and an expedited pathway to recovery. There are specific subsets of patients at higher risk for conversion during VATS procedures, particularly in cases where dissection is difficult due to fibrocalcified nodes, large tumor >3 cm, or prior induction therapy [16, 17]. In these cases, the advantages of robotics can be significant. The fundamental benefit of the robotic platform is that it simulates open techniques but with the advantages of smaller incision surgery. RATS procedures utilize insufflation to help maximize exposure, 3-dimensional optics to help define important structures and their relationship to adjacent structures, 10× magnification rather to improve visualization, and the ability to reach farther into the chest with longer instruments while still performing fine dissection work, all without losing out on the ergonomics associated with open surgery. This includes the ability to use robotic stapling devices which are similar to open and VATS variants, bipolar energy devices that articulate, vessel sealing devices that articulate, and fluorescence imaging in cases where tumor localization or performance of segmental resection is preferred. Not only does this provide open-only surgeons with an easier opportunity to incorporate MIS into their technical portfolio but affords a larger number of patients with the opportunity to undergo minimally invasive lung resection when appropriate.

An additional advantage is the ease in which segmental resection can be performed. RATS visualization and the precision in which segmental anatomy can be dissected has helped improve the adoption of segmentectomy in the United States [18]. As new data becomes available regarding the advantage of segmental resection over wedge, and potentially the equivalence of segmentectomy to lobectomy for subsets of early stage NSCLC either <2 cm or in patients with non-solid nodules, the utilization of techniques to improve rates of segmentectomy will become more important. While VATS segmentectomy is both well described and widely performed, it remains a technical challenge for many surgeons to adopt with proficiency required that can be significantly more complex than superior segmentectomy. RATS segmentectomy may be an opportunity for lobectomy only surgeons to increase their success with segmentectomy given these advantages. Previously data has demonstrates that surgical outcomes are comparable between RATS and VATS segmentectomy, both in terms of oncologic outcome and the adequacy of lymph node evaluation [19]. This principle is important to keep in mind as there is no scenario in which the size of an incision is more important than achieving an appropriate and adequate lung cancer resection.

2.1 Patient selection

MIS allows surgeons to select patients who would otherwise be unable to tolerate open pulmonary resection. The morbidity of a thoracotomy precludes many patients from benefitting from surgery with otherwise resectable cancers, leading to suboptimal treatments and decreased survival. In these cases, some institutions may turn to a more liberal use of radiation therapy as a means of local control. However, many studies have demonstrated the increased risk of local recurrence and inferior 5-year survival that makes radiation a less desirable choice for subsets of NSCLC patients, even in early stage cancers [1, 20, 21]. The decision to pursue surgery and in what format requires clinical judgment and cannot be determined by looking a one particular clinical parameter (ex. FEV1/DLCO, performance status, specific comorbidities alone). For example, a patient with less than perfect but acceptable pulmonary reserve, a history of cardiac disease who is medically optimized with a negative stress test, and in a motivated patient with reasonable performance status, surgical resection is likely to be well tolerated and preferable to other local therapy options (ex. SBRT or ablation). In this subset, MIS has obvious benefits compared to open resection. For example, in patients who underwent minimally-invasive thorascopic surgery, preoperative FEV1 < 60% was noted to be significantly associated with a lower risk for postoperative compilations compared to thoracotomy patients [12]. Although this concept may have seemed novel at the time, there is clearly an association between postoperative pain control, patient ambulation and participation with pulmonary toilet, and risk for postoperative complications following lung resection. Therefore, in patients who might be viewed as medically more marginal, MIS provides these patients with an opportunity for a curative resection and the benefits of lung cancer survival identified in the lung cancer study group with a lower complication profile [22].

Elderly patients are also at risk of receiving suboptimal treatment due to a perception of high-risk associated with surgery. When evaluating the surgical candidacy of this group, it is critical to determine both: 1) preoperative cardiac fitness and performance status as well as 2) competing causes of death. In the current era, it is reasonable to consider MIS as a curative procedure for early stage NSCLC in patients in their 80's or even in their 90's. Without a competing cause of death, it is reasonable to consider surgical resection for early-stage NSCLC in this age group. However, thoracotomy is a physiologically demanding procedure, and in elderly patients, MIS should be strongly considered when possible. Previous reports have demonstrated that post-operative outcomes remain superior in RATS and VATS compared to open thoracotomy for elderly patients. One propensity score-adjusted analysis examining 2,766 patients over the age of 65 with stage I to IIIa NSCLC in the Surveillance, Epidemiology, and End Results (SEER)-Medicare database found lower overall surgical complication rates in RATS versus thoracotomy, as well as lower rates of blood transfusion, shorter ICU stay, and a significant decrease in overall length of stay [23]. In the same study, both VATS and RATS were found to have lower complication rates, adequate lymph node evaluation, and equivalent lung cancer specific survival [23].

Obese patients pose unique challenges for thoracic surgery. While studies show obese patients may have similar risk for complications and long-term outcomes compared to patients with normal body mass index (BMI), severely overweight patients (BMI greater than or equal to 40 kg/m2) face an increased risk of any major postoperative complication, including atelectasis requiring bronchoscopy, pneumonia, ARDS, extended ventilatory support, reintubation, and tracheostomy [24]. In addition to consideration for postoperative pain control, adequate pulmonary toilet, the ability to transfer patients from bed to chair, and the need for postoperative patients to ambulate aggressively, a question that arises is an obese patient's tolerability of a longer surgical case. This may be even more important when for RATS lung resection, especially for surgeons early in their learning curve where operative times may be longer than VATS procedures When we look to literature and evaluate best available data to help develop a recommendation, the use of RATS in obese patients has not been shown to be associated with a significantly higher risk of postoperative complications, longer hospital length-of-stay (LOS), and is associated with similar 5-year survival compared to open lobectomy, suggesting that a robotic approach remains safe in this patient population [25]. While the outcomes of RATS lung resection in the obese population may be similar to VATS, the technical advantages of performing an anatomic lung resection in this population remain significant. To date, no large database or single institution data has defined an association between BMI and inferior outcomes in obese patients that require conversion due to vascular injury or technical challenges associated with lung resection.

2.2 Perioperative complications

Patients undergoing RATS experience a similar or lower rate of perioperative complications compared to those who undergo open thoracotomy or VATS. Post-operative complications after robotic lung resection were seen in 10–39% of patients in a review which included five case series and four comparative studies [26]. The most common postoperative complications included prolonged air leaks and atrial fibrillation [26, 27]. Pooled analysis of several studies did not show a prolonged air leak risk that was significantly higher following robotic surgery compared to thoracotomy [28].

Major complications including acute respiratory distress, reoperation for air leak, pulmonary embolism, or arrhythmia requiring pacemaker placement were rare, seen in approximately 2.4% of patients [27]. The rate of major complication in robotic surgery appears lower than thoracotomy, with fewer instances of respiratory failure, hemorrhage, or reoperation [29, 30]. Currently, perioperative mortality at high volume centers where most robotic surgeries are performed is lower in RATS compared to open resection [31]. Although this outcome metric is difficult to interpret as mortality is low for all lung resection regardless of surgical technique, it should be expected than as more centers adopt robotics for minimally invasive resection, the morbidity and mortality of RATS should remain at a comparable level to open and VATS resection.

Conversion from RATS to an open procedure is also low. Recent studies demonstrated a conversion rate of 6.5–9.2% [27, 29, 32]. The most common indications for conversion were technical limitations, inability to achieve an adequate oncologic resection, and bleeding [27]. The learning curve for RATS proficiency appears to be in the range of 20–25 cases, after which the risk for conversion can be expected to go down significantly. Unlike VATS conversions, where the surgeon is present at the bedside and can more easily perform a thoracotomy expeditiously, RATS conversions require a coordinated and well planned 'fire drill' to ensure patient safety. This includes a bedside assist that can hold pressure on a bleeding structure via a non-robot port, that the robot arms can be moved away to allow for better access to the chest, and that the staff in the room are prepared to open instruments that are needed to complete the case. Although these processes may be unfamiliar to the novice robotic surgeon, adequate preparation for case should include discussion of these scenarios with the operating and anesthesia staff. When compared to VATS, there were no differences in conversion rates in recent independent studies or meta-analyses [28, 29].

Robotic surgery holds several key advantages with regards to post-operative outcomes when directly comparing VATS and RATS techniques. In one retrospective propensity score-matched study of 774 patients undergoing anatomical segmentectomy at a single academic institution, there were no significant differences in operative time, blood loss, risk for postoperative complication, or length of stay between RATS and VATS [33]. In another study examining 50 RATS and 80 VATS segmentectomies for patients with stage IA lung cancer at the Shanghai Chest Hospital, there was a shorter mean operative time and lower blood loss with RATS during anatomic resection and mediastinal lymphadenectomy [34]. For centrally located tumors which may be more difficult to access through VATS, robotic surgery was found to be associated with less bleeding, shorter operative times, and reduced volume of chest tube drainage and days with a chest tube, while having comparable oncologic outcomes including disease-free survival [35]. In a meta-analysis of ten studies by Emmert examining perioperative outcomes of minimally invasive thoracic surgery, tube drainage duration, length of hospitalization, and mortality were lower in patients undergoing RATS compared to VATS [36]. Therefore, it is reasonable to consider that the technical advantages associated with the robotic platform, including enhanced visualization and use of articulating instructions, are responsible for the low complication rates seen in RATS lung resection, and that with proficiency the outcomes of this technique can be equivalent to VATS.

2.3 Patient outcomes

One important area of scrutiny associated with the adoption of robotic surgery has been that VATS outcomes are already significantly better than open surgery, and that an expensive minimally invasive alternative with surgeon only advantages is a challenge to justify. As with any new technology, are the important outcomes the same or better? This is a fundamental necessity in cancer surgery. These concerns have been expressed since the introduction of the first robot in 2001, particularly with respect to adoption of both VATS and RATS approaches. When studied well, it is clear that both VATS and RATS are associated with excellent oncologic outcomes, equivalent to open surgery particularly with respect to lymph node evaluation and adequacy of resection, and that depending on the platform chosen, a proficient surgeon can be expected to have outcomes that meet or exceed their open surgery experience.

Several studies have examined and compared margin status, recurrence, disease-specific survival, and overall survival in open thoracotomy, VATS, and RATS. A study of the National Cancer Database found similar positive margin status (2%) after robotic surgery as compared to open resection, which is considerable given the lack of haptic feedback associated with RATS [37]. Other series also describe similar R0 resection rates of 97% [38]. Five-year disease recurrence has reported to be from 3% to 24.9% depending on cancer stage, which is also comparable to open surgery for appropriately matched patients [32, 39]. In this series and others, overall and disease-free survival at three and five years did not differ between RATS and either open surgery or VATS [32, 37, 38, 40–43]. These results all suggest that robotic lung resection is a non-inferior alternative to prior surgical options.

The data on nodal evaluation during lung resection is heterogenous for robotic surgery. Some studies report no advantage in nodal stations examined or nodal harvest when compared to open surgery or VATS [28, 29, 44, 45]. One study found that fewer lymph nodes were examined with RATS compared to VATS [14]. Others report improved lymph node examination and retrieval [30, 33, 37, 46, 47]. In particular, one study found N1 (hilar) lymph nodes were better evaluated by robotic surgery as compared to VATS, both in terms of the number (4 vs. 3) and stations (3 vs. 2) examined [33]. The experience of these authors and others are that the technical advantages of robotic surgery allow for an equivalent lymph node dissection to VATS, with some significant advantages including improved hemostasis and thoroughness of lymph node resection performed during mediastinal lymphadenectomy. The use of articulating bipolar instruments allows for complete lymph node packet resection, while improved visualization helps to define lymph node associations to adjacent structures. This is clearly an advantage over VATS, were ring clamps or non-articulating instruments can be used to grasp lymph nodes and non-articulating energy devices are used to free lymph nodes from surrounding structures. Whether these technical advantages translate into differences in short or long-term outcomes is unknown. However, no study to date has demonstrated that taking fewer lymph nodes or an incomplete lymph node evaluation is better than comprehensive lymphadenectomy. Additionally, as surgical outcomes become more heavily scrutinized, particularly with respect to the adequately of lymph node dissection, the use of this platform is likely to help facilitate a comprehensive hilar and mediastinal lymphadenectomy to meet these expectations.

2.4 Technical considerations

The true advantage of robotic surgery appears to be the technical advantages conferred to the surgeon, specifically the enhanced visualization and improved dexterity of the instruments. While comparisons between robotic and open thoracotomy appear to have similar rates of complications, outcomes of VATS versus RATS are less uniform. Robotic surgery, in some series, is associated with less bleeding, shorter operative time, and shorter tube drainage duration [35]. These studies are largely retrospective and do not offer a definitive answer as to the causation for these improvements. However, one factor that likely contributes to these perceived results are the ergonomics of the robotic system. Robotic instruments moved with seven degrees of freedom, and as a result the surgeon in control at the console can mimic natural motions of the hand and wrist in the handling of tissue. This allows a surgeon to perform more complex functions in a safer fashion, reducing the risk of inadvertent injury while maintaining the oncologic standards. Important moves during anatomic lung resection, including thorough performance of lymphadenectomy and circumferential mobilization of critical vascular structures, can be performed with improved hemostasis, improved visualization, and reduced risk of injury.

2.5 Conclusions

Overall, the literature supports RATS as an alternative to open surgery and VATS. Fewer perioperative complications, improved quality of life, and similar oncologic outcomes have been established following RATS lung resection, bringing minimally invasive surgical options to a wider range of patients. While the advantages of RATS over VATS are certainly up for debate and are more informed by surgeon preference, the ability to improve minimally invasive lung resection availability to patients across the United States helps to drive interest in outcomes related to RATS procedures. The literature clearly demonstrates that surgeons facile with VATS lung resection provide patients with an oncologically sound operation and survival/recurrence expectations that rival results demonstrated in the LCSG. However, this skillset is challenging to learn and the highest standards for technical excellence are not as reproducible as open surgical techniques. In this space, RATS lung resection continues to evolve as adoption of minimally invasive lung resection grows.

3. What makes robotic surgery adoption different than VATS?

While robotic surgery has key advantages compared to open and VATS techniques, it has not been uniformly adopted. As compared to VATS, this technology requires a significant capital investment, is associated with its own learning curve, and requires robotically trained support staff for a surgeon to have a successful robotic lung resection practice. All of these characteristics can be overcome but require stakeholders from surgery and the operating room to commit to the success of this platform.

3.1 Cost

The cost of robotic surgery is one of its main points of contention. There are two aspects of robotic surgery which contributes to this cost. The first is the initial investment in the robotic system. The second includes intra-operative costs, consisting of the use of consumables and longer operative times associated with RATS [28, 33, 45]. As the second is modifiable, it has garnered more attention in the literature. One study using patients from the SEER-Medicare database found the total cost of lung resection was similar between RATS and thoracotomy ($54,702 vs. $57,104, $p = 0.08$) [23]. Much of the variability in cost associated with robotic surgery likely stems from the difference in post-operative complications when compared to open resection. In particular, overall length of stay after RATS is significantly shorter than open surgery [29, 31, 38, 47, 48], and may be similar or better than VATS (4 days vs. 5 days) [40]. Therefore, although the cost of the operation may be higher in RATS, the direct associated cost may not be significantly different compared to open or VATS [49]. In time, as familiarity with the robotic platform increases and operating room efficacy is improved to rival VATS procedures, further cost savings can offset the increased initial investment and operative costs.

3.2 Learning curve

Another concern for surgeons unfamiliar with robotic surgery is training and familiarization with a new surgical platform. In fact, one of the early difficulties with the transition from VATS to open surgery was the steep learning curve. Laparoscopic instruments are relatively inflexible compared to the dexterity a surgeon is accustomed to during open surgery. Circumferential mobilization of important blood vessels requires dissection facilitated by subtle changes in how one engages the tissue, and these techniques are both important and challenging to learn for a novice VATS surgeon. Additionally, the VATS camera is limited to 3.5x magnification, images are shown in only 2 dimensions, and the camera needs to be held and constantly adjusted by the surgeon assistant. At 10× magnification, with 3D imaging, and a fixed camera that is not subject to fatigue or the concept of 'guess what I am thinking and look where I want you to look', getting used to robotic optics is fairly quick. The learning curve for a robotic lobectomy is approximately twenty cases [26, 50]. In this regard, mastery of robotic surgery appears to easier than VATS, owing to the more natural movements afforded by the robot.

Efficiency of RATS does rely more heavily on the familiarity of supporting operating room staff and the surgeon's bedside assistant than VATS procedures. As the surgeon is seated at a console away from the sterile field, a bedside assistant must assist in exchanging instruments and repositioning robotic arms as needed. Thus, in addition to surgeon training, it is imperative that adequate training be provided to dedicated staff supporting the surgeon in order to maintain a safe working environment and maximum efficiency.

3.3 Choosing robotic surgery

In our experience, a surgeon who gains robotic proficiency prefers the robot for a majority of their cases unless the platform is unavailable. Technically, VATS offers little advantage over RATS for the operating surgeon. Few instances exist where cost and time to set up outweighs the benefit. We utilize VATS for short cases such as decortications and pleurodesis, but favor RATS for most pulmonary resections. For technically challenging cases such as pneumonectomies, open surgery may be preferred, however, some case series describe successful RATS applications in pneumonectomy [51, 52].

4. Conclusions

In conclusion, robotic surgery represents the latest innovation for lung cancer surgery and an important opportunity for general and thoracic surgeons who still perform open lung resection. RATS procedures are associated with comparable or better outcomes than open surgery or VATS, and over the past two decades has been shown to be a safe platform with which lung cancer procedures can be performed. RATS procedures have significant technical advantages for the surgeon, namely the 3D vision, 10× magnification, and articulating instruments that mimics open surgery and allows for the performance of critical components of an operation safely. Although the advantages of RATS for patients are similar to VATS procedures, the adoption of RATS by open surgeons allows for a larger number of lung cancer patients in the United States to undergo minimally invasive procedures than ever before, which further realizes the patient specific advantages of minimally invasive techniques in this often medically complex population. A lower complication rate and better tolerability increases access to a definitive resection for NSCLC, optimizing 5-year survival. In time, as the volume of robotic surgery increases, the capital investment associated with adoption is likely to decrease. Additionally, with increased surgeon experience, operative times, risks for air leak, and overall hospital length of stay are also expected to decrease, allowing for improved utilization of hospital resources and efficiency.

Conflict of interest

Justin D. Blasberg, MD MPH is a proctor for Intuitive Surgical.

Notes/thanks/other declarations

None.

Author details

Andrew X. Li and Justin D. Blasberg*
Section of Thoracic Surgery, Department of Surgery, Yale School of Medicine, New Haven, Connecticut, United States of America

*Address all correspondence to: justin.blasberg@yale.edu

References

[1] Cornwell LD, Echeverria AE, Samuelian J, Mayor J, Casal RF, Bakaeen FG, et al. Video-assisted thoracoscopic lobectomy is associated with greater recurrence-free survival than stereotactic body radiotherapy for clinical stage I lung cancer. J Thorac Cardiovasc Surg. 2018;155(1):395-402.

[2] Hristov B, Eguchi T, Bains S, Dycoco J, Tan KS, Isbell JM, et al. Minimally Invasive Lobectomy Is Associated With Lower Noncancer-specific Mortality in Elderly Patients: A Propensity Score Matched Competing Risks Analysis. Ann Surg. 2019;270(6):1161-1169.

[3] Kumar A, Deng J, Raman V, Okusanya O, Baiu I, Berry MF, et al. A National Analysis of Minimally Invasive vs Open Segmentectomy for Stage IA Non-small-cell Lung Cancer. Semin Thorac Cardiovasc Surg. 2020.

[4] Gaudet MA, D'Amico TA. Thoracoscopic Lobectomy for Non-small Cell Lung Cancer. Surg Oncol Clin N Am. 2016;25(3):503-513.

[5] Nachira D, Meacci E, Margaritora S, Ismail M. Level of evidence on long-term results after VATS lobectomy: state of the art. J Thorac Dis. 2019;11(6):2192-2194.

[6] Lewis RJ, Caccavale RJ, Sisler GE, Mackenzie JW. One hundred consecutive patients undergoing video-assisted thoracic operations. Ann Thorac Surg. 1992;54(3):421-426.

[7] McKenna RJ, Jr. Thoracoscopic lobectomy with mediastinal sampling in 80-year-old patients. Chest. 1994;106(6):1902-1904.

[8] Nagai S, Imanishi N, Matsuoka T, Matsuoka K, Ueda M, Miyamoto Y. Video-assisted thoracoscopic pneumonectomy: retrospective outcome analysis of 47 consecutive patients. Ann Thorac Surg. 2014;97(6):1908-1913.

[9] Xie D, Deng J, Gonzalez-Rivas D, Zhu Y, Jiang L, Jiang G, et al. Comparison of video-assisted thoracoscopic surgery with thoracotomy in bronchial sleeve lobectomy for centrally located non–small cell lung cancer. The Journal of Thoracic and Cardiovascular Surgery. 2020.

[10] Dal Agnol G, Oliveira R, Ugalde PA. Video-assisted thoracoscopic surgery lobectomy with chest wall resection. J Thorac Dis. 2018;10(Suppl 22):S2656-S2S63.

[11] Blasberg JD, Seder CW, Leverson G, Shan Y, Maloney JD, Macke RA. Video-Assisted Thoracoscopic Lobectomy for Lung Cancer: Current Practice Patterns and Predictors of Adoption. Ann Thorac Surg. 2016;102(6):1854-1862.

[12] Ceppa DP, Kosinski AS, Berry MF, Tong BC, Harpole DH, Mitchell JD, et al. Thoracoscopic lobectomy has increasing benefit in patients with poor pulmonary function: a Society of Thoracic Surgeons Database analysis. Ann Surg. 2012;256(3):487-493.

[13] Phillips JD, Bostock IC, Hasson RM, Goodney PP, Goodman DC, Millington TM, et al. National practice trends for the surgical management of lung cancer in the CMS population: an atlas of care. J Thorac Dis. 2019;11(Suppl 4):S500-S5S8.

[14] Rajaram R, Mohanty S, Bentrem DJ, Pavey ES, Odell DD, Bharat A, et al. Nationwide Assessment of Robotic Lobectomy for Non-Small Cell Lung Cancer. Ann Thorac Surg. 2017;103(4):1092-1100.

[15] Wightman SC, Lui NS. Overview of robotic surgery for lung cancer. Video-Assisted Thoracic Surgery. 2020;5.

[16] Augustin F, Maier HT, Weissenbacher A, Ng C, Lucciarini P, Öfner D, et al. Causes, predictors and consequences of conversion from VATS to open lung lobectomy. Surg Endosc. 2016;30(6):2415-2421.

[17] Byun CS, Lee S, Kim DJ, Lee JG, Lee CY, Jung I, et al. Analysis of Unexpected Conversion to Thoracotomy During Thoracoscopic Lobectomy in Lung Cancer. Ann Thorac Surg. 2015;100(3):968-973.

[18] Perroni G, Veronesi G. Robotic segmentectomy: indication and technique. Journal of Thoracic Disease. 2020;12(6):3404-3410.

[19] Liang H, Liang W, Zhao L, Chen D, Zhang J, Zhang Y, et al. Robotic Versus Video-assisted Lobectomy/Segmentectomy for Lung Cancer: A Meta-analysis. Ann Surg. 2018;268(2):254-259.

[20] Bryant AK, Mundt RC, Sandhu AP, Urbanic JJ, Sharabi AB, Gupta S, et al. Stereotactic Body Radiation Therapy Versus Surgery for Early Lung Cancer Among US Veterans. Ann Thorac Surg. 2018;105(2):425-431.

[21] Shirvani SM, Jiang J, Chang JY, Welsh J, Likhacheva A, Buchholz TA, et al. Lobectomy, sublobar resection, and stereotactic ablative radiotherapy for early-stage non-small cell lung cancers in the elderly. JAMA Surg. 2014;149(12):1244-1253.

[22] Ginsberg RJ, Rubinstein LV. Randomized trial of lobectomy versus limited resection for T1 N0 non-small cell lung cancer. Lung Cancer Study Group. Ann Thorac Surg. 1995;60(3):615-622; discussion 22-3.

[23] Veluswamy RR, Whittaker Brown SA, Mhango G, Sigel K, Nicastri DG, Smith CB, et al. Comparative Effectiveness of Robotic-Assisted Surgery for Resectable Lung Cancer in Older Patients. Chest. 2020;157(5):1313-1321.

[24] Williams T, Gulack BC, Kim S, Fernandez FG, Ferguson MK. Operative Risk for Major Lung Resection Increases at Extremes of Body Mass Index. Ann Thorac Surg. 2017;103(1):296-302.

[25] Casiraghi M, Sedda G, Diotti C, Mariolo AV, Galetta D, Tessitore A, et al. Postoperative outcomes of robotic-assisted lobectomy in obese patients with non-small-cell lung cancer. Interact Cardiovasc Thorac Surg. 2020;30(3):359-365.

[26] Louie BE. Robotic lobectomy for non-small cell lung cancer. Indian J Surg Oncol. 2013;4(2):125-131.

[27] Casiraghi M, Galetta D, Borri A, Tessitore A, Romano R, Diotti C, et al. Ten Years' Experience in Robotic-Assisted Thoracic Surgery for Early Stage Lung Cancer. Thorac Cardiovasc Surg. 2019;67(7):564-572.

[28] Guo F, Ma D, Li S. Compare the prognosis of Da Vinci robot-assisted thoracic surgery (RATS) with video-assisted thoracic surgery (VATS) for non-small cell lung cancer: A Meta-analysis. Medicine (Baltimore). 2019;98(39):e17089.

[29] Kneuertz PJ, D'Souza DM, Richardson M, Abdel-Rasoul M, Moffatt-Bruce SD, Merritt RE. Long-Term Oncologic Outcomes After Robotic Lobectomy for Early-stage Non-Small-cell Lung Cancer Versus Video-assisted Thoracoscopic and Open Thoracotomy Approach. Clin Lung Cancer. 2020;21(3):214-224 e2.

[30] Nelson DB, Mehran RJ, Mitchell KG, Rajaram R, Correa AM, Bassett RL, Jr., et al. Robotic-Assisted Lobectomy for Non-Small Cell Lung Cancer: A Comprehensive Institutional

Experience. Ann Thorac Surg. 2019;108(2):370-376.

[31] Tchouta LN, Park HS, Boffa DJ, Blasberg JD, Detterbeck FC, Kim AW. Hospital Volume and Outcomes of Robot-Assisted Lobectomies. Chest. 2017;151(2):329-339.

[32] Cerfolio RJ, Ghanim AF, Dylewski M, Veronesi G, Spaggiari L, Park BJ. The long-term survival of robotic lobectomy for non-small cell lung cancer: A multi-institutional study. J Thorac Cardiovasc Surg. 2018;155(2):778-786.

[33] Zhang Y, Chen C, Hu J, Han Y, Huang M, Xiang J, et al. Early outcomes of robotic versus thoracoscopic segmentectomy for early-stage lung cancer: A multi-institutional propensity score-matched analysis. J Thorac Cardiovasc Surg. 2020.

[34] Zhou Q, Huang J, Pan F, Li J, Liu Y, Hou Y, et al. Operative outcomes and long-term survival of robotic-assisted segmentectomy for stage IA lung cancer compared with video-assisted thoracoscopic segmentectomy. Transl Lung Cancer Res. 2020;9(2):306-315.

[35] Qiu T, Zhao Y, Xuan Y, Qin Y, Niu Z, Shen Y, et al. Robotic sleeve lobectomy for centrally located non-small cell lung cancer: A propensity score-weighted comparison with thoracoscopic and open surgery. J Thorac Cardiovasc Surg. 2020;160(3):838-46 e2.

[36] Emmert A, Straube C, Buentzel J, Roever C. Robotic versus thoracoscopic lung resection: A systematic review and meta-analysis. Medicine. 2017;96(35):e7633-e.

[37] Tang A, Raja S, Bribriesco AC, Raymond DP, Sudarshan M, Murthy SC, et al. Robotic Approach Offers Similar Nodal Upstaging to Open Lobectomy for Clinical Stage I Non-small Cell Lung Cancer. Ann Thorac Surg. 2020;110(2):424-433.

[38] Park BJ, Yang HX, Woo KM, Sima CS. Minimally invasive (robotic assisted thoracic surgery and video-assisted thoracic surgery) lobectomy for the treatment of locally advanced non-small cell lung cancer. J Thorac Dis. 2016;8(Suppl 4):S406–S413.

[39] Spaggiari L, Sedda G, Maisonneuve P, Tessitore A, Casiraghi M, Petrella F, et al. A Brief Report on Survival After Robotic Lobectomy for Early Stage Lung Cancer. J Thorac Oncol. 2019;14(12):2176-2180.

[40] Li C, Hu Y, Huang J, Li J, Jiang L, Lin H, et al. Comparison of robotic-assisted lobectomy with video-assisted thoracic surgery for stage IIB-IIIA non-small cell lung cancer. Transl Lung Cancer Res. 2019;8(6):820-828.

[41] Sesti J, Langan RC, Bell J, Nguyen A, Turner AL, Hilden P, et al. A Comparative Analysis of Long-Term Survival of Robotic Versus Thoracoscopic Lobectomy. Ann Thorac Surg. 2020;110(4):1139-1146.

[42] Turner SR, Latif MJ, Park BJ. Robotic assisted VATS lobectomy for loco-regionally advanced non-small cell lung cancer. Video Assist Thorac Surg. 2017;2.

[43] Yang HX, Woo KM, Sima CS, Bains MS, Adusumilli PS, Huang J, et al. Long-term Survival Based on the Surgical Approach to Lobectomy For Clinical Stage I Nonsmall Cell Lung Cancer: Comparison of Robotic, Video-assisted Thoracic Surgery, and Thoracotomy Lobectomy. Ann Surg. 2017;265(2):431-437.

[44] Louie BE, Farivar AS, Aye RW, Vallières E. Early experience with robotic lung resection results in similar operative outcomes and morbidity when

compared with matched video-assisted thoracoscopic surgery cases. Ann Thorac Surg. 2012;93(5):1598-1604; discussion 604-5.

[45] Louie BE, Wilson JL, Kim S, Cerfolio RJ, Park BJ, Farivar AS, et al. Comparison of Video-Assisted Thoracoscopic Surgery and Robotic Approaches for Clinical Stage I and Stage II Non-Small Cell Lung Cancer Using The Society of Thoracic Surgeons Database. Ann Thorac Surg. 2016;102(3):917-924.

[46] Li JT, Liu PY, Huang J, Lu PJ, Lin H, Zhou QJ, et al. Perioperative outcomes of radical lobectomies using robotic-assisted thoracoscopic technique vs. video-assisted thoracoscopic technique: retrospective study of 1,075 consecutive p-stage I non-small cell lung cancer cases. J Thorac Dis. 2019;11(3):882-891.

[47] Novellis P, Bottoni E, Voulaz E, Cariboni U, Testori A, Bertolaccini L, et al. Robotic surgery, video-assisted thoracic surgery, and open surgery for early stage lung cancer: comparison of costs and outcomes at a single institute. J Thorac Dis. 2018;10(2):790-798.

[48] Lazar JF, Spier LN, Hartman AR, Lazzaro RS. Standardizing Robotic Lobectomy: Feasibility and Safety in 128 Consecutive Lobectomies Within a Single Healthcare System. Innovations (Phila). 2017;12(2):77-81.

[49] Kneuertz PJ, Singer E, D'Souza DM, Abdel-Rasoul M, Moffatt-Bruce SD, Merritt RE. Hospital cost and clinical effectiveness of robotic-assisted versus video-assisted thoracoscopic and open lobectomy: A propensity score-weighted comparison. J Thorac Cardiovasc Surg. 2019;157(5):2018-2026 e2.

[50] Lee EC, Lazzaro RS, Glassman LR, Singh VA, Jurado JE, Hyman KM, et al. Switching from Thoracoscopic to Robotic Platform for Lobectomy: Report of Learning Curve and Outcome. Innovations (Phila). 2020;15(3):235-242.

[51] Spaggiari L, Galetta D. Pneumonectomy for Lung Cancer: A Further Step in Minimally Invasive Surgery. The Annals of Thoracic Surgery. 2011;91(3).

[52] Louie BE. Robotic Pneumonectomy. Thoracic Surgery Clinics. 2014;24(2):169-175.

Section 3

Radiotherapeutic and Ablative Technology

Chapter 4

Radiotherapy: An Alternative to Surgery

Paul Van Houtte, Charlier Florian, Luigi Moretti and Dirk Van Gestel

Abstract

Many major technical developments have occurred during the last decades in radiotherapy: our efficacy has improved with less toxicity. Nowadays, it allows us to challenge the role of surgery as a local modality for lung cancer both for early, advanced and even metastatic disease. In the present paper, we will mainly discuss the role of SBRT for stage I lung cancer, the place of conventional radiotherapy for stage III and we will review the current treatment of small cell lung cancer from a radiation oncologist perspective.

Keywords: SBRT, trimodality stage III, small cell lung cancer chest RT, PCI

1. Introduction

Radiation oncology is an important player in the treatment of lung cancer either alone taking advantage of the new technological developments (stereotactic radiotherapy, intensity modulated radiotherapy, image guide radiotherapy) or with surgery and systemic treatment (chemotherapy, immunotherapy, targeted drugs). To-day, radiotherapy may even challenge surgery as the loco-regional treatment both for stage I and III non-small cell lung cancer (NSCLC) and is the local treatment for small cell lung cancer (SCLC). In the present chapter, we will discuss those different clinical situations and presenting the current knowledge.

2. Stage I lung cancer: radiotherapy as an alternative to surgery

2.1 Stereotactic radiotherapy for early stage lung cancer (SBRT)

Surgery is the treatment of reference for early stage lung cancer and a lobectomy or an anatomical segmentectomy in selected cases coupled with a lymph node dissection is the preferred approach [1]. For early stages, surgery is generally technically less complex and associated with less toxicity and mortality than for more advanced stages. Still, some patients cannot undergo surgery due to medical comorbidities. In the past, conventional (long course) radiotherapy or even no treatment was often proposed to those patients; the outcome was very poor: in a review, the 2-year survival rates range from 22 to 72% and the 5-year survival rates from 0 to 42% [2].

In early 1990's, a new radiotherapy technique emerged in Europe and Japan, built on the experience with intracranial stereotactic treatments, called stereotactic hypofractionated radiotherapy, stereotactic irradiation (STI), or extracranial stereotactic radioablation (ESR), and now more commonly referred to Stereotactic Body Radiation Therapy (SBRT) or Stereotactic Ablative Radiotherapy (SABR) [3, 4]. This is a novel form of high-precision, image-guided radiotherapy and aims to deliver higher radiation doses in a reduced number of fractions resulting in a higher Biologically Effective Dose (BED) than "conventional RT", i.e. a higher biological impact for a given physical dose. This approach treats only the tumour without any coverage of the hilar or mediastinal lymph nodes.

Several retrospective studies observed encouraging results for early stage lung cancers and in 2006, the results of a prospective phase II trial testing SBRT for inoperable patients was published by Timmerman et al.: encouraging oncological outcomes were confirmed with 60 Gy or 66 Gy delivered in 3 fractions for T1 or T2 tumours [5–7]. However, the trial also showed an 11-fold increase in high grade toxicity, including even death. This was associated with the treatment of perihilar/centrally located tumours, those in a region close to the proximal bronchial tree that was later referred to as the "no-fly-zone".

In 2010, the phase II trial NRG Oncology Radiation Therapy Oncology Group (RTOG) 0236 reported a 97.6% 3-year local control (LC) rate (95% CI 84.3–99.7) for a cohort of 55 patients with a T1–T2N0M0 peripheral lesion (tumour diameter less than 5 cm) treated with 3 fractions of 18 Gy [8]. Toxicity was limited with 2 grade 4 events and no grade 5. This trial updated results was reported in 2018 with a median follow-up of 48 months: recurrences at the primary site were rare at 5 years (7.3%) but the 5-year disease-free survival and overall survival (OS) rates were respectively 25.5% and 40.0% [9]. If SBRT is very effective to treat a specific lesion, occult spread may already occur and impact prognosis as well as intercurrent death related to the patient comorbidity. Data from larger cohorts and many other phase 2 trials also confirmed that SBRT is an effective and safe approach for inoperable patients but some studies also included medically operable patient who had refused a surgery [10–13]. The latter group showed a better outcome due to less intercurrent death with even long term survival data close to the surgical series [14]. Furthermore, in the US National Cancer Data Base, Nanda et al. reported better survival for elderly patients (70 years or older) treated with SBRT than no treatment and this was still valid regardless of patient age [15]. Last but not least, SBRT was compared to conventional RT in two randomised trials: a better outcome was observed with less toxicity and was more convenient for the patients by reducing the travels to the radiotherapy department [16, 17].

2.2 Central tumours

Central tumours represent a challenge after the toxicity reported by the RTOG phase II trial [7]. Different groups have tried to identify treatment possibilities for these patients, mainly with different dose-fractionation schemes or with lower doses to the periphery of the planning target volume (PTV) than 3 fractions of 20 Gy [18–21]. With more data available from many centres, a distinction was necessary within the central tumours located within the no-fly-zone: the distance to the bronchial tree and the oesophagus was crucial in determining the toxicity risk and leading to the definition of ultra-central tumours (UC): meaning the PTV overlaps the proximal bronchial tree or the oesophagus [21, 22]. A systematic review published in 2019 reported on the results of nine trials with at least 5 UC tumours, for a total of 291 patients but all studies have a slightly different definition for an UC [23]. SBRT treatments delivered a BED (for a α/β ratio of 10 Gy, $BED_{10\,Gy}$) of 67.2 Gy (48 Gy in 12 fractions) to 112.5 Gy (50 Gy in 4 fractions). Grade 3 toxicity or more ranged from 0% in two smaller-sized trials up to 55.5% at 2 years including 10 deaths in a cohort of 47 patients. In this particular trial there was no dose limit to the trachea and main bronchi and there was a great difference between the prescribed dose and the maximum dose delivered. In total, 8 studies reported grade 5 complications, mostly due to haemorrhage (15 of 22 cases). All studies reporting statistical comparisons of outcomes did not find differences in OS (6 studies) or LC (4 studies) between central and ultra-central tumours. Furthermore, six trials described a statistical comparison of toxicity rates without any significant difference.

The question of the best radiation management for non-peripheral tumours is currently still open and being examined by the LungTech and SUNSET trials, respectively investigating central and ultra-central localizations [24, 25]. In current clinical practice, SBRT is commonly performed for central tumours or isolated mediastinal lymph nodes at lower doses than peripheral tumours. In Onishi experience, a $BED_{10\,Gy} > 100$ Gy was decisive to obtain a high local control and survival with SBRT [6]. For (ultra-)central tumours, this cannot always be achieved, but at the same time, dose constraints for central airways and oesophagus can be observed to avoid severe toxicity but at the price of a lower efficacy.

2.3 SBRT vs. surgery

Since the early 2010's, SBRT is accepted as a standard treatment for patients medically inoperable or refusing surgery. As comorbidities can also prevent a safe biopsy, SBRT is now accepted for the management of lesions highly suspicious of lung cancer without necessary a histological confirmation. SBRT has a favourable toxicity profile and a good local efficacy and SBRT may challenge surgery. Survival outcomes of SBRT could seem somewhat poor when compared to surgical series. However, most patients treated with SBRT present severe comorbidities or were older and such a direct comparison of survival is not appropriate. These comorbidities could dramatically impact prognosis by influencing further treatments, non-cancer related survival...

Several studies performed propensity score matching to compare surgical and SBRT patients' outcomes with controversial results. A meta-analysis of propensity score matched studies was published in 2019 including 15 studies [26]. The results seemed to confirm a better 3-year OS after surgery but these results were questionable as unbalance remained in the matchings, meaning that patients were not similar after all. When restricting the analyses to studies with comparable covariates, no statistically significant difference in OS was found anymore. Selection biases seem inevitable in clinical practice, and so the need for randomised trials is generally recognised.

Several phase III trials randomised patients for SBRT or surgery and were initiated by different groups. STARS (registered as NCT00840749 on ClinicalTrials.gov), started in 2008 in the United States, aiming to identify a difference in 3-year OS, which required enrolment of 1030 patients over an expected period of 7 years. After having recruited 36 patients in 4 years, enrolment was prematurely closed. The ROSEL trial (NCT00687986) that started in the Netherlands, also in 2008, faced a similar situation as only 22 of the 900 patients planned could be enrolled.

A pooled analysis of the STARS and ROSEL cohorts was published in 2015 [27]. These trials were quite similar in terms of inclusion criteria and interventions, although central tumours were eligible in the STARS trial only (two were included). For the 58 patients enrolled, 31 were treated with SBRT (20 in STARS, 11 in ROSEL) and 27 with surgery. All surgical patients had hilar lymph node dissection and either dissection or sampling of several mediastinal nodal levels. Radiotherapy treatments for peripheral lesions were 54 Gy in three 18 Gy fractions in both trials but could also have been 60 Gy in five fractions in ROSEL trial (which happened for 5 patients), based on the practice of treating centres. It should be noted that, as often the case in RT, the prescription corresponded to technically slightly different treatments between the two trials.

Although based on few patients, the Chang analysis showed a statistically significant difference in OS with estimated survival rates at 1 and 3 years of 100% (95% CI 100–100) and 95% (85–100) in the SBRT arm for 88% (95% CI 77–100) and 79% (95% CI 64–97) in the surgical group (log rank p = 0.037, HR 0.34, 95% CI 0.017–1.19). Only seven deaths were reported: one patient in the SBRT group who died of cancer progression and six patients in the surgery group (three from lung cancer including a second primary, two from comorbidities and one from attributed to the surgical treatment). Both the STARS and ROSEL trials surgical groups included patient treated with the older thoracotomy technique and not the more actual and less morbid Video-Assisted Thoracoscopy (VATS).

To put things into perspective, a meta-analysis based on 40 SBRT studies (10 prospective, 30 retrospective) and 23 surgery studies (all retrospective), for respectively 4850 and 7071 patients, reported unadjusted 3-year OS for SBRT, lobectomy and sublobar resections of 56.6%, 80.7%, and 77.8%, respectively [28]. After adjustment for suitability for surgery (which integrates comorbidities and age), the estimated survival rates were higher for SBRT patients, although not statistically different, with 89% (95% CI 76–95) vs. 81% (95% CI 76–85) for lobectomy and 80% (95% CI 76–86) for limited lung resection. Currently, the Veteran administration is running a large phase III trial comparing surgery to SBRT (VALOUR trial) [29]. Interesting, the trial includes operable patients with tissue confirmation of NSCLC, staging with FDG-PET/CT, and biopsies of all hilar and/or mediastinal lymph nodes >10 mm that have a SUV >2.5. SBRT doses depend on the tumour location: peripheral tumours will receive either 18 Gy x 3,14 Gy x 4, or 11.5 Gy x 5 fractions, while central tumours will be treated with 10 Gy x 5. The surgery will be either a lobectomy or anatomic pulmonary resection (a segmentectomy) and mediastinal lymph node sampling.

If indeed new decisions regarding patients' management cannot be made based on a post-hoc analysis of two very small sample trials and observational data, the superiority of the surgical approach might not be certain anymore and randomising large numbers of patients is still necessary to provide level-I evidence to answer the question.

The major accrual problem in these trials was attributed to the lack of equipoise in the physicians' minds, or maybe to financial considerations. The two treatment modalities are very different, which can have strong impact on both patients and physicians limiting the acceptability of leaving the treatment choice to chance. Surgery is performed on in-patient basis. As the tumour is removed, it is easier to identify local recurrences. Mediastinal nodal dissection or sampling also allows to identify false negative of PET/CT staging and to guide the decision for an adjuvant treatment. In many SBRT series, the mediastinal evaluation is often limited to the CT or the PET-CT with fewer patients having a mediastinal sampling with Endobronchial Ultrasonography – Transbronchial Needle Aspiration (EBUS–TBNA). Even though an operable patient could be safely operated for salvage in the rare cases of regional relapse, it is probably better to provide the most exhaustive staging possible before choosing the treatment modality.

Another issue is the extra-thoracic failure suggesting to add a systemic treatment. The patients treated currently with a SBRT have often many co-morbidities and are not the good candidate for adjuvant chemotherapy due to the acute toxicity. An answer may be immunotherapy following the impressive positive results for more advanced stages: pembroluzimab, durvalumab and atezolumab are tested in different trials (KEYNOTE-867, PACIFIC-4, SWOG S1914) as an adjuvant treatment or concurrently with SBRT. An important issue will be the tolerance and the toxicity in this elderly population.

In conclusion, SBRT is an effective treatment modality and a very acceptable alternative to surgery for patients at high surgical risk. For fit patients, a large scale randomised trial is still considered necessary to answer the question: can SBRT replace safely surgery?

3. Stage III non-small cell lung cancer

To-day, most fit patients with a stage III NSCLC are treated with a program of chemoradiotherapy favouring a concurrent approach (CRT) [30]. The results remain far from satisfactory in term of overall survival. This is due to distant metastases and loco-regional failure. Using all our technological developments (IMRT, image guided radiotherapy, PET-CT based planning), local failure is still a major challenge even after doses in excess of 60 Gy. In the recent trial conducted by the RTOG comparing 60 to 74 Gy, the 5 year local failure rates are 49.7% after 60 Gy and 55.4% after 74 Gy [31]. Adding a third modality, surgery, is an appealing approach already proposed many years ago by Strauss and Sugerbacker in their literature review [32]. From a theoretical point of view, there is a clear synergism between radiotherapy and surgery: failure after radiotherapy is often observed in the bulk of the tumour, an area of hypoxia less sensitive to radiation while for surgery, local relapses occur at the margins of resection. Another approach is to improve the systemic treatment by adding immunotherapy.

There are several ways of combining the three modalities: induction chemoradiotherapy (concurrent or sequential) followed by surgery or a sequential approach with an induction chemotherapy followed by surgery and postoperative radiotherapy (PORT). The latter has the advantage to have less toxicity, the ability to evaluate the response to the chemotherapy especially the possible downstaging of mediastinal nodes allowing selecting the best candidate for surgery, the use of full dose of chemotherapy, to treat the possible micro metastatic spread and to have a full pathological evaluation. The drawback is that PORT will be less efficient due to the poor vascularization and the loss of lung volume especially in case of a pneumonectomy. The former allows taking advantage of the radiosensitizing properties of many drugs to obtain a higher rate of tumour response including pathologic complete response but at the price off more surgical complications and more toxicity. The ultimate goal of a three-modality approach is to improve survival while local control and progression free survival (PFS) are only surrogate endpoints.

3.1 Induction chemoradiotherapy before surgery

Many phase II trials reported a higher response rate, more downstaging and pathologic complete response but also more postoperative complications with CRT compared to chemotherapy alone. Using the National Cancer database including more than 11,000 patients with stage III NSCLC, the trimodality approach let to a better outcome with a 5-year survival around 32% [33]. In another analysis from the same database, 1936 patients with a T1, T2 N2 disease were treated with preoperative CRT or induction chemotherapy [34]. The pathologic complete response was higher after CRT (14.2% vs. 4%) but with an increased perioperative mortality and no improvement in OS. One problem with databases even a large one is certainly all the possible biases of patient selections but also the difference in local medical facilities. Indeed, academic facilities were more likely to treat patient with the trimodality than in a community hospital [35]. This is well illustrated by a recent paper including more than 83,000 patients presenting a stage III NSCLC treated in 1319 facilities. Those treated in a high volume centre (more than 15 patients) were more likely to have surgery or a trimodality and had significantly a lower risk of death [36]. This is one reason to look more to randomised trials to answer the question.

The role of surgery after a concurrent CRT compared to an exclusive CRT approach was tested by two trials conducted in Germany and in the US [37, 38]. Both trials did not observe any difference in OS but only a better local control after a surgical resection or a better PFS. Do we need to include radiotherapy in an induction program? The main advantage of avoiding RT is to reduce the acute toxicity and the surgical complications. Three randomised trials compared induction chemotherapy to a CRT approach for patients presenting with N2 disease initially considered resectable. The Swiss trial is the largest one and the most recent [39]. 232 patients were randomised between induction chemotherapy followed 4 weeks later by surgery and induction chemotherapy followed by RT (44 Gy in 22 fractions and 3 weeks) without any chemotherapy and surgery 3 to 4 weeks later. PFS and OS were not found different between the two arms. A R0 resection was observed in 91% and 81% in the arm with or without RT respectively. The pathologic complete responses were very similar with respectively 16 and 12%. Interestingly, no operative mortality was reported after RT. The main criticism is the use of a sequential approach perhaps explaining the low rate of pathological complete response. Recently, our Spanish colleague reported 99 patients treated with either preoperative CRT or induction chemotherapy. CRT significantly increased the pathologic complete response rate and nodal down staging and reduced the loco-regional recurrence; unfortunately, this did not translate in any survival benefit [40].

PreCRT is a commonly used strategy in patients with superior sulcus tumours. In two phase II trials including 110 and 76 patients, a CRT delivered 45 Gy combined with cisplatin, etoposide or cisplatin, vindesine, mitomycin chemotherapy. A N2 disease was an exclusion criterion. The 5-year survival rates were 44% and 56%, respectively [41, 42]. Important prognostic factors were R0 resection and pathologic complete response. One drawback is the relatively low RT dose in case of no surgery or incomplete resection. Another approach is to deliver a full RT dose. In a Dutch series, 49 patients treated with CRT before surgery (19 patients) or as a definitive treatment (30 patients) [43]. 5-year survival was 33% for the three modalities and 18% for the definitive RT. Clearly, patients selected for the trimodality were highly selected.

3.2 Induction chemotherapy followed by surgery and postoperative radiotherapy

Most trials evaluating PORT were carried out in an era of old radiation technique and not after induction chemotherapy. The meta-analysis showed a detrimental effect of PORT especially for stage I and II disease [44]. Another meta-analysis stratified the trials according to the use of a cobalt 60 unit or a linear accelerator [45]. PORT carried out with a linear accelerator increased OS and local control for stage III disease. Many retrospective analyses from single centre or from large data base look at the impact of PORT for stage III: if local control was improved, the impact on survival led to conflicting results.

RT technique is a key factor to avoid an excessive toxicity. The radiation plans used in the trials included in the meta-analysis were compared to our current RT techniques [46]. The older technique led to poor target coverage and an excessive toxicity. The target coverage reached only 65% and the heart $V30_{Gy}$ and the lung $V20_{Gy}$ were higher with the technique used in the randomised trials. A Polish study evaluated the cardio-respiratory functions in patients who did and did not receive modern PORT technique: they observed no increase in non-cancer radiation-induced mortality or deterioration of lung functions [47].

Currently, another issue is the role of PORT after induction chemotherapy for N2 disease since local relapse is a common feature as observed in several prospective phase II series. The cumulative loco regional recurrence rose even to 60% in the Betticher trial including 75 patients treated with upfront chemotherapy followed by surgery [48]. Persistent N2 disease after ICT is a pejorative factor but several questions on PORT remain: the place of PORT according to the pathologic response ypN0 versus ypN2 and PORT only or with sequential or concurrent chemotherapy. The data were coming from retrospective studies but the results of the LungArt trial were just presented at the ESMO congress: this phase III trial compared mediastinal PORT (54 Gy in 27–30 fractions) to no PORT. Patients included had a complete resection with nodal exploration, proven N2 disease and neo or adjuvant chemotherapy. PORT was associated with a non- statistically significant 15% increase in DFS at 3 years but without an OS benefit [49].

3.3 Discussion

All those trials have a major problem: they were conducted many years ago and are not in agreement with our current practice due to technological developments in diagnostic procedure (MR, PET-CT), in radiotherapy and in surgery and to the new drugs available including target agents and immunotherapy. Clearly, those data do not help us to choose between a trimodality and a concurrent chemoradiotherapy as the results suggest similar outcome in term of survival. Furthermore, stage III is a very heterogeneous group of tumours and the TNM has evolved over the years with different stage grouping both for the T and the N components in the different UICC classifications. Many trials have only included N2 patients or stage IIIA while other also included stage IIIB.

Nevertheless, there are a few lessons we have learned. One concern using induction chemotherapy before a local treatment is the delay between its termination and the start of the local treatment: accelerated repopulation of cancer cells and tumour regrowth can occur [50]. This is even more valid when the decision to do the surgery is taken after the induction treatment to see the possibility of a resection with free margins. In case of no resection or incomplete resection, the patient may have not an optimal curative treatment as the preoperative RT dose is often too low to achieve a good local control. Moreover, the addition of a boost delivered after several weeks of RT interruption is not very effective due to tumour repopulation.

The decision between both approaches should be discuss on individual base after a careful patient evaluation with a full staging including PET-CT and brain MR to avoid a futile treatment and an evaluation of patient fitness to undergo surgery or even radiotherapy. Many patients have a long history of tobacco smoking and are suffering from many co-morbidities increasing the risk of complications or even not allowing a surgical resection. The decision is to be taken during a tumour board involving all specialties: the feasibility of a complete resection with free margins should be evaluated; an incomplete resection is by definition a futile thoracotomy and salvage treatments have limited efficacy. Another issue is the possibility to deliver a full course of radiotherapy with concurrent chemotherapy. This implies to be able to deliver doses in excess of 60 Gy or a biological equivalent dose taken into account the tolerance of the different organs at risk including the normal lung but also the heart. Finally yet importantly, an essential parameters are the local treatment facilities and the local clinical expertise but also the discussion with the patient of the pros and cons.

3.4 Immunotherapy with anti PDL1 drugs

If immunotherapy approach was in the past not very successful especially the vaccination strategies; the current approach is to play on T-cell activation or modulation in the tumour or microenvironment using anti-PD-1/PD-L1 drugs. Those drugs have fully changed the pattern of care for stage IV NSCLC with marked improved survival. It was often consider that RT had an immunosuppressive effect. Nowadays, there is a body of evidence suggesting that RT may increase the immune response both locally and systematically [51]. RT may act through a spectrum of cellular and molecular alterations and through the release of tumour-associated antigen. There are now a lot of observations suggesting a synergistic action of RT with anti-immune-checkpoint blockades with anti-PD-(L)1. Experimental data showed an increase in the expression of PD-L1 at the surface of tumoral cells after RT, improving the survival [52].

An interesting observation was seen in the phase I trial with pembrolizumab in stage IV NSCLC: in the phase I trial Keynote-001, patients treated with radiotherapy prior to pembrolizumab had a better survival regardless of the site irradiated [53]. In case of chest RT, 3 patients out of 24 developed a grade 3 lung toxicity after prior RT compared to one 1 out of 73 for pembroluzimab.

PACIFIC is a large scale phase III trial comparing durvalumab (an anti-PD-L1 antibody) to a placebo as a consolidation treatment after chemoradiotherapy [54]. Patients had to have received two cycles of cisplatin-based chemotherapy and a response or stable disease. The randomisation was performed 1 to 42 days after the end of radiotherapy. Few data are available regarding the initial chemoradiotherapy. Durvalumab was administered every 2 weeks for up to 12 months. The three year OS was 66.3% versus 43.5% for the placebo arm, results highly statistically significant. The PD-L1 status was not known for all patients but a post hoc analysis found similar results regardless of PD-L1 status. The lung toxicity was 13% after durvalumab and 8% in the placebo arm but grade 3 pneumonitis rates were very similar (3.4% vs. 2.6%). It is also not easy to compare the observed survival to others series as randomisation in PACIFIC is done after initial chemoradiotherapy, excluding those patients progressing or not tolerating the initial treatment. Nevertheless, this trial has changed our daily practice by adding durvalumab quickly after the end of chemoradiotherapy in locally advanced NSCLC.

The question of finding the best combination of immunotherapy and radiotherapy remains. Experimental data suggest better results when the drug is given during radiotherapy rather after its end: this was seen in an experimental study conducted on mice with colon carcinoma CT26 tumours [52]. One concern is the risk of increased toxicity especially at the level of lungs and heart: pneumonia is a classical complication of anti-PD-L1 drugs but also after chest radiotherapy. The NICOLAS phase II trial was designed specifically to answer this question [55]. Patients were treated with three cycles of a cisplatin-based chemotherapy and radiotherapy started with the second cycle together with nivolumab given up to 1 year. The endpoint was grade 3 or more pneumonitis observed during 6 months after the end of RT. Amongst the 80 patients included, 8 developed grade 3 pneumonitis after radiotherapy.

Radiation may also release tumoral antigens allowing a better recognition by the immune system but also acting against tumour cells outside the radiation field (the so called "abscopal effect"). In the Pembroluzimab-RT phase II trial, patients with stage IV NSCLC were randomised between pembroluzimab alone and pembroluzimab given after SBRT to a single metastatic site [56]. The goal was to test if SBRT increases the response rate: 17 patients out of 36 presented a response with the combined approach vs. 9 out of 40 patients in the pembroluzimab alone arm. The disease control rates at 12 weeks were respectively 63% vs. 40%. A retrospective study included 117 patients: 54 received SBRT with concurrent immune checkpoint inhibition and 63 SBRT alone. The risk of grade 3 radiation pneumonitis was higher in the combined approach (10.7% vs. 0%) [57]. In patients with a oligometastatic disease, the addition of a local treatment such as SBRT is a very exciting approach but a close monitoring for pneumonitis should be considered. Several trials are currently on-going.

Ultimately, there are a lot of unresolved questions: what is the optimal dose (low or high as the one used with SBRT), the actual volume to be treated, the timing...? Clearly, it is not easy to use a SBRT approach in stage III NSCLC as it is done for smaller metastatic lesions in stage IV NSCLC; the total volume to irradiate in stage III disease is much larger and could potentially lead to an excessive toxicity. Another issue lies in the volume of circulating immune cells during RT: the current technique to irradiate stage III NSCLC uses IMRT techniques delivering very low doses spread across large normal tissue volumes which may decrease the lymphocytes counts (a very sensitive cell to low RT dose), and subsequently the immune response. A retrospective study has observed a lower survival in case of lower absolute lymphocyte blood count [58]. So, blood-containing organs such as great vessels, heart and bone marrow may become a new organ at risk to spare in the future. Ideally, there is an urgent need to find a biomarker allowing to better select patients candidate for a combined approach in order to avoid futile treatments and also to decrease the expenses of those new treatments.

4. Small cell lung cancer (SCLC)

SCLC accounts for around 15% of all diagnosed lung cancers worldwide [59]. It is a highly aggressive, undifferentiated neoplasia characterised by a high proliferation rate and early metastatic spread. Although SCLC is very responsive to initial chemotherapy and radiotherapy, early recurrences are common and the prognosis of SCLC remains poor with 5-year overall survival rates of under 10% [60].

In the late 60's, SCLC was staged as limited disease to the thorax (LS) or extensive stage (ES) according to the Veterans' Affairs Lung Study Group classification and later modified by the International Association for the Study of Lung (IASLC) [61, 62]. Interestingly, limited disease include tumour confined to the ipsilateral hemithorax and regional lymph nodes in order to be encompassed in a radiation field. More recently, the IASLC recommends to use the revised TNM staging classification for lung cancer (American Joint Committee on Cancer AJCC 7th edition) for clinical decision making and clinical trials instead of the LS- and ES-categories, as it better discriminate the prognostic impact [63, 64].

4.1 Limited stage-small cell lung cancer (LS-SCLC)

CRT is the current standard of care [65]. In the early 90's two meta-analyses have outlined the benefit of adding chest RT to chemotherapy [66, 67]. The Pignon meta-analysis was the most interesting due to the utilisation of the patient individual data from 13 randomised trials: chest RT improved the OS by 5.4% at 3 years but at the price of more esophagitis [67]. The benefit was greater for patients under 55 years (the relative risk of death was 0.72), than for those over 70 years. Two meta-analyses of randomised controlled trials have looked to the timing of chemotherapy and RT: concurrent CRT should start as early as the 1st or 2nd cycle of platinum-based chemotherapy to be more effective in terms of survival, compared to delaying the start of RT to the 3rd cycle or later [68, 69].

Another question was the optimal dose and fractionation. In the Intergroup 0096 trial, 471 patients were randomised between 45 Gy in 30 fractions twice daily (BiD), in a total of 3 weeks and 45 Gy in 25 fractions, once a day in 5 weeks. In both arm, RT started with the first of the 4 cycles of chemotherapy (cisplatin and etoposide) [70]. Overall survival rates at 2 and 5 years were respectively 41 vs. 47%, and 16 vs. 26% ($p = 0.04$) in favour of the BiD treatment. The drawback was more acute toxicity, mainly grade 3–4 esophagitis, from 16–32% with the BiD but without any increase in the risk of grade 3 or higher pneumonitis (6% in both arms). Given the highly proliferative nature of SCLC, a shorter time between RT fractions and a shorter overall treatment time (3 weeks instead of 5) could explain the better results of BiD fractionation against tumour repopulation. However, the major limitation in the design of the Turrisi trial is that the two arms have not the same biologically equivalent dose, a higher dose for the BiD arm. Nevertheless, this pivotal trial confirmed the impact of a better local turning in a benefit of survival and cure. However, many radiation oncology centres did not use the BiD fractionation because of the increased oesophageal toxicity and the inconvenience for the patient linked to have two treatments on the same day with an interval of minimum 6 h between the 2 fractions but also for busy radiation facilities [71].

The Japan Clinical Oncology group JCO 9104 phase III trial compared a concurrent CRT to a sequential CRT and included 231 patients. Chest RT was delivered with the first of the 4 cycles of chemotherapy (cisplatine and etoposide) or one month after the last cycle. The chest RT was a BiD delivering 45 Gy in 30 fractions over 3 weeks [72]. The median OS was significantly better for the concurrent arm compared to the sequential one (27.2 vs. 19.7 months, $p = 0.02$ after adjustment for performance status, age, and stage in a Cox model). The oesophageal toxicity was quite similar between the two arms (4% vs. 9% for sequential vs. concurrent, respectively) but the haematological toxicity was increased with the concurrent treatment (grade 3–4 leukopenia: 88% vs. 54%, $p < 0.001$).

The CONVERT trial designed to answer the question rose by the Turrisi trial and included 547 patients [73]. The trial compared a BiD approach (45 Gy delivered in 30 fractions over 3 weeks) to an escalated daily RT (66 Gy in 33 fractions over 6.5 weeks). The study was designed to show superiority for the once daily experimental arm over the control BiD arm. While there was no difference in toxicity and OS between the two groups, the BiD arm showed a trend toward an improved median OS (30 vs. 25 months, $p = 0.14$), leading to the conclusion that BiD remains the standard of care. Still, a lot of radiotherapy centres prefer to use the more convenient once daily fractionation (at the total dose of 66 Gy) since survival and toxicity were similar in both arms [74]. A recent Scandinavian randomised phase II trial presented at the annual ASCO meeting randomised between high-dose BiD CRT of 60 Gy in 40 fractions (4 weeks) vs. 45 Gy in 30 fractions (3 weeks), both arms with 4 courses of platinum. The survival rate at 2 years were in favour of the 60 Gy arm (73% vs. 46%, $p = 0.001$), and they had a significantly longer median OS (42 months vs. 23 months; HR 0.63, $p = 0.031$) without any significant differences in term of toxicity (esophagitis or grade 3–4 pneumonitis) [75]. Those promising results need a confirmation through a phase III trial including more than the 160 patients. The RTOG is conducting a three arm trial comparing 70 Gy in 7 weeks, 61.2 Gy delivered with one fraction daily of 1.8 Gy for 16 days followed by 1.8 Gy BiD for 9 days to the classical 45 Gy in 3 weeks BiD (RTOG 0538 trial); the second arm was prematurely closed.

Durvalumab has also showed activity for extensive SCLC and is tested as adjuvant treatment for limited disease with or without tremalimumab (The

Adriatic trial). In a phase III trial, Atezolumab is delivered concurrently with chest RT and cisplatine-etoposide(NRG-LU005). The results of the Stimuli trial were presented at the last ESMO congress. After the end of chemoradiotherapy including also PCI, patients were randomised to receive ipilinumab and nivolumab for 12 months. No difference was observed in PFS neither in OS but increase the toxicity [76].

There is also the question of the target volume for radiotherapy: an elective nodal irradiation including the full mediastinum to treat the possible microscopic nodal sites was typically used in the past but at the cost of increased toxicity, an era of no PET-CT. In several prospective studies, the RT volume was limited to the known macroscopic disease as seen on a PET-CT and failures outside were a rare event: 3% and 2% in two different series of 60 patients from the Netherlands and the USA [77, 78].

Currently, the indications for surgery are limited to the very limited disease mainly stage I and II disease for fit patients and adjuvant chemotherapy is then necessary.

4.2 Extensive stage-small cell lung cancer (ES-SCLC)

The treatment cornerstone is a platinum-based chemotherapy regimens including cisplatin or carboplatin and etoposide combined with immunotherapy. This first line treatment yields often excellent initial responses and improved survival. However, recurrent or persistent intrathoracic disease is observed in more than 75% patients and local control remains a major problem during the first year of follow-up. A phase III study compared chest radiotherapy (54 Gy in 38 fractions over 18 days with concurrent cisplatin/etoposide) to only additional cycles of chemotherapy [79]. Patients had to have obtained a complete response at the metastatic sites and a complete or partial response in the thorax. The combined approach led to a better survival: median survival time of 17 months vs. 11 months and a 5-year survival rate of 9.1% vs. 3.7%.

The CREST trial randomised 498 patients to evaluate the benefit in term of OS by adding chest RT (30 Gy in 10 fractions over 2 weeks) as a local consolidation after first line cisplatin-based chemotherapy [80]. Although the study failed to achieve its initial endpoint of survival at 1-year, an interesting observation is certainly the slight survival improvement seen at 2 years: 13% vs. 3%, ($p = 0.004$). Importantly, RT allowed a marked 50% reduction in loco-regional recurrences. The radiation target volumes included the post-chemotherapy tumour and the nodal stations initially involved before the start of first line chemotherapy. These results lead to consider consolidative chest RT as a standard treatment after a response to chemotherapy, in addition to prophylactic cranial radiotherapy. Nevertheless, this is now questionable: two trials have showed a survival improvement by adding atezolumab to a platinum doublet [81, 82]. A trial is now on-going to evaluate the role of consolidative radiotherapy to up to 5 sites after a partial response or stable disease after a doublet of cisplatinum with atezolumab (Raptor trial).

4.3 Prophylactic cranial irradiation (PCI)

Brain metastases (BM) represent a major challenge in the management of SCLC, with an incidence as high as 50% at 2 years. The brain is considered a sanctuary site due to the blood brain barrier and the limited access for most available drugs. Based on prior experiences in leukaemia, Heine Hansen introduced in 1973 the concept of PCI for SCLC [83]. The aim of PCI is to prevent BM, avoiding the potential neurological complications, and ultimately to improve survival.

Several randomised trials demonstrated that PCI decreased the incidence of BM and Auperin's meta-analysis using the individual data of 987 SCLC patients from 7 randomised trials confirmed clearly the survival benefits (both OS survival and PFS): PCI reduced by 25% the incidence of BM and increased the survival by 5,4% at 3 years (20,7% vs. 15,3%) [84–86]. Most patients had a limited-stage disease (85%) considered in complete response to the initial chemotherapy. A more recent meta-analysis including 1983 patients from 16 randomised trials showed a similar survival benefit without any impact of disease extent [87]. One problem with many trials is the lack of brain imaging in the initial staging and the CR evaluation: BM incidence is reduced by PCI from 53–40% in the absence of brain imaging while it reduces BM from 33 to 10% in case of brain CT-scan [88]. Today, MRI has increased the detection rate of BM from 10 to 24%. Importantly, the patients detected with BM by CT scan were often symptomatic while they had no symptoms in case of brain MRI.

The optimal radiation dose for PCI was tested by the large Intergroup PCI99–01 trial: 720 patients were randomised between 25 Gy in 10 fractions in 2 weeks vs. 36 Gy in 18 daily fractions or 24 BiD fractions [89]. This study failed to show any benefit with a higher radiation dose, neither on the incidence of BM or in survival; furthermore, the incidence of brain metastases remained high (35% at 3 years). Therefore, the recommended radiation schedule for PCI remains 25 Gy in 10 fractions delivered in 2 weeks.

Toxicity remains a major concern: acute (hair loss, fatigue,..) or late (hearing and cognitive impairment, dementia, leukoencephalopathy,...). The cognitive functions were evaluated before, at 6 and 12 months after PCI with the self-reported cognitive functions tests of EORTC: a threefold cognitive decline was observed at 6 months as well as at 12 months after PCI [90]. Those neurocognitive functions are highly depending on the hippocampus area. Currently trials are on-going to evaluate the efficacy and safety of a PCI using a hippocampus avoidance technique. Most guidelines recommend PCI for patients in complete response but it is also challenge by a close brain MRI follow-up [91, 92].

For patients presenting an extensive disease, PCI is also proposed after a response to platinum-based chemotherapy. This is based on the results of the EORTC phase III trial: patients with any response to chemotherapy were randomised between PCI and no PCI. PCI reduced the incidence of BM from 40–16% at one year, leading to a significant survival increase (13–27%) [93]. A pooled analysis of the North Central Cancer Treatment Group (NCCTG) trials including 421 patients observed similar results [94].

In contrast, a recent Japanese phase III trial randomised patients between PCI (25 Gy in 10 fractions) or no PCI after any response to initial chemotherapy and a recent MRI showing no BM [95]. The observation arm required to have brain MRI at 3-month intervals up to 12 months and at 18 and 24 months after enrolment. PCI reduced the incidence of BM but without any overall survival benefit: median survival was 11.6 months in the PCI group and 13.7 months in the observation group (HR = 1.27, 95% CI = 0.96–1.68; p = 0.094). Consequently, the Japan Lung Cancer Society removed PCI from their treatment guidelines in ES-SCLC. In those two trials, the patient population is quite different just by looking to the difference in survival. This trial and the concerns on PCI toxicity have led the SWOG to launch a trial comparing PCI to a MRI surveillance for extensive but also limited small cell lung cancer.

5. Conclusion

Over the past few years, major improvements have been made in the management of lung cancer due to the introduction of SBRT and immunotherapy. Both have changed the daily practice not only of early stage lung cancer but also for stage IV diseases. A major development in the future will be to include (SB) RT in the management of metastatic lung cancer to promote the immune system but also to treat local lung tumours. So, there is still a long way to understand how to optimise those modalities for each individual patient but also to understand the disease.

Author details

Paul Van Houtte*, Charlier Florian, Luigi Moretti and Dirk Van Gestel
Department of Radiation Oncology, Institut Jules Bordet, Université Libre de Bruxelles, Belgium

*Address all correspondence to: paul.vanhoutte@bordet.be

References

[1] Ginsberg RJ, Rubinstein LV. Randomized trial of lobectomy versus limited resection for T1 N0 non-small cell lung cancer. Lung Cancer Study Group. Ann. Thorac. Surg. 1995;**60**:615-622

[2] Rowell NP, Williams CJ. Radical radiotherapy for stage I/II non-small cell lung cancer in patients not sufficiently fit or declining surgery (medically inoperable): a systematic review. Thorax. 2001;**56**:628-638

[3] Blomgren H, Lax I, Naslund I, Svanström R. Stereotactic high dose fraction radiation therapy of extracranial tumors using an accelerator: Clinical experience of the first thirty-one patients. Acta Oncologica. 1995;**34**:861-870

[4] Uematsu M, Shioda A, Tahara K, et al. Focal, high dose, and fractionated modified stereotactic radiation therapy for lung carcinoma patients. Cancer. 1998;**82**:1062-1070

[5] Nagata Y, Takayama K, Matsuo Y, et al. Clinical outcomes of a phase I/II study of 48 Gy of stereotactic body radiotherapy in 4 fractions for primary lung cancer using a stereotactic body frame. International Journal of Radiation Oncology, Biology, Physics. 2005;**63**:1427-1431

[6] Onishi H, Araki T, Shirato H, et al. Stereotactic hypofractionated high-dose irradiation for stage I non small cell lung carcinoma. Cancer. 2004;**101**:1623-1631

[7] Timmerman R et al. Excessive toxicity when treating central tumors in a phase II study of stereotactic body radiation therapy for medically inoperable early-stage lung cancer. Journal of Clinical Oncology. 2006;**24**:4833-4839

[8] Timmerman R et al. Stereotactic body radiation therapy for inoperable early stage lung cancer. JAMA. 2010;**303**:1070-1076

[9] Timmerman RD, Paulus R, Pass HI, et al. Long-term results of stereotactic body radiation therapy in medically inoperable stage I non–small cell lung cancer. JAMA Oncology. 2018;**4**:1287-1288

[10] Uematsu M, Shioda A, Suda A, et al. Computed tomography-guided frameless stereotactic radiotherapy for stage I non-small cell lung cancer: A 5-year experience. Int. J. Radiat. Oncol. Biol. Phys. 2001;**51**:666-670

[11] Nyman J, Johansson K-A, Hultén U. Stereotactic hypofractionated radiotherapy for stage I non-small cell lung cancer—Mature results for medically inoperable patients. Lung Ca. 2006;**51**:97-103

[12] Ricardi U, Filippi AR, Guameri A, et al. Stereotactic body radiation therapy for early stage non-small cell lung cancer: Results of a prospective trial. Lung Ca. 2010;**68**:72-77

[13] Nagata Y, Hiraoka M, Shibata T, et al. Prospective trial of stereotactic body radiation therapy for both operable and inoperable T1N0M0 non-small cell lung cancer: Japan clinical oncology group study JCOG0403. Int. J. Radiat. Oncol. Biol. Phys. 2015;**93**:989-996

[14] Onishi H, Shirato H, Nagata Y, Hiraoka M, Fujino M, Gomi K, et al. Hypo-fractionated stereotactic radiotherapy (HypoFXSRT) for stage I non-small-cell-lung cancer: Updated results of 257 patients in a Japanese multiinstitutional study. J. Thorac. Oncol. 2007;**2**:94-100

[15] Nanda R, Liu Y, Gillepsie TW, et al. Stereotactic body radiation therapy versus no treatment for early stage non-small cell lung cancer in medically

inoperable elderly patients: a national cancer data base analysis. Cancer. 2015;**121**:4222-4230

[16] Nyman J, Hallqvist LJA, et al. Space SPACE - A randomized study of SBRT vs conventional fractionated radiotherapy in medically inoperable stage I NSCLC. Radiother Oncol. 2016;**121**:1-8

[17] Ball D, Mai GT, Shalini V, et al. Stereotactic ablative radiotherapy versus standard radiotherapy in stage 1 non-small-cell lung cancer (TROG 09.02 CHISEL): a phase 3, open-label, randomised controlled trial. Lancet Oncol. 2019;**20**:494-503

[18] Chang JY, Balter PA, Dong L, et al. Stereotactic body radiation therapy in centrally and superiorly located stage I or isolated recurrent non–small-cell lung cancer. Int. J. Radiat.Oncol.Biol. Phys. 2008;**72**:967-971

[19] Bral S, Gevaert T, Linthout N, et al. Prospective, risk-adapted strategy of stereotactic body radiotherapy for early-stage non–small-cell lung cancer: Results of a phase II trial. Int.J. Radiat. Oncol.Biol.Phys. 2011;**80**:1343-1349

[20] Haasbeek CJA, Lagerwaard FJ, Slotman BJ, Sunan S. Outcomes of stereotactic ablative radiotherapy for centrally located early-stage lung cancer. Journal of Thoracic Oncology. 2011;**6**:2036-2043

[21] Bezjak A, Paulus R, Gaspar LE, et al. Safety and efficacy of a five-fraction stereotactic body radiotherapy schedule for centrally located non–small-cell lung cancer: NRG oncology/RTOG 0813 trial. J. Clinic.Oncol. 2019;**37**:1316-1325

[22] Shibamoto Y, Hashizume C, Baba F, et al. Stereotactic body radiotherapy using a radiobiology-based regimen for stage I nonsmall cell lung cancer. Cancer. 2012;**118**:2078-2084

[23] Rim CH, Kim Y, Kim CY, et al. Is stereotactic body radiotherapy for ultra-central lung tumor a feasible option? A systemic review and meta-analysis. International Journal of Radiation Biology. 2019;**95**:329-337

[24] Adebahr S, Collette S, Shash E, et al. LungTech, an EORTC phase II trial of stereotactic body radiotherapy for centrally located lung tumours: A clinical perspective. Brit.J. Radiology. 2015;**88**:20150036

[25] Giuliani M, Mathew AS, Bahig H, et al. SUNSET: Stereotactic radiation for Ultracentral non–small-cell lung cancer—A safety and efficacy trial. Clinical Lung Cancer. 2018;**19**:e529-e532

[26] Zhang Q, Shao L, Tian J, et al. Stereotactic body radiation therapy or surgery for stage I–II non-small cell lung cancer treatment?—Outcomes of a meta-analysis. Translational Cancer Research. 2019;**8**:1381-1394

[27] Chang, J.Y., Senan S., Paul M..A.et al., Stereotactic ablative radiotherapy versus lobectomy for operable stage I non-small-cell lung cancer: A pooled analysis of two randomised trials. The Lancet Oncology 2015; 16: 630-637.

[28] Zheng X, Shipper M, Kidwell K, et al. Survival outcome after stereotactic body radiation therapy and surgery for stage I non-small cell lung cancer: A meta-analysis. Int. J. Radiat.Oncol.Biol. Phys. 2014;**90**:603-611

[29] Moghanaki D, Hagan M. Strategic initiatives for veterans with lung cancer. Fed.Pract. 2020;**37**(suppl 4):s76-s80

[30] Auperin A, Le Péchoux C, Rolland E, et al. Meta-analysis of concomitant versus sequential radiochemotherapy in locally advanced non-small-cell lung cancer. Journal of Clinical Oncology. 2010;**28**:2181-2190

[31] Bradley JD, Hu C, Komaki R, et al. Long-term results of NRG oncology RTOG 0617: Standard-versus high-dose

chemoradiotherapy with or without Cetuximab for unresectable stage III non-small-cell lung cancer. J.Clin.Oncol. 2020;**38**:706-714

[32] Strauss GM, Langer MP, Elias AD, Skarin AT, Sugarbaker DJ. Multimodality treatment of stage IIIA non-small cell lung carcinoma: Acritical review of literature and strategies for future research. J.Clin.Oncol. 1992:829-838

[33] Koshy M, Fedewa SA, Malik R, et al. Improved survival associated with neoadjuvant chemoradiation in patients clinical stageIIIA(N2)non-small cell lung cancer. J.Thor.Onc. 2011;**8**:915-922

[34] Krantz SB, Mitzman B, Lutfi W, et al. Neoadjuvant chemoradiation shows no survival advantage to chemotherapy alone in Stage IIIA Patients. Ann.Thorac. Surg. 2018;**105**:1008-1016

[35] Behera M, Steuer C, Liu Y, et al. Trimodality therapy in the treatment of stage III N2-positive non-small cell lung cancer: A National Cancer Database analysis. The Oncologist. 2020;**25**:e964-e975

[36] Kommalapati A, Tella SH, Goyal G, et al. Association between facility volume, therapy types and overall survival in patients with stage IIIA non-small cell lung cancer. J.Natl Compr.Canc.Netw. 2019;**17**:229-236

[37] Albain KS, Swann RS, Rusch VW, et al. Radiotherapy plus chemotherapy with or without surgical resection for stage III non-small-cell lung cancer: A phase III randomised controlled trial. Lancet. 2009;**374**:379-386

[38] Eberhardt WE, Pöttgen C, Gauler TC, et al. Phase III Study of Surgery Versus Definitive Concurrent Chemoradiotherapy Boost in Patients With Resectable Stage IIIA(N2) and Selected IIIB Non-Small-Cell Lung Cancer After Induction Chemotherapy and Concurrent Chemoradiotherapy (ESPATUE). J. Clin. Oncol. 2015;**33**:4194-4201

[39] Pless M, Stupp R, Ris HB, et al. Induction chemoradiation in stage IIIA/N2 non-small-cell lung cancer: a phase 3 randomised trial. Lancet. 2015;**386**:1049-1056

[40] Pöttgen C, Eberhardt W, Stamatis G, Montemuino S, de Dios NR, Martin M, et al. High-dose neoadjuvant chemoradiotherapy versus chemotherapy alone followed by surgery in potentially- resectable stage IIIA-N2 NSCLC. A multi-institutional retrospective study by the Oncologic Group for the Study of Lung Cancer (Spanish Radiation Oncology Society). Reports of Practical Oncology and Radiotherapy. 2020;**25**:447-455

[41] Rusch VW, Giroux DJ, Kraut MJ, et al. Induction chemoradiation and surgical resection for superior sulcus non-small-lung carcinomas: Long-term results of southwest oncology group trial 9416 (intergroup trial 0160). J.Clin. Oncol. 2007;**25**:313-318

[42] Kunitoh H, Kato H, Tsuboi M, et al. Phase II trial of preoperative chemoradiotherapy followed by surgical resection in patients with superior sulcus non-small-cell lung cancer: Report of Japan clinical oncology group trial 9806. Journal of Clinical Oncology. 2008;**26**:644-649

[43] Kappers I, Klomp H, Koolen MG, et al. Concurrent high-dose radiotherapy with low-dose chemotherapy in patients with non-small cell lung cancer of the superior sulcus Radioth. Oncologia. 2011;**101**:278-283

[44] Burdett S., Rydzewska L., Tierney J., et al Postoperative radiotherapy for non-small cell lung cancer Cochrane Database Syst. Rev. 2016;Oct 11, 10 CD002142

[45] Billiet C, Decaluwé H, Peeters S, et al. Modern post-operative radiotherapy for stage III non-small cell lung cancer may improve local control and survival: A meta-analysis. Radiother. Oncol. 2014;**110**:3-8

[46] Abuodeh Y, Naghavi AO, Echevarria M, et al. Quantitative excessive normal tissue toxicity and poor target coverage in postoperative lung cancer radiotherapy meta-analysis. Clin Lung Cancer. 2018;**19**:e123-e130

[47] Kepka L, Bujko K, Orlowski TM, et al. Cardiopulmonary morbidity and quality of life in non-small cell lung cancer patients treated with or without postoperative radiotherapy Radiother. Oncologia. 2011;**98**:2310

[48] Betticher DC, Hsu Schmitz SF, Tötsch M, et al. Prognostic factors affecting long-term outcomes in patients with resected stage IIIA pN2 non-small-cell lung cancer: 5-year follow-up of a phase II study. British Journal of Cancer. 2006;**94**:1099-1106

[49] Le Pechoux C., Pourel N., Barlesi F. et al. An international randomized trial, comparing post-operative conformal radiotherapy (PORT) to no PORT in patients with completely resected non-small cell lung cancer (NSCLC) and mediastinal N2 involvement: Primary end-point analysis of LungART (IFCT-0503, UK NCRI, SAKK, NCT00410683) Ann. Oncol. 2020; 31 (suppl-4): S1142-1215. 10.106/annonc/annonc325

[50] Chen CP, Weinberg VK, Jahan TM, et al. Implications of delayed initiation of radiotherapy: Accelerated repopulation after induction chemotherapy for stage III non-small cell lung cancer. Journal of Thoracic Oncology. 2011;**6**:1857-1864

[51] Salam AK, Postow MA, Salama JK. Irradiation and immunotherapy: From concept to the clinic. Cancer. 2016;**122**:1659-1671

[52] Dovedi SJ, Adlard AL, Lipowska-Bhalla G, et al. Acquired resistance to fractionated radiotherapy can be overcome by concurrent PD-L1 blockade. Cancer Research. 2014;**74**:5458-5468

[53] Shaverdian N., Lisberg A.E., Bornazyan K. et al Previous radiotherapy and the clinical activity and toxicity of pembroluzimab in the treatment of non-small-cell lung cancer: a secondary analysis of the KEYNOTE-001 phase I trial Lancet Oncol. 2017; 18:895-903

[54] Gray J, Villegas A, Daniel D, et al. Three-year overall survival with Durvalumab after chemoradiotherapy in stage III NSCLC-update from PACIFIC. J.Thorac.Oncol. 2020;**15**:288-293

[55] Peters S., Felip E., Dafni U. et al Safety evaluation of nivolumab added concurrently to randiotherapy in a standard first line chemo-radiotherapy regimen in stage III non-small cell lung cancer-The ETOP NICOLAS trial Lung Ca 2019; 133:83-87

[56] Theelen W.S.M.S., Peulen H.M.U., Lalezari F. et al Effect of Pembroluzimab after stereotactic body radiotherapy vs pembroluzimab alone on tumor response in patients with advanced non-small cell lung cancer/ results of the PEMBRO-RT phase 2 randomizedclinical trial JAMA Oncol. 2019;5:1276-82

[57] Tian S., Swithchenko J.M., Buchwald Z.S. et al Lung stereotactic body radiation therapy and concurrent immunotherapy: a multicenter safety and toxicity analysis. Int.J.Radiat.Oncol. Biol.Phys. 2020; 108:304-&"

[58] Chen D, Patel RR, Verma V, et al. Interaction between lymphopenia radiotherapy technique, dosimetry and survival outcomes in lung cancer patients receiving combined

immunotherapy and radiotherapy. Radiother. Oncol. 2020;**150**:114-120

[59] Govindan R, Page N, Morgensztern D, et al. Changing epidemiology of small-cell lung cancer in the United States over the last 30 years: Analysis of the surveillance, epidemiologic, and end results database. Journal of Clinical Oncology. 2006;**24**:4539-4544

[60] Sant M, Allemani C, Santiaquilani M, et al. EUROCARE-4. Survival of cancer patients diagnosed in 1995-1999. Results and commentary. Eur. J. Cancer. 2009;**45**:931-991

[61] Green RA, Humphrey E, Close H, Patno ME. Alkylating agents in bronchogenic carcinoma. The American Journal of Medicine. 1969;**46**:516-525

[62] Stahel RA, Ginsberg R, Havemann K, et al. Staging and prognostic factors in small cell lung cancer: A consensus report. Lung Ca. 1989;**5**:119-126

[63] Shepherd FA, Crowley J, Van Houtte P, et al. The international association for the study of lung cancer lung cancer staging project: Proposals regarding the clinical staging of small cell lung cancer in the forthcoming (seventh) edition of the tumor, node, metastasis classification for lung cancer. Journal of Thoracic Oncology. 2007;**2**:1067-1077

[64] Lababede O, Meziane M, Rice T, et al. Seventh edition of cancer staging manual and stage grouping of lung cancer: Quick reference chart and diagrams. Chest. 2011;**139**:183-189

[65] Stahel R, Thatcher N, Früh MC, et al. 1st ESMO consensus conference in lung cancer; Lugano 2010: small-cell lung cancer. Ann. Oncologia. 2011;**22**:1973-1980

[66] Warde P, Payne D. Does thoracic irradiation improve survival and local control in limited-stage small-cell lung cancer? A meta-analysis. Journal of Clinical Oncology. 1992;**10**:890-895

[67] Pignon JP, Arriagada R, Ihde C, et al. A meta-analysis of thoracic radiotherapy for small-cell lung cancer. The New England Journal of Medicine. 1992;**327**:1618-1624

[68] Fried DB, Morris DE, Poole C, et al. Systematic review evaluating the timing of thoracic radiation therapy in combined modality therapy for limited-stage small-cell lung cancer. Journal of Clinical Oncology. 2004;**22**:4785-4793

[69] De Ruysscher D, Lueza B, Le Péchoux C, et al. Impact of thoracic radiotherapy timing in limited-stage small-cell lung cancer: Usefulness of the individual patient data meta-analysis. Annals of Oncology. 2016;**27**:1818-1828

[70] Turrisi AT, Kim K, Blum R, et al. Twice-daily compared with once-daily thoracic radiotherapy in limited small-cell lung cancer treated concurrently with cisplatin and etoposide. The New England Journal of Medicine. 1999;**340**:265-271

[71] Komaki R, Khalid N, Langer C, et al. Penetration of recommended procedures for lung cancer staging and management in the United States over 10 years: A quality research in radiation oncology survey. International Journal of Radiation Oncology, Biology, Physics. 2013;**85**:1082-1089

[72] Takada M, Fukuoka M, Kawahara T, et al. Phase III study of concurrent versus sequential thoracic radiotherapy in combination with cisplatin and etoposide for limited-stage small-cell lung cancer: Results of the Japan clinical oncology group study 9104. Journal of Clinical Oncology. 2002;**20**:3054-3060

[73] Faivre-Finn C, Snee M, Ashcroft L, et al. Concurrent once-daily versus twice-daily chemoradiotherapy in

patients with limited-stage small-cell lung cancer (CONVERT): An open-label, phase 3, randomised, superiority trial. The Lancet Oncology. 2017;**18**:1116-1125

[74] Glatzer M, Faivre-Finn C, De Ruysscher D, et al. Once daily versus twice-daily radiotherapy in the management of limited disease small cell lung cancer - decision criteria in routine practise. Radiotherapy and Oncology. 2020;**150**:26-29

[75] Henning Gronberg B., Toftaker Killingberg K, Fløtten O. et al. Randomized phase II trial comparing the efficacy of standard-dose with high-dose twice-daily thoracic radiotherapy (TRT) in limited disease small-cell lung cancer (LD SCLC). J. Clin. Onco.l 38: 2020 (suppl; abstr 9007). DOI:10.1200/JCO.2020.38.15_suppl.9007

[76] Peters S, Pujol J., Dafni U.et al Consolidation ipilimumab and nivolumab vs observation in limited stage SCLC after chemo-radiotherapy – results from the ETOP/IFCT 4-12 STIMULI trial – Ann Oncol 2020; 31(suppl 4): s1142-s1215 10.106 annonc/annonc 325

[77] Van Loon J, De Ruysscher D, Wanders R, et al. Selective nodal irradiation on basis of (18) FDG-PET scans in limited-disease small-cell lung cancer: A prospective study. International Journal of Radiation Oncology, Biology, Physics. 2010;**77**:329-336

[78] Shrivani SM, Komaki R, Heymach JV, et al. Positron emission tomography/computed tomography-guided intensity-modulated radiotherapy for limited-stage small-cell lung cancer. International Journal of Radiation Oncology, Biology, Physics. 2012;**82**:e91-e97

[79] Jeremic B, Shibamoto Y, Nikolic N, et al. Role of radiation therapy in the combined-modality treatment of patients with extensive disease small-cell lung cancer: A randomized study. Journal of Clinical Oncology. 1999;**17**:2092-2099

[80] Slotman BJ, van Tinteren H, Praag JO, et al. Use of thoracic radiotherapy for extensive stage small-cell lung cancer: A phase 3 randomised controlled trial. Lancet. 2015;**385**:36-42

[81] Paz-Ares L, Dvorkin M, Chen Y, et al. Durvalumab plus platinume-etoposide versus platinum-etopisde in first-line treatment of extensive-stage small-cell lung cancer (CASPIAN) : a phase randomised, controlled, open-label, phase 3 trial. Lancet. 2019;**394**:1929-1939

[82] Horn L, Mansfield AS, Szcesna A, et al. First-line Atezolizumab plus chemotherapy in extensive-stage small-cell lung cancer. NEJM. 2018;**379**:2220-2229

[83] Hansen H. Should initial treatment of small cell lung cancer carcinoma include systemic chemotherapy and brain irradiation ? Cancer Chemother. Rep. 1973;**4**:239-241

[84] Arriagada R, Le Chevalier T, Borie F, et al. Prophylactic cranial irradiation for patients with small-cell lung cancer in complete remission. J Natl. Cancer Inst. 1995;**87**:183-190

[85] Gregor A, Cull A, Stephens RJ, et al. Prophylactic cranial irradiation is indicated following complete response to induction therapy in small cell lung cancer: Results of a multicenter randomized trial (UKCCCR and EORTC). European Journal of Cancer. 1997;**33**:1752-1758

[86] Auperin A, Arriagada R, Pignon JP, et al. Prophylactic cranial irradiation for patients with small-cell lung cancer in complete remission. Prophylactic

cranial irradiation overview collaborative group. N. Engl. J. Med. 1999;**341**:476-484

[87] Viani GA, Boin AC, Ikeda VY, et al. Thirty years of prophylactic cranial irradiation in patients with small cell lung cancer: A meta-analysis of randomized clinical trials. Jornal Brasileiro de Pneumologia. 2012;**38**:372-381

[88] Seute T, Leffers P, ten Velde GP, et al. Detection of brain metastases from small cell lung cancer: Consequences of changing imaging techniques (CT versus MRI). Cancer. 2008;**112**:1827-1834

[89] Le Péchoux C, Dunant A, Senan S, et al. Standard-dose versus higher-dose prophylactic cranial irradiation (PCI) in patients with limited stage small cell lung cancer in complete remission after chemotherapy and thoracic radiotherapy (PCI99-01, EORTC22003-08004, RTOG0212 and IFCT99-01): A randomized clinical trial. The Lancet Oncology. 2009;**10**:467-473

[90] Gondi V, Paulus R, Bruner DW, et al. Decline in tested and self-reported cognitive functioning after prophylactic cranial irradiation in lung cancer: Pooled secondary analysis of radiation oncology group randomized trials 0212 and 0214. International Journal of Radiation Oncology, Biology, Physics. 2013;**86**:656-664

[91] Manapov F, Käsmann L, Roengvoraphoj O, et al. Prophylactic cranial irradiation in small-cell lung cancer: Update on patient selection, efficacy and outcomes. Lung Cancer (Auckl). 2018;**9**:49-55

[92] Rusthoven C.G., Kavanagh B.D. Prophylactic Cranial Irradiation (PCI) versus Active MRI Surveillance for Small Cell Lung Cancer: The Case for Equipoise. J. Thorac. Oncol. 2017;.12:1746-54.

[93] Slotman BJ, Faivre-Finn C, Kramer GW, et al. Prophylactic cranial irradiation in small-cell lung cancer. The New England Journal of Medicine. 2007;**357**:664-672

[94] Schild SE, Foster NR, Meyers JP, et al. Prophylactic cranial irradiation in small-cell lung cancer: Findings from a north central cancer treatment group pooled analysis. Annals of Oncology. 2012;**23**:2919-2924

[95] Takahashi T, Yamanaka T, Seto T, et al. Prophylactic cranial irradiation versus observation in patients with extensive-disease small-cell lung cancer: A multicentre, randomised, open-label, phase 3 trial. The Lancet Oncology. 2017;**18**:663-671

Chapter 5

Definitive Radiotherapy for Locally Advanced Non-Small Cell Lung Cancer: Current Status and Future Perspectives

Hiroshi Doi and Kozo Kuribayashi

Abstract

Lung cancer remains one of the most common cancers, and the mortality rate is still high. Radiotherapy plays an important role in radical treatment for locally advanced non-small cell lung cancer. Treatment outcomes in lung cancer have improved over the last few decades. Several treatment regimens have been shown to be effective and safe. Further, modern technological approaches of radiotherapy have been developed along with advanced imaging and immunotherapy in order to improve outcomes and minimize radiation-induced toxicity. This chapter summarizes the historical results of the key clinical studies that were conducted in the past with the focus on various regimens of chemoradiotherapy used. In addition, we discuss future perspectives of definitive radiotherapy for locally advanced non-small cell lung cancer.

Keywords: lung cancer, radiotherapy, chemoradiotherapy, intensity modulated radiation therapy, dulvalumab

1. Introduction

The lung cancer remains one of the most common cancers, and 80% of lung cancers account for non-small cell lung cancer (NSCLC) [1]. Patients diagnosed at a locally advanced stage represent 20 to 30%, and radical surgery is challenging for those patients [1]. Definitive chemoradiotherapy is a well-established treatment option for unresectable locally advanced NSCLC [2, 3]. Treatment outcomes in such patients have improved over the last few decades. Several treatment regimens have been shown to be effective and safe. Moreover, modern radiotherapy technologies have been developed along with the development of optimal chemotherapy and immunotherapy to improve outcomes and minimize radiation-induced toxicity. This chapter summarizes historical results of key clinical studies in the past in terms of various regimens of chemoradiotherapy. In addition, we discuss definitive radiotherapy, which is recommended for locally advanced NSCLC. Specifically, we address future perspectives of definitive radiotherapy for locally advanced NSCLC.

IntechOpen

2. History of the development of definitive radiotherapy for locally advanced NSCLC

Radiotherapy alone was a standard treatment for inoperable lung cancer up to the 1980s based on the results of a randomized controlled trial in the 1960s [4]. Perez et al. showed the dose–response efficacy up to 60 Gy, which had been a standard dose from the combined results of the RTOG 7101 and 73–02 study [5]. After the 1990s, definitive radiotherapy, using ≥60Gy in a conventional fractionated regimen, combined with chemotherapy, has been used as a standard treatment for unresectable locally advanced NSCLC. In the early 1990s, sequential cisplatin-based chemotherapy followed by radiotherapy had been proven to have a survival benefit over definitive radiotherapy alone and chemotherapy alone for unresectable stage III NSCLC [6–9]. Then, from the late 1990s to the 2000s, several randomized clinical trials revealed that the concurrent approach of chemoradiotherapy enhanced survival compared to the sequential approach [10–13]. After 2000, the usefulness of several new agents, such as paclitaxel, gemcitabine, vinorelbine, and docetaxel, which are called third-generation chemotherapy agents, have been studied. They have been usually administered in combination with platinum compounds, and demonstrated increased survival in patients with metastatic NSCLC [14, 15]. Although there has been no significant improvement in survival achieved with chemoradiotherapy using third-generation regimens, it has become a standard treatment with a favorable toxicity profile [16, 17].

Some clinical studies conducted between 1990s and 2000s showed that hyperfractionated, accelerated radiotherapy was superior to the conventional fractionated radiotherapy with a feasible toxicity [18–21]. However, the benefit of hyperfractionated, accelerated radiotherapy is controversial, with high risk of acute esophageal toxicity; and has been less accepted in clinical practice [2, 21, 22]. After 2000, the utility of consolidation chemotherapy following chemoradiotherapy has failed to prove a significant survival benefit [23–25]. A dose escalation of radiotherapy has been investigated because loco-regional tumor control might be associated with better survival; and there is a potential dose–response efficacy in the control of NSCLC using this approach [5, 26]. However, RTOG 0617 trial failed to prove benefits on overall survival (OS) and progression-free survival (PSF) using the escalated doses of 74 Gy compared to the standard dose of 60 Gy in an open-label randomized phase 3 study [27]. Volume prescriptions such as D95 using updated calculation algorithms in recent clinical trials could reveal a slightly escalated dose for the target, in comparison with the point prescription that has been used in previous studies. However, the standard regimen of definitive radiotherapy has been 60 Gy in 30 fractions.

As shown in **Figure 1**, the median survival time after treatment has improved with the development of chemoratiotherapy. However, the 5-year survival rate has been unsatisfactorily, reaching only up to 20%. Recently, immune checkpoint inhibitors (ICIs) have been applied in the treatment of advanced malignancies, including lung cancer [29]. ICIs block checkpoint proteins that can weaken immune responses by T cells to cancer cells. Recent systematic reviews have demonstrated the beneficial effects of ICIs on OS and PSF in advanced NSCLC [30]. The PACIFIC trial, a randomized, double-blind, placebo-controlled multi-center trial, has tested the efficacy of dulvalumab, which is a human monoclonal antibody directed against programmed cell death-ligand 1 (PD-L1), in patients with stage III NSCLC as sequential treatment following standard concurrent chemoradiotherapy [19–32]. Dulvalumab has brought a breakthrough in the treatment of locally advanced

NSCLC in decades, and median survival after treatment has not reached with a median follow-up of 33.3 months in a recent updated result [28]. The transition of standard definitive radiotherapy for locally advanced NSCLN and representative of the clinical outcomes of selected prospective clinical trials with time are shown in **Table 1** and **Figure 1**.

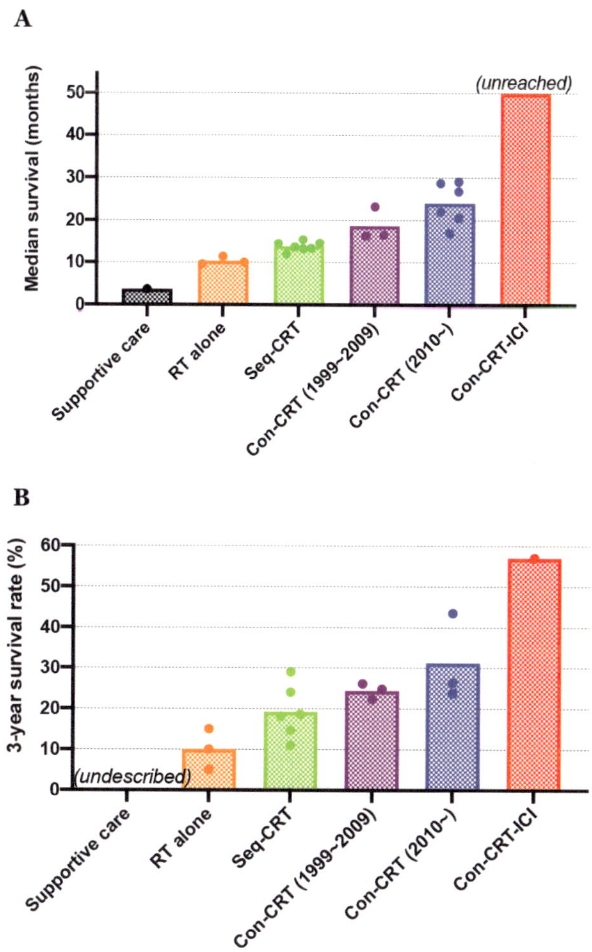

Figure 1.
Improvement of survival outcome of locally advanced NSCLN. (A) Median survival and (B) 3-year overall survival per selected prospective clinical studies and meta-analyses [4–13, 16, 17, 23, 24, 27, 28]. Each bar indicates the mean value of the results. Radiotherapy group included locally advanced NSCLC patients who underwent treatment with standard radiation doses such as ≥60Gy in a conventional schedule. Abbreviations: *Con-CRT, concurrent chemoradiotherapy; Con-CRT-ICI, concurrent chemoradiotherapy with consolidation immune checkpoint inhibitor; RT, radiotherapy; Seq-CRT, sequential chemoradiotherapy.*

~ 1980s	Radiotherapy alone
1990s	Sequential chemoradiotherapy
	Concurrent chemoradiotherapy (second-generation regimen)
2000s	Concurrent chemoradiotherapy (third-generation regimen)
2020~	Concurrent chemoradiotherapy followed by immune checkpoint inhibitor (dulvalumab)

Table 1.
Transition of standard definitive radiotherapy for locally advanced NSCLN.

3. Utility of intensity-modulated radiotherapy, learning from RTOG 0617 and PACIFIC trials

RTOG 0617 trial failed to demonstrate the benefit of dose-escalation of 74 Gy compared with 60 Gy, but also provided significant information for clinical practice, as it was the first phase III NSCLC study to allow intensity-modulated radiotherapy (IMRT) as a treatment modality for locally advanced NSCLC, and 46% of enrolled patients underwent IMRT [27, 33].

The disadvantage of IMRT in terms of dose distribution is increased volume of lungs receiving low-dose radiation, called "low-dose bath" because the IMRT plan is created using the increased number of beam angles [34]. Low-dose baths represented by large volumes of lung V5 (the volume of the lungs receiving ≥5 Gy) has been reported to increase the risk of acute and late pulmonary toxicity [34–36]. IMRT was used to treat larger and unfavorable tumors in RTOG 0617 [37]. Lung V5 was significantly higher in the IMRT group than in the 3D-CRT group. However, IMRT was associated with lower rates of severe pneumonitis in the RTOG 0617 prospective clinical trial. In addition, severe pneumonitis was predicted by lung V20, but not V5. Thus, V20 has been confirmed as a well-established risk factor of radiation pneumonitis with high reproducibility [38]. It is difficult to clarify the controversial meaning of V5 as a predictor of radiation pneumonitis. However, IMRT could improve target coverage and reduce the volume of normal lungs irradiated with intermediate doses such as V20 [34]. Grade ≥ 2 pneumonitis after chemoradiotherapy was a significant exclusion criterion in the PACIFIC trial [31]. The reduction of the risk of radiation pneumonitis by using IMRT might maximize the opportunity of receiving consolidation ICI based on the PACIFIC trial, although detailed data on radiotherapy was not collected in the PACIFIC trial [28, 31, 32, 37].

Higher doses to heart and esophagitis were associated with poor survival [37, 39]. In patients receiving heart V50 < 25% versus ≥25, the 1-year OS rates were 70.2% versus 46.8% and the 2-year OS rates were 45.9% versus 26.7% ($p < 0.0001$) [39]. Heart V40, which has been shown to be a prognostic factor for survival, can be substantially reduced with IMRT compared to 3D-CRT. In addition, the use of IMRT was associated with significantly less decline in quality of life [40]. These toxicities were potentially associated with poor survival in patients treated with escalated radiation doses of 74 Gy [27]. Furthermore, the correlation of institution accrual volume with the treatment outcomes is controversial but can be associated with other malignancies such as head and neck cancers [39, 41–43]. Quality assurance and institutional experience seem important in radical treatment of locally advanced NSCLC.

The benefits of proton therapy have been reported and included a better dose distribution to the lung and heart in treatment plan than in photon radiotherapy [44]. A randomized control study that compared the utility of proton therapy with that of IMRT showed no significant benefit in terms of the occurrence of radiation pneumonitis and local failure [45]. Modern proton techniques might improve clinical outcomes, but there is no significant evidence of a superiority of proton therapy over IMRT at this moment.

IMRT allows the treatment of challenging cases with dosimetric and clinical benefits. Therefore, IMRT is a current standard technique in the definitive radiotherapy for advanced NSCLC, as the use of IMRT has various advantages over 3D-CRT, which obviously outweighs the disadvantages.

4. Tips for using definitive radiotherapy for locally advanced NSCLC

4.1 Involved-field radiotherapy

The European Society for Radiotherapy and Oncology recommends that metastatic nodes and the applicable margin with no further elective lymph nodes should be included in clinical tumor volume (CTV) [46]. Radiotherapy has been prescribed to the intersection point of the treatment beams [18]. An initial radiotherapy was administered to the anteroposterior parallel–opposed pair of portals and then to a pair of oblique fields during the boosted radiotherapy [16]. Traditionally, definitive radiotherapy for locally advanced NSCLC targets the primary disease and nodal metastases as well as the mediastinum and ipsilateral hilum whether or not there is clinical involvement of all nodal stations [6, 7, 9–11, 13, 17, 18, 22]. This technique is known as elective nodal irradiation (ENI). Potential dose–response has been reported, and an increased radiation dose has been believed to improve survival in NSCLC before RTOG 0617 [5, 26]. Involved field radiotherapy (IFRT) is a radiation treatment techniquc that minimizes the radiation dose to uninvolved areas [47]. For example, **Figure 2** indicates the difference in planning target volume (PTV) between ENI and IFRT. IFRT allows radiation doses to be increased to the primary tumor and involves mediastinal lymph nodes. Thus, landmark clinical trials testing dose escalation adopted IFRT [27, 48, 49]. Although there are limited data directly comparing IFRT and ENI, the elective nodal failure rate after IFRT has been reported to be <10% in most reports [50–56]. Generally, EFRT can decrease the risk of severe toxicities, including acute esophagitis and pneumonitis, while showing no significant differences in elective nodal failure rate and survival outcomes in comparison with ENI [54–56]. Importantly, metastatic nodes should be defined with the guidance of PET images [46, 57]. Thereafter, CTV is generated by adding 5 to 10 mm to the gross tumor volume (GTV) of the primary tumor (typically 8 mm and 6 mm for adenocarcinoma and squamous carcinoma, respectively) and 3 mm for GTV of metastatic nodes of <20 mm [46, 58, 59].

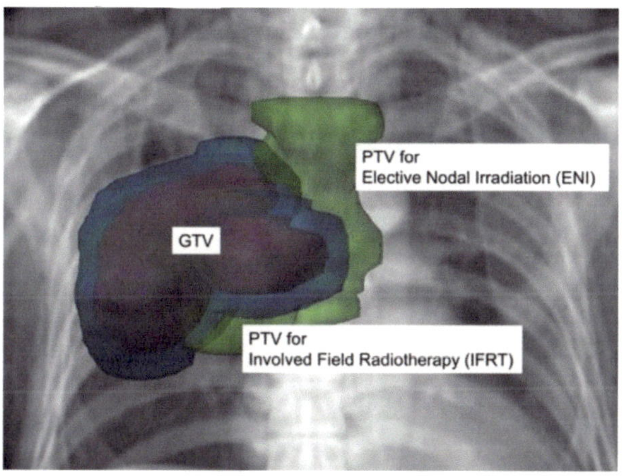

Figure 2.
Differences in radiotherapy target selection in elective nodal irradiation and involved field radiotherapy. Squamous cell carcinoma in the upper lobe of the right lung with nodal metastases (cT3N2M0). Red, green, and blue indicates gross tumor volume (GTV), planning target volume (PTV) for elective nodal irradiation (ENI), and that for involved field radiotherapy (IFRT), respectively. The clinical target volume (CTV) for ENI including the upper mediastinum enlarges the size of the PTV.

4.2 Respiratory management in locally advanced NSCLC

An important challenge for lung cancer radiotherapy treatment is the management of physiological movements related to breathing. The lung tumors can move during breathing. Usually, to ensure adequate dose delivery to the tumor, an appropriate margin is added around the tumor. Four-dimensional computed tomography (4DCT) is a technique that allows to quantify the movement of the tumor with the use of respiratory reduction equipment such as an abdominal compression device. The internal target volume (ITV) is delineated on the 4DCT scan in order to account for tumor motion, and an additional margin is added to generate PTV. However, the target is large as it covers the entire tumor motion, especially in tumors in the lower lobe of the lung [60].

The breath-hold technique has been used to minimize the target volume, which must be irradiated with high-dose radiation and can help to reduce risk of radiation pneumonitis (**Figure 3**). In particular, the deep inspiration breath hold (DIBH) technique provides an advantage to a free-breathing treatment and could reduce the dosimetric parameters of normal organs such as the lung in dose-volume histograms [61]. DIBH gating has been clinically used in thoracic and upper abdominal radiotherapy [62]. In addition, it has recently been reported that compliance and reproducibility of DIBH was sufficiently high, with a reported compliant rate of 72% in a prospective clinical study [63]. DIBH has a high potential as a standard treatment in definitive radiotherapy for locally advanced NSCLC.

4.3 Image-guided radiotherapy in locally advanced NSCLC

In recent years, advancements in image-guided radiotherapy (IGRT) technology have enabled more accurate positioning and precise radiotherapy. IGRT is an essential companion to IMRT and allows the treatment to account for daily changes in target anatomy, motion, and positioning. Megavoltage (MV) portal imaging had been conventionally used to correct the setup errors and limited to verification of bony anatomy. In recent years, the X-ray source for imaging has been evolving from MV imaging to kilovoltage (kV) imaging, and from two-dimensional to three- dimensional

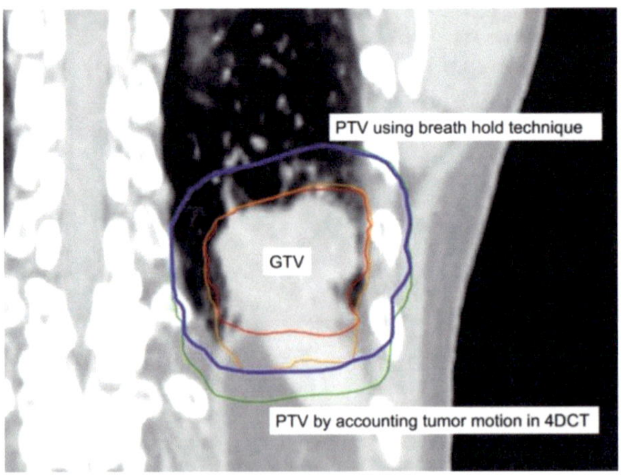

Figure 3.
Breath hold technique can minimize a target volume. Non-small cell lung cancer in the lower lobe of the left lung. Red, orange blue, and green indicate gross tumor volume (GTV), accumulated GTV on four-dimensional computed tomography (4DCT), planning target volume (PTV) using the breath-hold technique (exhale), and PTV, which was generated by accounting tumor motion in 4DCT, respectively. The breath-hold technique reduces the target volume.

imaging. Modern IGRT is performed with either gantry mounted MV or kV cone beam computed tomography (CBCT) or room-mounted kV systems for tracking during treatment. IGRT allows for easier and improved accuracy leading more frequent positioning changes with leading to a therapeutic advantage. Kilburn et al. has reported that IGRT using daily CBCT improved locoregional tumor control than radiotherapy using weekly MV portal images [64].

Three-dimensional images in CBCT are used not only for positioning but also for the evaluation of the radiotherapy planning by dose calculation on the CBCT images. It has recently been reported that dose distribution and dose volume histogram were accurately calculated on CBCT images with a deformable imaging registration [65].

Further, acquired images from CBCT can be used for individualized treatment, called adaptive radiotherapy (ART). Since there are possibe changes of tumor and surround tissues during the treatment courses due to tumor shrinking and anatomical changes, it is necessary to modify the radiotherapy plan with accounting the appropriate margin, positioning, and tumor. CBCT provides significant three-dimensional information to evaluate if the patient would benefit from a re-scanning and re-planning. Indeed, ART can improve locoregional tumor control over radiotherapy without ART [66].

Daily IGRT with CBCT and ART has been reported to reduce toxicity and probably increase tumor response due to a better tumor localization and reduction of an interfraction target miss due to anatomical changes [64, 66, 67]. Further studies should be conducted in order to establish the optimal systemic replanning technique.

5. Future perspectives of definitive radiotherapy for locally advanced NSCLC

5.1 Failure pattern and potential salvage after definitive radiotherapy

Approximately 40% and 50% of locally advanced NSCLC patients experience locoregional and distant failures two years after the definitive chemoradiotherapy [27]. Consolidation ICI has been proven to reduce disease progression in both the intrathoracic and extrathoracic areas [32, 68]. Time to death or distant metastasis was longer, and the frequency of new lesions was lower with the use of durvalumab in comparison with placebo [32]. Notably, distant failure occurred in one or two lesions (66.6% in durvalumab arm) in a single organ (95.2% in durvalumab arm) at first progression in both arms of durvalumab and placebo with a median follow-up of 25.2 months [68]. Therefore, there seems to be a window of opportunity for treating these limited failures as a salvage, which might lead to a longer survival [69–71]. Cutting-edge radiotherapies, such as stereotactic radiotherapy and particle therapy, have the potential to be a prospective option as a salvage modality.

The results of the PACIFIC clinical trial have led to the design of several clinical trials combining radiotherapy with ICIs, including PACIFIC-2 study, where a chemoradiotherapy plus durvalumab arm is currently studied (NCT03519971). In addition, combining chemotherapy, radiotherapy, and ICIs with surgical resection is also under investigation in clinical trials (NCT03694236, NCT03237377, NCT04073745, NCT03348748).

There are oncological differences between pathological subtypes in NSCLC, as widely known in metastatic diseases [72]. Ito et al. showed that adenocarcinoma and squamous cell carcinoma tended to develop distant and locoregional failures, respectively, after chemoradiotherapy for locally advanced NSCLC [73].

In addition, non-squamous cell carcinoma tends to benefit more from adding durvalumab than squamous cell carcinoma, although there is a lack of direct comparison analysis [32]. The effects of histopathological and oncological differences in NSCLC on definitive chemoradiotherapy should be investigated with the aim of developing a precision treatment for locally advanced NSCLC.

5.2 Immune enhancement and preservation in radiotherapy

Recent developments in immunotherapy have started a new era in the treatment of various malignancies, including NSCLC [29, 30, 74]. Induction of the expression of immune checkpoint molecules such as PD-L1 results in the inhibition of T cell function and immune tolerance of tumors.

Radiation may cause immune activation through cytokine signaling and tumor antigen release [75, 76]. However, PD-L1 expression in tumors has been reported to be upregulated by radiation exposure in both pre-clinical and clinical settings and can suppress the immunogenic effect on tumors [75–78]. ICIs block the immunosuppressive mechanisms of cancer cells and have a synergistic effect in combination with radiotherapy [75, 77]. The addition of durvalumab was proven to benefit disease control and survival after definitive chemoradiotherapy for locally advanced NSCLC [28, 31, 32]. The density of CD8+ tumor-infiltrating lymphocytes was significantly associated with favorable survival in locally advanced NSCLC patients undergoing chemoradiotherapy [79]. In their report, PD-L1 expression, which could be blocked by ICIs, was associated with inferior survival. In addition, radiation-induced lymphopenia has been reported to be associated with inferior survival [80, 81]. Therefore, radiotherapy will be

ClinicalTrials.gov identifier	Study design	Brief of treatment
NCT04432142	Phase 2	Immune changes after concurrent chemoradiation followed by durvalumab
NCT03589547	Phase 2	Durvalumab and consolidation SBRT following chemoradiation
NCT04092283	Phase 3	Durvalumab as concurrent and consolidative therapy or consolidative therapy alone
NCT03801902	Phase 1	Accelerated or conventionally fractionated radiotherapy combined with durvalumab
NCT03663166	Phase 1, 2	Chemoradiotherapy with ipilimumab followed by nivolumab
NCT04310020	Phase 2	Hypofractionated radiotherapy followed by atezolizumab
NCT03693300	Phase 2	Durvalumab following sequential chemotherapy and radiotherapy
NCT04249362	Phase 2	Durvalumab following radiotherapy (standard or hypofractionated bioequivalent dose)
NCT04392505	Phase 2	Investigating biomarkers related to chemoradiation followed by durvalumab
NCT04505267	Phase 1	Reirradiation with NBTXR3 for locoregional recurrence

Searched for: radiotherapy, immune | Recruiting, Not yet recruiting Studies | Non-small Cell Lung Cancer Stage III at https://clinicaltrials.gov with excluding trials including surgery on Sep. 7, 2020.

Table 2.
Ongoing phase 1 to 3 clinical trials for locally advanced NSCLN in terms of definitive radiotherapy and immune therapy.

modified to enhance the immune response to tumors. Hypofractionated regimens might have less immunosuppressive effects and are more appropriate than conventional fractionated regimens in terms of immune preservation [82, 83]. A clinical trial has been designed to test the addition of durvalumab to two schedules of radiotherapies of conventional and hypofractionated schedules (NCT03801902). Ongoing clinical trials in terms of definitive radiotherapy combined with ICIs are summarized in **Table 2**.

PTV size can be associated with circulating blood, including the leukocytes [84]. Thus, IFRT is appropriate in terms of not only reducing the risk of pneumonitis but also preservation of the host immune system. Ladbury et al. have presented a predictive model of the estimated dose of radiation to immune cells, which was calculated using the radiation doses for heart, lung, body, and number of fractions, and was associated with cancer-specific outcomes [85]. Thereafter, sparing the host immune system will be discussed, and new optimizing theory for IMRT should be investigated in the future. Radio-immune therapy strategy is giving a new direction to radiotherapy and is warranted to explore future definitive radiotherapy for locally advanced NSCLC.

6. Conclusions

In this chapter, the historical improvement and the current recommendation of definitive radiotherapy for locally advanced NSCLC are described. The current standard treatment for locally advanced NSCLC is definitive radiotherapy, concurrently combined with chemotherapy, followed by anti-PD-L1 treatment. In order to improve outcomes and minimize radiation-induced toxicity, IMRT using an involved-field under modern management of respiration is a present recommendation in this chapter. An optimal combination of radiotherapy and immunotherapy should be warranted in a future investigation.

Acknowledgements

This work was supported by JSPS KAKENHI Grant Number JP20K08093.

Author details

Hiroshi Doi[1]* and Kozo Kuribayashi[2]

1 Department of Radiation Oncology, Kindai University Faculty of Medicine, Osaka-Sayama, Osaka, Japan

2 Division of Respiratory Medicine, Department of Internal Medicine, Hyogo College of Medicine, Nishinomiya, Hyogo, Japan

*Address all correspondence to: h-doi@med.kindai.ac.jp

References

[1] Walters S, Maringe C, Coleman MP, et al. Lung cancer survival and stage at diagnosis in Australia, Canada, Denmark, Norway, Sweden and the UK: a population-based study, 2004-2007. Thorax. 2013;68:551-564.

[2] NCCN Clinical Practice Guidelines in Oncology (NCCN Guidelines®) Non-Small Cell Lung Cancer Version 6. 2020 https://www.nccn.org/professionals/physician_gls/pdf/nscl.pdf [Accessed: 2020-Aug-01]

[3] Park K, Vansteenkiste J, Lee KH, Pentheroudakis G, Zhou C, Prabhash K, et al. Pan-Asian adapted ESMO Clinical Practice Guidelines for the management of patients with locally-advanced unresectable non-small-cell lung cancer: a KSMO-ESMO initiative endorsed by CSCO, ISMPO, JSMO, MOS, SSO and TOS. Ann Oncol. 2020;31:191-201.

[4] Roswit B, Patno ME, Rapp R, Veinbergs A, Feder B, Stuhlbarg J, et al. The Survival of Patients with Inoperable Lung Cancer: A Large-Scale Randomized Study of Radiation Therapy Versus Placebo. Radiology. 1968;90:688-697.

[5] Perez CA, Pajak TF, Rubin P, Simpson JR, Mohiuddin M, Brady LW, et al. Long-term observations of the patterns of failure in patients with unresectable non-oat cell carcinoma of the lung treated with definitive radiotherapy. Report by the Radiation Therapy Oncology Group. Cancer. John Wiley & Sons, Ltd; 1987;59:1874-1881.

[6] Le Chevalier T, Arriagada R, Quoix E, Ruffle P, Martin M, Tarayre M, et al. Radiotherapy Alone Versus Combined Chemotherapy and Radiotherapy in Nonresectable Non-Small-Cell Lung Cancer: First Analysis of a Randomized Trial in 353 Patients. JNCI Journal of the National Cancer Institute. 1991;83:417-423.

[7] Kubota K, Furuse K, Kawahara M, Kodama N, Yamamoto M, Ogawara M, et al. Role of radiotherapy in combined modality treatment of locally advanced non-small-cell lung cancer. Journal of Clinical Oncology. 1994;12:1547-1552.

[8] Dillman RO, Herndon J, Seagren SL, Eaton WL, Green MR. Improved Survival in Stage III Non-Small-Cell Lung Cancer: Seven-Year Follow-up of Cancer and Leukemia Group B (CALGB) 8433 Trial. JNCI Journal of the National Cancer Institute. 1996;88:1210-1215.

[9] Sause W, Kolesar P, Taylor S IV, Johnson D, Livingston R, Komaki R, et al. Final results of phase III trial in regionally advanced unresectable non-small cell lung cancer: Radiation Therapy Oncology Group, Eastern Cooperative Oncology Group, and Southwest Oncology Group. Chest. 2000;117:358-364.

[10] Furuse K, Fukuoka M, Kawahara M, Nishikawa H, Takada Y, Kudoh S, et al. Phase III Study of Concurrent Versus Sequential Thoracic Radiotherapy in Combination With Mitomycin, Vindesine, and Cisplatin in Unresectable Stage III Non–Small-Cell Lung Cancer. Journal of Clinical Oncology. 1999;17:2692-2699.

[11] Fournel P, Robinet G, Thomas P, Souquet P-J, Lena H, Vergnenégre A, et al. Randomized phase III trial of sequential chemoradiotherapy compared with concurrent chemoradiotherapy in locally advanced non-small-cell lung cancer: Groupe Lyon-Saint-Etienne d'Oncologie Thoracique-Groupe Français de Pneumo-Cancérologie NPC 95-01 Study. Journal of Clinical Oncology. 2005;23:5910-5917.

[12] Auperin A, Le Pechoux C, Rolland E, Curran WJ, Furuse K, Fournel P, et al. Meta-Analysis of

Concomitant Versus Sequential Radiochemotherapy in Locally Advanced Non–Small-Cell Lung Cancer. Journal of Clinical Oncology. 2010;28:2181-2190.

[13] Curran WJ, Paulus R, Langer CJ, Komaki R, Lee JS, Hauser S, et al. Sequential vs Concurrent Chemoradiation for Stage III Non-Small Cell Lung Cancer: Randomized Phase III Trial RTOG 9410. JNCI Journal of the National Cancer Institute. 2011;103:1452-1460.

[14] Schiller JH, Harrington D, Belani CP, et al: Comparison of four chemotherapy regimens for advanced non-small-cell lung cancer. N Engl J Med. 2002;346:92-98.

[15] Bunn PA Jr, Kelly K: New chemotherapeutic agents prolong survival and improve quality of life in non-small cell lung cancer: A review of the literature and future directions. Clin Cancer Res. 1998;4:1087-1100.

[16] Segawa Y, Kiura K, Takigawa N, Kamei H, Harita S, Hiraki S, et al. Phase III Trial Comparing Docetaxel and Cisplatin Combination Chemotherapy With Mitomycin, Vindesine, and Cisplatin Combination Chemotherapy With Concurrent Thoracic Radiotherapy in Locally Advanced Non–Small-Cell Lung Cancer: OLCSG 0007. Journal of Clinical Oncology. 2010;28:3299-3306.

[17] Yamamoto N, Nakagawa K, Nishimura Y, Tsujino K, Satouchi M, Kudo S, et al. Phase III Study Comparing Second- and Third-Generation Regimens With Concurrent Thoracic Radiotherapy in Patients With Unresectable Stage III Non–Small-Cell Lung Cancer: West Japan Thoracic Oncology Group WJTOG0105. Journal of Clinical Oncology. 2010;28:3739-3745.

[18] Saunders M, Dische S, Barrett A, Harvey A, Griffiths G, Palmar M. Continuous, hyperfractionated, accelerated radiotherapy (CHART) versus conventional radiotherapy in non-small cell lung cancer: mature data from the randomised multicentre trial. CHART Steering committee. Radiotherapy and Oncology. 1999;52:137-148.

[19] Nyman J, Friesland S, Hallqvist A, Seke M, Bergström S, Thaning L, et al. How to improve loco-regional control in stages IIIa-b NSCLC? Results of a three-armed randomized trial from the Swedish Lung Cancer Study Group. Lung Cancer. 2009;65:62-67.

[20] Haslett K, Pöttgen C, Stuschke M, Faivre-Finn C. Hyperfractionated and accelerated radiotherapy in non-small cell lung cancer. J Thorac Dis. 2014;6:328-335.

[21] Mauguen A, Le Pechoux C, Saunders MI, Schild SE, Turrisi AT, Baumann M, et al. Hyperfractionated or accelerated radiotherapy in lung cancer: an individual patient data meta-analysis. J Clin Oncol. 2012;30:2788-2797.

[22] Baumann M, Herrmann T, Koch R, Matthiessen W, Appold S, Wahlers B, et al. Final results of the randomized phase III CHARTWEL-trial (ARO 97-1) comparing hyperfractionated-accelerated versus conventionally fractionated radiotherapy in non-small cell lung cancer (NSCLC). Radiotherapy and Oncology. 2011;100:76-85.

[23] Hanna N, Neubauer M, Yiannoutsos C, McGarry R, Arseneau J, Ansari R, et al. Phase III Study of Cisplatin, Etoposide, and Concurrent Chest Radiation With or Without Consolidation Docetaxel in Patients With Inoperable Stage III Non–Small-Cell Lung Cancer: The Hoosier Oncology Group and U.S. Oncology. Journal of Clinical Oncology. 2008;26:5755-5760.

[24] Ahn JS, Ahn YC, Kim J-H, Lee CG, Cho EK, Lee KC, et al. Multinational

Randomized Phase III Trial With or Without Consolidation Chemotherapy Using Docetaxel and Cisplatin After Concurrent Chemoradiation in Inoperable Stage III Non–Small-Cell Lung Cancer: KCSG-LU05-04. Journal of Clinical Oncology. 2015;33:2660-2666.

[25] Tsujino K, Kurata T, Yamamoto S, Kawaguchi T, Kubo A, Isa S, et al. Is consolidation chemotherapy after concurrent chemo-radiotherapy beneficial for patients with locally advanced non-small-cell lung cancer? A pooled analysis of the literature. J Thorac Oncol. 2013;8:1181-1189.

[26] Martel M. Estimation of tumor control probability model parameters from 3-D dose distributions of non-small cell lung cancer patients. Lung Cancer. 1999;24:31-37.

[27] Bradley JD, Paulus R, Komaki R, Masters G, Blumenschein G, Schild S, et al. Standard-dose versus high-dose conformal radiotherapy with concurrent and consolidation carboplatin plus paclitaxel with or without cetuximab for patients with stage IIIA or IIIB non-small-cell lung cancer (RTOG 0617): a randomised, two-by-two factorial phase 3 study. Lancet Oncol. 2015;16:187-199.

[28] Gray JE, Villegas A, Daniel D, Vicente D, Murakami S, Hui R, et al. Three-Year Overall Survival with Durvalumab after Chemoradiotherapy in Stage III NSCLC-Update from PACIFIC. J Thorac Oncol. 2020;15:288-293.

[29] Granier C, De Guillebon E, Blanc C, Roussel H, Badoual C, Colin E, et al. Mechanisms of action and rationale for the use of checkpoint inhibitors in cancer. ESMO Open. 2017;2:e000213.

[30] Wagner G, Stollenwerk HK, Klerings I. Efficacy and safety of immune checkpoint inhibitors in patients with advanced non–small cell lung cancer (NSCLC): a systematic literature review. OncoImmunology. 2020;9:1.

[31] Antonia SJ, Villegas A, Daniel D, Vicente D, Murakami S, Hui R, et al. Durvalumab after Chemoradiotherapy in Stage III Non–Small-Cell Lung Cancer. N Engl J Med. 2017;377:1919-1929.

[32] Antonia SJ, Villegas A, Daniel D, Vicente D, Murakami S, Hui R, et al. Overall Survival with Durvalumab after Chemoradiotherapy in Stage III NSCLC. N Engl J Mcd. 2018;379:2342-2350.

[33] Bradley JD, Hu C, Komaki RR, Masters GA, Blumenschein GR, Schild SE, et al. Long-Term Results of NRG Oncology RTOG 0617: Standard-Versus High-Dose Chemoradiotherapy With or Without Cetuximab for Unresectable Stage III Non-Small-Cell Lung Cancer. J Clin Oncol. 2020;38:706-714.

[34] Yom SS, Liao Z, Liu HH, Tucker SL, Hu C-S, Wei X, et al. Initial Evaluation of Treatment-Related Pneumonitis in Advanced-Stage Non–Small-Cell Lung Cancer Patients Treated With Concurrent Chemotherapy and Intensity-Modulated Radiotherapy. International Journal of Radiation Oncology*Biology*Physics. 2007;68:94-102.

[35] HU Y, LI J, SU X. Fatal pneumonitis associated with postoperative intensity-modulated radiotherapy in lung cancer: Case report and review. Oncol Lett. 2012;5:714-716.

[36] Tsujino K, Hashimoto T, Shimada T, Yoden E, Fujii O, Ota Y, et al. Combined Analysis of V20, VS5, Pulmonary Fibrosis Score on Baseline Computed Tomography, and Patient Age Improves Prediction of Severe Radiation Pneumonitis After Concurrent Chemoradiotherapy for Locally Advanced Non–Small-Cell Lung

Cancer. Journal of Thoracic Oncology. 2014;9:983-990.

[37] Chun SG, Hu C, Choy H, Komaki RU, Timmerman RD, Schild SE, et al. Impact of Intensity-Modulated Radiation Therapy Technique for Locally Advanced Non-Small-Cell Lung Cancer: A Secondary Analysis of the NRG Oncology RTOG 0617 Randomized Clinical Trial. J Clin Oncol. 2017;35:56-62.

[38] Palma DA, Senan S, Tsujino K, Barriger RB, Rengan R, Moreno M, et al. Predicting Radiation Pneumonitis After Chemoradiation Therapy for Lung Cancer: An International Individual Patient Data Meta-analysis. International Journal of Radiation Oncology*Biology*Physics. 2013;85:444-450.

[39] Speirs CK, DeWees TA, Rehman S, Molotievschi A, Velez MA, Mullen D, et al. Heart Dose Is an Independent Dosimetric Predictor of Overall Survival in Locally Advanced Non-Small Cell Lung Cancer. J Thorac Oncol. 2017;12:293-301.

[40] Movsas B, Hu C, Sloan J, Bradley J, Komaki R, Masters G, et al. Quality of Life Analysis of a Radiation Dose-Escalation Study of Patients With Non-Small-Cell Lung Cancer: A Secondary Analysis of the Radiation Therapy Oncology Group 0617 Randomized Clinical Trial. JAMA Oncol. 2016;2:359-367.

[41] Eaton BR, Pugh SL, Bradley JD, Masters G, Kavadi VS, Narayan S, et al. Institutional Enrollment and Survival Among NSCLC Patients Receiving Chemoradiation: NRG Oncology Radiation Therapy Oncology Group (RTOG) 0617. J Natl Cancer Inst. 2016;108: djw034.

[42] Tan MY, Fisher R, Ball D. Does institutional patient accrual volume impact overall survival in patients with inoperable non-small-cell lung cancer receiving radical (chemo)radiation? A secondary analysis of TROG 99.05. Journal of Medical Imaging and Radiation Oncology. 2020;64:556-562.

[43] Wuthrick EJ, Zhang Q, MacHtay M, Rosenthal DI, Nguyen-Tan PF, Fortin A, et al. Institutional clinical trial accrual volume and survival of patients with head and neck cancer. J Clin Oncol. 2015;33:156-164.

[44] Harada H, Murayama S. Proton beam therapy in non-small cell lung cancer: state of the art. Lung Cancer (Auckl). 2017;8:141-145.

[45] Liao Z, Lee JJ, Komaki R, Gomez DR, O'Reilly MS, Fossella FV, et al. Bayesian Adaptive Randomization Trial of Passive Scattering Proton Therapy and Intensity-Modulated Photon Radiotherapy for Locally Advanced Non-Small-Cell Lung Cancer. J Clin Oncol. 2018;36:1813-1822.

[46] Nestle U, De Ruysscher D, Ricardi U, Geets X, Belderbos J, Pöttgen C, et al. ESTRO ACROP guidelines for target volume definition in the treatment of locally advanced non-small cell lung cancer. Radiotherapy and Oncology. 2018;127:1-5.

[47] Grills IS, Yan D, Martinez AA, Vicini FA, Wong JW, Kestin LL. Potential for reduced toxicity and dose escalation in the treatment of inoperable non–small-cell lung cancer: A comparison of intensity-modulated radiation therapy (IMRT), 3D conformal radiation, and elective nodal irradiation. International Journal of Radiation Oncology*Biology*Physics. 2003;57:875-890.

[48] Schild SE, McGinnis WL, Graham D, Hillman S, Fitch TR, Northfelt D, et al. Results of a Phase I trial of concurrent chemotherapy and escalating doses of radiation for unresectable non–small-cell lung

cancer. International Journal of Radiation Oncology*Biology*Physics. 2006;65:1106-1111.

[49] Bradley JD, Bae K, Graham MV, Byhardt R, Govindan R, Fowler J, et al. Primary analysis of the phase II component of a phase I/II dose intensification study using three-dimensional conformal radiation therapy and concurrent chemotherapy for patients with inoperable non-small-cell lung cancer: RTOG 0117. J Clin Oncol. 2010;28:2475-2480.

[50] Rosenzweig KE, Sim SE, Mychalczak B, Braban LE, Schindelheim R, Leibel SA. Elective nodal irradiation in the treatment of non-small-cell lung cancer with three-dimensional conformal radiation therapy. Int J Radiation Oncology Biol Phys. 2001;50:681-685.

[51] Rosenzweig KE, Sura S, Jackson A, Yorke E. Involved-field radiation therapy for inoperable non small-cell lung cancer. J Clin Oncol. 2007;25:5557-5561.

[52] Sulman EP, Komaki R, Klopp AH, Cox JD, Chang JY. Exclusion of elective nodal irradiation is associated with minimal elective nodal failure in non-small cell lung cancer. Radiat Oncol. 2009;4:5.

[53] De Ruysscher D, Wanders S, van Haren E, Hochstenbag M, Geeraedts W, Utama I, et al. Selective mediastinal node irradiation based on FDG-PET scan data in patients with non-small-cell lung cancer: a prospective clinical study. Int J Radiation Oncology Biol Phys. 2005;62:988-994.

[54] Yuan S, Sun X, Li M, Yu J, Ren R, Yu Y, et al. A Randomized Study of Involved-Field Irradiation Versus Elective Nodal Irradiation in Combination With Concurrent Chemotherapy for Inoperable Stage III Nonsmall Cell Lung Cancer. American Journal of Clinical Oncology. 2007;30:239-244.

[55] Chen M, Bao Y, Ma H-L, Hu X, Wang J, Wang Y, et al. Involved-Field Radiotherapy versus Elective Nodal Irradiation in Combination with Concurrent Chemotherapy for Locally Advanced Non-Small Cell Lung Cancer: A Prospective Randomized Study. BioMed Research International. 2013;2013:1-7.

[56] Fernandes AT, Shen J, Finlay J, Mitra N, Evans T, Stevenson J, et al. Elective nodal irradiation (ENI) vs. involved field radiotherapy (IFRT) for locally advanced non-small cell lung cancer (NSCLC): A comparative analysis of toxicities and clinical outcomes. Radiotherapy and Oncology. 2010;95:178-184.

[57] Nestle U, Schimek-Jasch T, Kremp S, Schaefer-Schuler A, Mix M, Küsters A, et al. Imaging-based target volume reduction in chemoradiotherapy for locally advanced non-small-cell lung cancer (PET-Plan): a multicentre, open-label, randomised, controlled trial. Lancet Oncol. 2020;21:581-592.

[58] Giraud P, Antoine M, Larrouy A, Milleron B, Callard P, De Rycke Y, et al. Evaluation of microscopic tumor extension in non-small-cell lung cancer for three-dimensional conformal radiotherapy planning. Int J Radiation Oncology Biol Phys. 2000;48:1015-1024.

[59] Yuan S, Meng X, Yu J, Mu D, Chao KSC, Zhang J, et al. Determining optimal clinical target volume margins on the basis of microscopic extracapsular extension of metastatic nodes in patients with non–small-cell lung cancer. International Journal of Radiation Oncology, Biology, Physics. 2007;67:727-734.

[60] Seppenwoolde Y, Shirato H, Kitamura K, Shimizu S, van Herk M, Lebesque JV, et al. Precise and real-time

measurement of 3D tumor motion in lung due to breathing and heartbeat, measured during radiotherapy. Int J Radiation Oncology Biol Phys. 2002;53:822-834.

[61] Giraud P, Morvan E, Claude L, Mornex F, Le Pechoux C, Bachaud J-M, et al. Respiratory gating techniques for optimization of lung cancer radiotherapy. J Thorac Oncol. 2011;6:2058-2068.

[62] Boda-Heggemann J, Knopf A-C, Simeonova-Chergou A, Wertz H, Stieler F, Jahnke A, et al. Deep Inspiration Breath Hold-Based Radiation Therapy: A Clinical Review. Int J Radiat Oncol Biol Phys. 2016;94:478-492.

[63] Mirjana Josipovic, et al. Deep inspiration breath hold in locally advanced lung cancer radiotherapy: validation of intrafractional geometric uncertainties in the INHALE trial. Br J Radiol. 2019;92:20190569.

[64] Kilburn JM, Soike MH, Lucas JT, Ayala-Peacock D, Blackstock W, Isom S, et al. Image guided radiation therapy may result in improved local control in locally advanced lung cancer patients. Practical Radiation Oncology. 2016;6:e73–e80.

[65] Giacometti V, King RB, Agnew CE, Irvine DM, Jain S, Hounsell AR, et al. An evaluation of techniques for dose calculation on cone beam computed tomography. Br J Radiol. 2019;92:20180383.

[66] Tvilum M, Khalil AA, Møller DS, Hoffmann L, Knap MM. Clinical outcome of image-guided adaptive radiotherapy in the treatment of lung cancer patients. Acta Oncol. 2015;54:1430-1437.

[67] Lozano Ruiz FJ, Ileana Pérez Álvarez S, Poitevin Chacón MA, Maldonado Magos F, Prudencio RR, Cabrera Miranda L, et al. The importance of image guided radiotherapy in small cell lung cancer: Case report and review of literature. Reports of Practical Oncology and Radiotherapy. 2020;25:146-149.

[68] Raben D, Rimner A, Senan S, et al. Patterns of disease progression with durvalumab in stage III non-small cell lung cancer (PACIFIC). Int J Radiation Oncology Biol Phys. 105:683.

[69] Taugner J, Eze C, KÄSMANN L, Roengvoraphoj O, Gennen K, Karin M, et al. Pattern-of-failure and salvage treatment analysis after chemoradiotherapy for inoperable stage III non-small cell lung cancer. Radiation Oncology; 2020;15:148.

[70] Schreiner W, Dudek W, Lettmaier S, Fietkau R, Sirbu H. Long-Term Survival after Salvage Surgery for Local Failure after Definitive Chemoradiation Therapy for Locally Advanced Non-small Cell Lung Cancer. Thorac cardiovasc Surg. 2018;66:135-141.

[71] Palma DA, Olson R, Harrow S, Gaede S, Louie AV, Haasbeek C, et al. Stereotactic ablative radiotherapy versus standard of care palliative treatment in patients with oligometastatic cancers (SABR-COMET): a randomised, phase 2, open-label trial. Lancet. 2019;393:2051-2058.

[72] Socinski MA, Obasaju C, Gandara D, Hirsch FR, Bonomi P, Bunn P, et al. Clinicopathologic Features of Advanced Squamous NSCLC. J Thorac Oncol. 2016;11:1411-1422.

[73] Ito H, Matsuo Y, Ohtsu S, Nishimura T, Terada Y, Sakamoto T, et al. Impact of histology on patterns of failure and clinical outcomes in patients treated with definitive chemoradiotherapy for locally advanced non-small cell lung cancer. Int J Clin Oncol.2019;25:274-281.

[74] Sanmamed MF, Chen L. A Paradigm Shift in Cancer Immunotherapy: From Enhancement to Normalization. Cell. 2018;175:313-326.

[75] Grassberger C, Ellsworth SG, Wilks MQ, Keane FK, Loeffler JS. Assessing the interactions between radiotherapy and antitumour immunity. Nat Rev Clin Oncol. 2019;16:729-745.

[76] Le Q-T, Shirato H, Giaccia AJ, Koong AC. Emerging Treatment Paradigms in Radiation Oncology. Clin Cancer Res. 2015;21:3393-3401.

[77] Deng L, Liang H, Burnette B, Beckett M, Darga T, Weichselbaum RR, et al. Irradiation and anti–PD-L1 treatment synergistically promote antitumor immunity in mice. J Clin Invest. 2014;124:687-695.

[78] Yoneda K, Kuwata T, Kanayama M, Mori M, Kawanami T, Yatera K, et al. Alteration in tumoural PD-L1 expression and stromal CD8-positive tumour-infiltrating lymphocytes after concurrent chemo-radiotherapy for non-small cell lung cancer. Br J Cancer. 2019;121:490-496.

[79] Tokito T, Azuma K, Kawahara A, Ishii H, Yamada K, Matsuo N, et al. Predictive relevance of PD-L1 expression combined with CD8+ TIL density in stage III non-small cell lung cancer patients receiving concurrent chemoradiotherapy. Eur J Cancer. 2016;55:7-14.

[80] Tang C, Liao Z, Gomez D, Levy L, Zhuang Y, Gebremichael RA, et al. Lymphopenia association with gross tumor volume and lung V5 and its effects on non-small cell lung cancer patient outcomes. Int J Radiat Oncol Biol Phys. 2014;89:1084-1091.

[81] Wang W, Huang L, Jin J-Y, Jolly S, Zang Y, Wu H, et al. IDO Immune Status after Chemoradiation May Predict Survival in Lung Cancer Patients. Cancer Research. 2018;78:809-816.

[82] Wang W, Huang L, Jin J-Y, Pi W, Ellsworth SG, Jolly S, et al. A Validation Study on IDO Immune Biomarkers for Survival Prediction in Non-Small Cell Lung Cancer: Radiation Dose Fractionation Effect in Early-Stage Disease. Clin Cancer Res. 2020;26:282-289.

[83] Crocenzi T, Cottam B, Newell P, Wolf RF, Hansen PD, Hammill C, et al. A hypofractionated radiation regimen avoids the lymphopenia associated with neoadjuvant chemoradiation therapy of borderline resectable and locally advanced pancreatic adenocarcinoma. Journal for ImmunoTherapy of Cancer. 2016;4:45.

[84] Yovino S, Kleinberg L, Grossman SA, Narayanan M, Ford E. The etiology of treatment-related lymphopenia in patients with malignant gliomas: modeling radiation dose to circulating lymphocytes explains clinical observations and suggests methods of modifying the impact of radiation on immune cells. Cancer Invest. 2013;31:140-144.

[85] Ladbury CJ, Rusthoven CG, Camidge DR, Kavanagh BD, Nath SK. Impact of Radiation Dose to the Host Immune System on Tumor Control and Survival for Stage III Non-Small Cell Lung Cancer Treate d with Definitive Radiation Therapy. International Journal of Radiation Oncology*Biology*Physics. 2019;105:346-355.

Chapter 6

Image-Guided Ablative Therapies for Lung Tumors

Joyce W.Y. Chan, Rainbow W.H. Lau and Calvin S.H. Ng

Abstract

While the gold standard for early stage lung cancers is still surgical resection, many patients have comorbidities or suboptimal lung function making surgery unfavorable. At the same time, more and more small lung nodules are being incidentally discovered on computer tomography (CT), leading to the discovery of pre-malignant or very early stage lung cancers without regional spread, which could probably be eradicated without anatomical surgical resection. Various ablative energies and technologies are available on the market, including radiofrequency ablation, microwave ablation, cryoablation, and less commonly laser ablation and irreversible electroporation. For each technology, the mechanism of action, advantages, limitations, potential complications and evidence-based outcomes will be reviewed. Traditionally, these ablative therapies were done under CT guidance with percutaneous insertion of ablative probes. Recently, bronchoscopic ablation under ultrasound, CT, or electromagnetic navigation bronchoscopy guidance is gaining popularity due to improved navigation precision, reduced pleural-based complications, and providing a true "wound-less" option.

Keywords: radiofrequency ablation, microwave ablation, cryoablation, percutaneous ablation, bronchoscopic ablation, electromagnetic navigation bronchoscopy

1. Introduction

With the increasing availability of computer tomography (CT) scans and enlarging body of evidence for low-dose CT screening in high risk populations, a rising number of lung nodules are discovered incidentally. Many of them are small, sub-solid, and harbor pre-malignant or early stage cancers. Local therapies for these lesions are gaining evidence support, especially in patients with high surgical risks or decline surgery. Sublobar resection has been shown to confer similar 5-year survival rates, especially in older patients, tumor smaller than 2 cm, and pure bronchoalveolar carcinoma [1–3]. Stereotactic body radiation therapy (SBRT) is targeted toward patients with stage I or II non-small cell lung carcinoma (NSCLC) without lymph node involvement and who are medically inoperable. SBRT has a local control rate of more than 80% in multiple retrospective series [4], and disease-free survival of 26% and overall survival of 40% at 4 years in a multicentre phase II study [5]. However, sublobar resection still carries surgical risks while SBRT has up to 22.3% risk of radiation pneumonitis and pneumonia. Since the early 2000s, percutaneous ablation of lung tumors has been attempted [6] following reports of efficacy of local ablation in liver cancers. The subsequent decade saw the blossom

IntechOpen

of image-guided local ablative therapies of lung tumors, first with radiofrequency ablation (RFA), later with microwave ablation (MWA) and cryoablation. In this chapter, we discuss the preparation and procedure of lung ablative therapies, the various energy used, their pros and cons, evidence for safety and efficacy, and a glimpse into the future with a special section on bronchoscopic ablation.

2. Patient and nodule selection

Image-guided lung ablation is best suited for patients who have high surgical risks, either due to underlying medical comorbidities, or due to inadequate respiratory reserve, for instance significant chronic obstructive pulmonary disease (COPD) or previous contralateral lobectomy or pneumonectomy making intra-operative one-lung ventilation difficult. In general, there are no lower limits of lung function requirement for ablation candidates [7], but patients should be expected to tolerate sedation or general anesthesia at supine, lateral decubitus or semi-prone position for at least an hour. Contraindications for ablation include severe interstitial lung disease (ILD), where exacerbation of ILD may lead to severe pulmonary failure and death [8].

When ablation is intended for local control of early stage lung cancer, the tumor should ideally be small enough to be covered by the expected ablation zone with adequate margin, and there should be no nodal or extrathoracic metastasis based on pre-operative imaging. Ablation with palliative intent is best suited for lung cancers with tumor-related symptoms, for example pain and airway obstruction. Tumor size must be considered, and numerous lung ablation studies have demonstrated increased risk of local recurrence for increasing size of tumors, with cut-off of 2 cm [9] and 3 cm [10, 11] reported. In case of larger tumors, double ablation may be required, which either involves re-ablating in the same position, after pull-back of electrode, or after repositioning of electrode. Alternatively, ablation catheters with multiple electrodes can be used to generate a larger ablation zone.

Tumor location is also important to consider before submitting patient to thermal ablation. Nodules which are not suitable candidates for CT-guided biopsy are generally not recommended for percutaneous ablation, for example those shielded by the bony scapula, very close to diaphragm or hilar structures. Tumors located close to medium to large blood vessels are susceptible to heat-sink effects and ablation efficacy may be reduced. Ablation of tumors close to the apex or mediastinal structures may risk thermal injury to brachial plexus, phrenic nerve and adjacent organs such as the heart and esophagus, although hydro-dissection or artificial pneumothorax to protect surrounding structures have been reported with success [12].

3. Procedure and planning

Pre-procedure workup includes CT imaging ideally within 4 weeks of the planned ablation date. Patients were fasted overnight before ablation to reduce risk of sedation-induced nausea and aspiration. Anti-coagulation or anti-platelet medications were stopped as per regional guidelines for invasive procedures. Implantable cardiac devices like pacemakers or defibrillators are susceptible to interference from certain ablation modalities, and should be interrogated and programed by cardiac electrophysiologist to automatic pacing modes, or by placing a magnet over the device, while defibrillation should be turned off during ablation. Grounding pads should be placed to guide the flow of current away from the cardiac device and electrodes should be inserted at least 5 cm away from pacemaker or defibrillator leads. External pacing and defibrillator system should be readily available in case of emergency.

Most ablation strategies are performed percutaneously, and nearly all are done under CT guidance. The great majority of ablation are performed with conscious sedation, while general anesthesia is reserved for pediatric patients or patients who cannot tolerate sedation alone, although some authors have reported higher feasibility rates and lower peri-procedural pain with general anesthesia [13]. For certain ablation energies, a reference electrode or grounding pad is necessary, which is attached to patient's skin usually on the opposite chest wall or thigh. Initial scout CT images are acquired; the skin entry site is determined and cross-marked on the skin by laser lights from the CT gantry. Following sterile preparation and draping, local anesthesia is injected along the tract from skin to the level of pleura. A spinal needle is advanced according to the planned trajectory with CT and/or fluoroscopy guidance, which is then exchanged to the ablation electrode after confirmation of correct placement.

The aim of all ablation modalities is to create a zone of tissue necrosis that encompasses both the tumor and a margin of normal parenchyma surrounding it. The choice of electrode length, active tip length and the number of electrodes is determined by the size and location of tumor. The actual ablation zone size may differ from the predicted size. Factors include the heat-sink effect [14], which refers to the fact that medium to large blood vessels or airways carry heat away leading to asymmetrical or truncated ablation zones. Depending on the energy used, the lung's conductivity, impedance and density also play a role in affecting the eventual ablation zone volume. In general, microwave is able to produce a larger ablation zone than radiofrequency due to its mechanism of energy deposition [15], with explanation detailed later in the chapter. After the initial ablation, a CT evaluation of ablation effect should be performed. In case of inadequate ablation volume, re-ablation with several overlapping ablation zones, or exchange to larger and more powerful electrodes can be performed.

After ablation and removal of electrode, CT images are acquired to evaluate technical success and rule out any complications, for example pneumothorax and bleeding. Patients are observed for 2–4 hours and a repeat chest x-ray confirms the absence of pneumothorax. Most patients are discharged the same day if no complications arise. Median length of stay was 1 day in a nation-wide review [16].

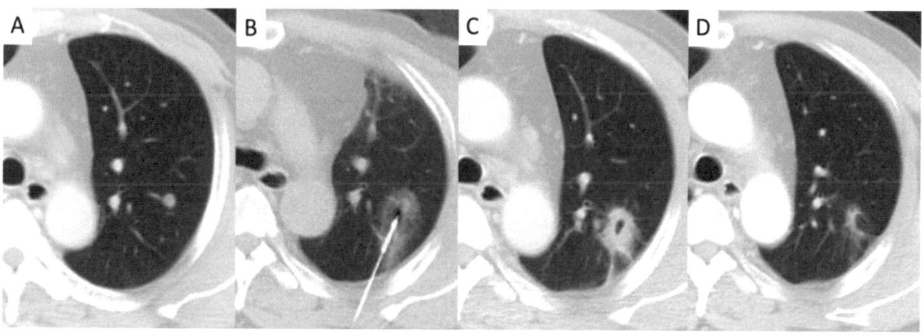

Figure 1.
(A) CT scan shows a biopsy proven left upper lobe lung metastasis in a patient with stage III colonic cancer who was treated with colectomy and chemoradiation previously. (B) CT-guided radiofrequency ablation of the lung metastasis was performed with ablation catheter in-situ and an area of surrounding ground glass opacities (GGO). (C)The ablated area evolved into a denser GGO with central cavitation at 1 month after ablation. (D) CT scan at 6 months after ablation showed evolution of the ablated area into a smaller contracted scar with no signs of recurrence.

Subsequent follow up required interval CT scans for evaluation of treatment response, usually every 3 months although no international guideline exists [17]. Typical early CT appearances following heat-based thermal ablation (eg. RFA, MWA) include ground glass opacities (GGO) or cavities, with or without soft tissue components. The GGO is typically concentric with three layers, the central consolidation represents ablated tumor tissue, the middle layer of faint GGO represents necrotic surrounding parenchyma, and an outer rim of denser GGO contains congested lung tissue and hemorrhage than may retain viability [17]. Cavitation, which is considered a positive response, is most likely to appear in the intermediate phase (1 week to 2 months after ablation). At 3 to 6 months post-ablation, the ablated area continues to involute and shrink down to a linear or nodular scar, or even a thin-walled cavity. Enlarging ablation zone beyond 6 months is highly suggestive for tumor recurrence. Central enhancement >10 mm or > 15HU suggests progression of incompletely ablated disease on contrast CT scans [18], while increased metabolic

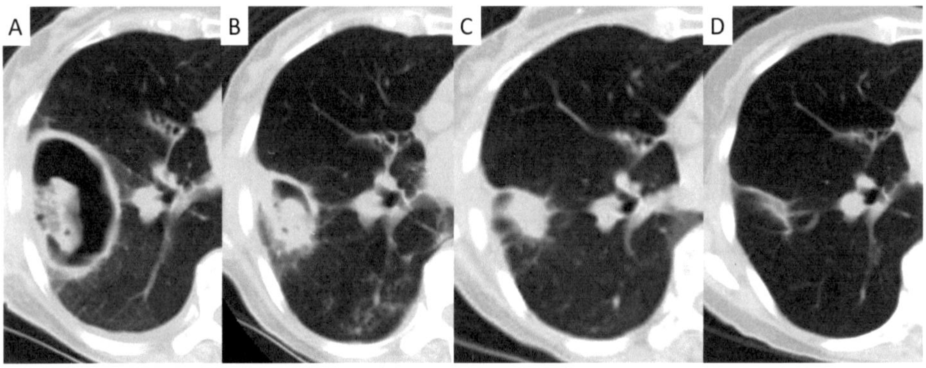

Figure 2.
(A): At 2 weeks after microwave ablation of a small right lower lobe lung tumor, there was a larger-than-expected cavity noted in chest x-ray upon follow up. CT showed a large thick-walled cavity with central soft tissue likely representing necrotic lung and tumor tissue. There was no pneumothorax. (B) CT scan at 3 months post-ablation showed reduction in size of the cavity and soft tissue component. (C) CT scan at 6 months post-ablation showed disappearance of cavity and further reduction in overall size of the ablated area, now consisting of soft tissue density. (D) CT scan at 9 months post-ablation showed a contracted scar representing good treatment response.

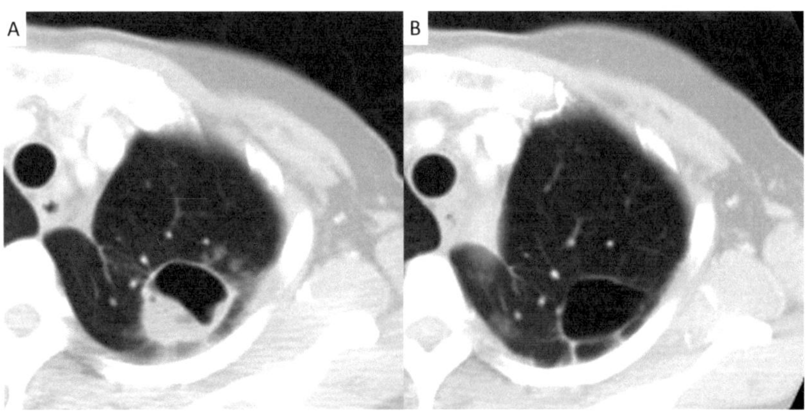

Figure 3.
(A) A cavity with soft tissue component surrounded by patchy ground-glass consolidations at 1 month after microwave ablation of a left upper lobe lung cancer. (B) Complete response as the ablation zone turned into a thin-walled cavity without soft tissue component at 6 months after ablation, which persisted with static appearance thereafter.

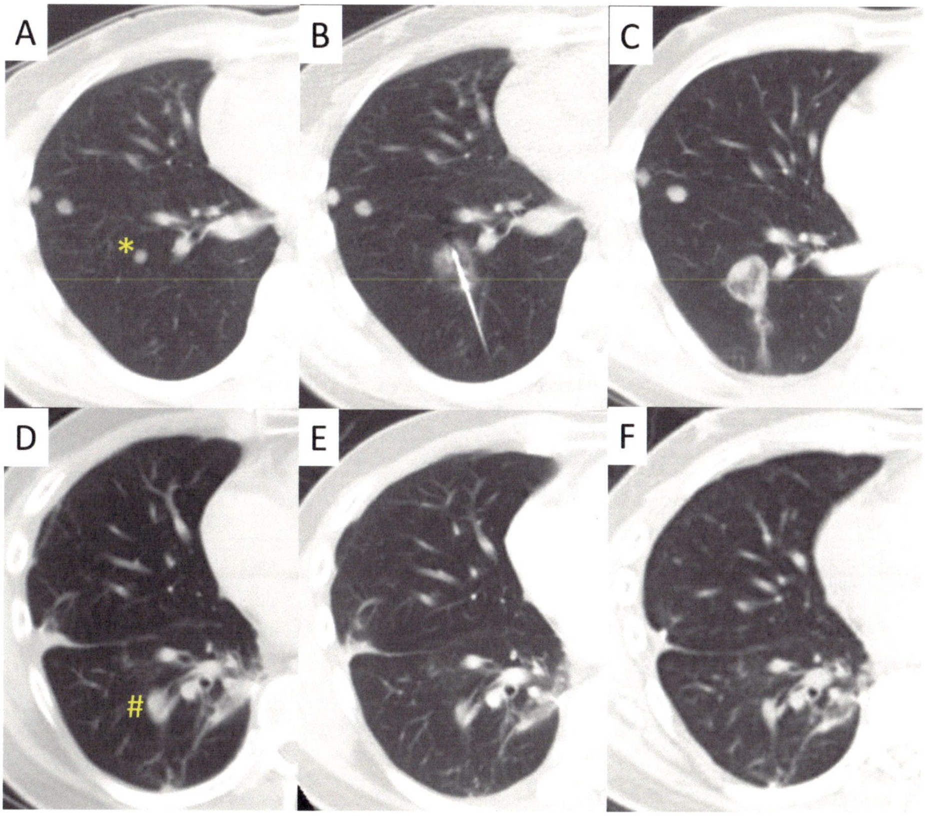

Figure 4.
(A) A 43 year old patient had curative resection of a hepatocellular carcinoma, but was found to have 5 lung metastases on surveillance CT, 3 of which in the right lower lobe (RLL) (as shown), and 2 more in the right middle lobe (not shown). The deepest lung metastasis in the RLL (*) would be difficult to palpate intra-operatively, making wedge resection difficult. Patient was keen for lung-preserving treatment, thus a combined strategy of CT-guided ablation and surgical wedge resection was planned. (B) CT guided radiofrequency ablation of the deepest RLL lung metastasis was performed. (C) The ablation zone evolved into a well-demarcated ground glass opacity with soft tissue component 2 weeks after ablation. (D) Wedge resection of the remaining 4 lung metastases located in peripheral right lower and middle lobe was performed with video-assisted thoracoscopic surgery. CT scan at 3 months after ablation showed contraction of the ablation zone (#) and disappearance of the other 2 RLL lung metastases after surgery. (E) CT scan at 7 months after ablation showed further contraction of the ablated area. (F) CT scan at 1 year after ablation showed a small contracted lobulated scar remaining at the ablated area, and no recurrence of lung metastasis.

activity or new uptake inside the ablation zone beyond 2 months post-ablation are worrisome of recurrence on PET/CT scans [19]. Patients with local recurrence can undergo repeated ablation to improve local control. **Figures 1–3** show the typical appearance of successfully ablated lung tumors over serial CT imagings. CT-guided ablation of centrally located metastasis can be combined with surgical resection of other more peripheral lung metastases as part of lung-preserving strategy, as illustrated in **Figure 4**.

4. Ablation energies

Ablation techniques can be divided into thermal or non-thermal ablations (e.g. irreversible electroporation). Among thermal ablations, heat-based techniques include radiofrequency ablation, microwave ablation and laser ablation, while cold-based technique includes cryoablation. **Table 1** shows the comparison of thermal ablation modalities in the lung.

	Radiofrequency ablation	Microwave Ablation	Cryoablation
Mechanism of action	Frictional heating from electron collisions under oscillating electric field	Frictional heating from rapidly realigning polar water molecules under oscillating electric field	Ultracold temperature when pressurized argon gas expands (Joule Thomson effect)
History of application in lung cancer	Since early 2000s	Since mid 2000s	Since mid 2000s
Temperature (°C)	60 to 100	Around 150	−20 to −40
Grounding pad	Required	Not required	Not required
Ablation zone size	Smaller	Larger	Larger
Dependence on impedance	Yes	No	No
Affected by tissue charring	Yes	No	No
Ablation time per ablation	Medium (10–15 minutes)	Shortest (2–10 minutes)	Longest (25 minutes)
Visibility on CT/MRI	Fair (concentric GGO)	Fair (concentric GGO)	Best (iceballs)
Heat sink effect	Larger	Smaller	—
Preservation of bronchovascular structures	Fair	Fair	Best
Procedural pain	Fair	Less	Least

GGO, ground glass opacity.

Table 1.
Comparison between different modalities of lung cancer thermal ablation.

4.1 Radiofrequency ablation (RFA)

Radiofrequency ablation is the most widely used ablative modality in the lung, and utilizes heat as a form of thermal ablation. Radiofrequency refers to a section in the electromagnetic spectrum with frequency ranging between 20 kHz to 30 MHz, but most clinically available devices function in the 375-500KHz range. A grounding pad or reference electrode is required in RFA, while the active electrode placed inside the tumor is coupled to an RF generator. The RF generator establishes a voltage between the active electrode and reference electrode, producing electric field lines that oscillate with alternating current. At the area closest to the applicator, electrons collide with adjacent molecules under the influence of oscillating electric field, inducing frictional heating [20]. Immediate cell death occurs at temperatures greater than 60°C. RF electrodes have an internal thermocouple that measures the temperature at the tip. Charring and desiccation at the electrode increases impedance and reduces heat conduction, thus most commercially available electrodes are coupled with infusion pumps that pump cold saline to internally cool the electrode tip. Treatments usually range between 4 and 12 minutes, and RFA electrodes may be single-tip applicators or cluster electrodes.

Multiple RFA systems are commercially available (Boston Scientific, Watertown, MA, USA; StarBurst (RITA) Medical Systems, Mountain View, CA, USA; Cool-Tip, Covidien, Boulder, CO, USA). The first two use a deployable radiofrequency array electrode with 4–16 small wires tines through a 14- to 17-gauge needle. The third system consists of a single or triple cluster (3 electrodes spaced 5 mm apart) electrode perfused with saline, and a switching controller allow for simultaneous placement of up to three separate single electrodes to create a greater volume of thermocoagulation in a single application.

4.1.1 Efficacy of radiofrequency ablation

The local control and survival rates of RFA have been examined in a handful of non-randomized single-institutional series and a few multicenter trials. The RAPTURE study published in 2008 is a prospective, intention-to-treat, multicenter trial involving seven centres in Europe, USA and Australia [21]. It included 106 patients with 183 biopsy-proven lung tumors, although there was a mixture of NSCLC and lung metastases. Technical success rate was 99%, and a confirmed complete response lasting at least 1 year was achieved in 88% of patients. For patients with NSCLC, overall survival was 70% at 1 year and 48% at 2 years, cancer-specific survival was 92% at 1 year and 73% at 2 years. Selecting those with stage 1 NSCLC, the 2-year overall survival was 75% and cancer-specific survival was 92%. More recently, another multicenter trial, the ALLIANCE Trial, was published in 2015 [9]. The overall survival was 86.3% at one year and 69.8% at two years, while local recurrence-free rate was 68.9% at one year and 59.8% at two years.

Regarding long term efficacy, a retrospective study revealed that for stage I NSCLC, the overall survival rate was 36% and 27% at 3 and 5 years respectively [10]. In another prospective intention-to-treat study, the complete response rate was 59.3% at a mean follow-up of 47 months, with a mean local recurrence interval of 25.9 months [22]. Median overall survival and cancer-specific survival were 33.4 and 41.4 months respectively, while cancer-specific actuarial survival was 59% at 3 years and 40% at 5 years [22].

Tumor diameter was found to be a negative prognostic factor. The difference between survival curves associated with large (>3 cm) and small (<=3 cm) lung tumors was significant (p = 0.002, 10], and there was a trend toward better efficacy for tumors smaller than 2 cm in diameter (p = 0.066, 23]. Tumor size less than 2 cm was associated with a statistically significant improved survival of 83% at two years in the ALLIANCE Trial [9]. In another study, complete necrosis was attained in all tumors less than 3 cm but only in 23% of larger tumors, and the mean survival of patients with complete necrosis was significantly better than that with partial necrosis [11]. An ablation area of at least 4 times larger than initial tumor was reported to be predictive of complete ablation treatment [23].

To date, there are no properly powered prospective trials comparing one RFA system with another or comparing RFA with other treatment modalities. There has been a propensity-matched analysis comparing RFA and surgery for stage 1 NSCLC, and the mean survival duration of RFA group and surgery group was 33.2 +/− 7.9 and 45.4 +/− 7.2 months respectively, although the difference is not statistically significant [24]. A large propensity-matched retrospective study comparing thermal ablation (mostly RFA) with SBRT using the National Cancer Database reported no significant difference in overall survival at a mean follow up of 52.4 months, however unplanned hospital readmission rates were high in the thermal ablation group [25]. In a systemic analysis and pooled review, the local control rate was significantly lower in the RFA group compared to SBRT, although the overall survival remained similar [26].

4.2 Microwave ablation (MWA)

Microwave ablation for lung tumors has been gaining increasing momentum since the mid-2000s. Microwave occupies a much higher frequency range in the electromagnetic spectrum between 300 MHz to 300 GHz. Compared to radiofrequency, microwave energy is able to create a much larger zone of active heating due to broader deposition of energy. Clinically available microwave applicators generally operate in the 900-245 MHz range [27]. MWA directly heats tissue to lethal temperatures greater than 150°C through dielectric hysteresis, which is a process in which the polar water molecules realign with the oscillating electric field generating kinetic energy, which is then transferred to neighboring tissues [28]. Being completely independent from electrical conductance, microwave energy deposition is less susceptible to tissue impedance, and is able to produce faster, larger and more predictable ablation zones than RFA [15]. The aerated lung has a relatively high impedance among all solid organs, thus making MWA a better modality than RFA in lungs [15, 29]. Heat-sink effect is also smaller with microwave [28].

There are 7 microwave systems commercially available in the United States and Europe, using either 915 MHz or 2450 MHz generators [30]. The antennae are generally straight, ranging from 14 to 17 gauge, with varying active tips of 0.6–4.0 cm in length. Five out of seven systems require perfusion of antenna shaft with room-temperature fluid or carbon dioxide to reduce conductive heating of the non-active portion of the antennae, which protects the skin and other tissues from thermal damage.

4.2.1 *Efficacy of microwave ablation*

The majority of evidence supporting the efficacy of MWA comes from retrospective data. The earlier studies reported an actuarial survival of 65% at 1 year, 55% at 2 years and 45% at 3 years, while cancer-specific survival was 83%, 73% and 61% at 1, 2 and 3 years respectively [31]. A more recent retrospective study reported cancer-specific survival of 69%, 54% and 49% at 1, 2 and 3 years respectively, and the mean survival was 27.8 months [32]. Local control rate was 84.4% at a mean follow-up of 446 days in another retrospective series [33]. A larger retrospective review of 108 patients reported that the median time to tumor recurrence was 62 months, and recurrence rates were 22%, 36% and 44% at 1, 2 and 3 years respectively [34]. It should be noted that the majority of the studies include both primary and secondary lung tumors, and results for NSCLC may not be separately reported. Longer term results were reported in a study involving large NSCLC (mean tumor size of 5.0+/− 1.8 cm). Owing to the larger tumor size, only 44.6% of cases achieved complete tumor ablation after first ablation, and 18.5% required a re-do MWA session. The 3- and 5-year cancer-specific survival rates were 42.1% and 30.0% respectively, and the median cancer-specific survival was 25 months [35].

Similar to RFA, tumor size is associated with poorer prognosis. For every millimeter increase in tumor maximal diameter, the odds of not attaining technical success increased by 7% [34]. Tumor size >4 cm is a significant predictor for local tumor progression and poorer survival [35]. Recurrence rate was 17% for tumors smaller than 3 cm, and increased to 31% for those greater than 3 cm [34]. A risk-factor analysis demonstrated that local tumor progression was significantly correlated with tumor diameter of more than 15.5 mm, irregular shape of index tumor, pleural contact and low energy deployed per unit volume of index tumor [36]. On the other hand, cavitation was associated with reduced cancer-specific mortality [31].

Again, there are no prospective studies comparing one MWA system with another, or with other modalities. There was a propensity-score matched analysis comparing MWA with lobectomy for stage I NSCLC, which reported no significant difference in overall survival and disease free survival (1,3 and 5-year disease free survival of 98.1%, 79.6% and 37.0% for MWA group and 98.1%, 81.5% and 29.6%

for lobectomy group) [37]. The complication rate in MWA group was significantly lower than lobectomy group (p = 0.008). However, the power of this study is undermined by the relatively poor results in lobectomy group when compared to international standard, probably due to poor patient premorbid. In a best evidence topic review, the best available evidence for MWA (7 studies) was compared to that for SBRT (5 studies) [38]. The 3-year survival was 29.2–84.7% for MWA and 42.7–63.5% for SBRT, while the median survival was 35–60 months for MWA and 32.6–48 months for SBRT. The authors concluded that MWA appears comparable to SBRT in terms of local control and survival rates. In the randomized controlled LUMIRA trial, 52 patients with stage IV lung tumors were recruited, and there was no significant difference in survival between the MWA group and RFA group, but MWA was found to produce less intraprocedural pain and a more significant reduction in tumor mass [39].

4.3 Percutaneous Cryoablation

Cryoablation makes use of the Joule-Thomson effect by distributing pressured argon gas to an area of lower pressure and reaching ultracold temperatures when the gas expands [40]. As low as −140°C can be achieved, although living tissue destruction already happens at −40°C. Cryogenic destruction occurs via a number of mechanisms, including protein denaturation, cell rupture due to osmotic shifts, and tissue ischemia from microvascular thrombosis [41]. Meanwhile, the term "cryosurgery" includes cryoablation performed through endobronchial, direct intrathoracic or percutaneous routes.

Traditionally, each cryoablation consists of a dual freeze cycle, involving a 10-minute freeze, followed by 8-minute helium thaw and another 10-minute freeze. Early animal models suggest that air leaks and bleeding could be reduced with this protocol [42]. Current commercially available cryoablation devices (for example Cryocare CS® system, Endocare, Irvine, CA, USA) use a faster cycle of 3-minute freeze, 3-minute thaw, 7-minute freeze, 7-minute thaw and a final 5-minute freeze. These systems allow placement of 1–10 individual 1.5–2.4 mm diameter cryoprobes, and one freeze–thaw–freeze cycle at a single probe position usually suffice. The faster cycle produces interstitial fluid in adjacent lung tissue and improves margin control. Radiologically, a visible "ice ball" and surrounding edematous changes can be seen on CT and serve as an estimation of ablation zone. The true volume of tissue necrosis has been shown to be 3-7 mm from the ice-ball edge [43], and should be taken into consideration when determining cytotoxic ice margin clearance.

Compared with heat-based thermoablation like RFA and MWA, cryoablation has the advantage of larger ablation volumes, availability of multiple applicators, a highly visible ablation zone (a clearly defined ice ball as opposed to concentric ground glass opacities in RFA or microwave), and less pain due to analgesic effect of freezing [44]. Another benefit is its safety near vasculature or bronchi due to the ability to preserve collagenous tissue and cellular architecture in frozen tissue [45]. Disadvantages of cryoablation include a longer procedural time (25 minutes per freeze–thaw–freeze cycle compared to roughly 5 to 10 minutes per ablation in MWA) and a higher incidence of pneumothorax up to 62% [46]. The latter can be tackled with fibrin glue tract coagulation or radiofrequency thermocoagulation of needle tract provided by one of the cryoablation systems.

4.3.1 Efficacy of Cryoablation

A retrospective review of 25 stage I NSCLC treated with cryoablation reported 3-year overall survival of 88% and mean overall survival of 62+/−4 months [47].

Another study involving 27 cryoablated stage I NSCLC demonstrated 3-year survival of 77%, 3-year cancer-specific survival of 90.2% and cancer-free survival of 45.6% [48]. In a study comprising of cryoablation of both primary and secondary lung tumors, the 1-, 2- and 3-year local progression free rates were reported to be 80.4%, 69.0% and 67.7% respectively [49]. In a long-term analysis of 47 stage I NSCLC treated with cryoablation, the 5-year cancer-specific survival rate was 56.6+/−16.5% and 5-year progression free survival rate was 87.9+/−9% [50]. There were two randomized controlled trials, the ECLIPSE trial [51] and SOLSTICE trial [52], evaluating cryoablation of metastatic lung tumors, which report favorable safety and efficacy, but are out of the scope of this chapter.

Cryoablation has been performed for stage IV lung cancer for palliation of symptoms. In a comparative study between cryoablation and palliative treatment alone, the overall survival of the cryoablation group was significantly longer, with median survival of 14 months compared to 7 months [53]. The same group has performed cryosurgery in various stages of NSCLC yielding an overall survival of 64%, 45% and 32% at 1, 2 and 3 years respectively [54].

Few studies have compared cryoablation with other treatment modalities. In 64 patients with stage I NSCLC deemed medically unfit for lobectomy, 25 were treated with sublobar resection, 12 with RFA and 27 with cryoablation. The 3-year survival rate was similar for the three groups (87.1% for sublobar resection, 87.5% for RFA and 77% for cryoablation) [48]. In a comparative study for stage IIIB or IV NSCLC treated with cryoablation or MWA, the overall survival and progression-free survival were similar for tumors ≤3 cm in diameter, but were poorer in tumors greater than 3 cm which are treated with cryoablation [44].

4.4 Percutaneous laser ablation

Laser ablation is a thermal technique where light energy is converted into heat by interaction with sources such as an Nd: YAG laser. Typically, energy is transmitted through a flexible fiberoptic cable which is percutaneously inserted into the lung through an outer sheath. Cooling of the fiberoptic cable enables greater energy deposition and a 50 percent increase in size of thermocoagulation [55], as the size of ablation zone is limited by tissue carbonization near the applicator. To date, there have been limited reports on the efficacy of laser ablation in humans [56]. A long term analysis of laser ablation for lung metastases reported 1-, 3- and 5-year survival of 81%, 44% and 27% respectively [57], with a relatively high rate of pneumothorax (38%). No data is available for primary lung cancers.

4.5 Irreversible electroporation (IRE)

Electroporation is a phenomenon in which cell membrane permeability to ions and macromolecules is increased by exposure to high voltage electric pulses. It can be reversible or irreversible, with the latter leading to cell death from loss of homeostasis and osmotic effects. Since IRE is a non-thermal ablation modality, its theoretical advantage includes overcoming the heat-sink effect [58] and preservation of structural integrity of nearby bronchovascular structures [59]. Although there have been reports on its efficacy in animal models [60] and in other organs such as the liver [61], there were few reports on its use in human lungs [62]. In fact, in the multicenter phase II ALICE trial for treatment of primary and secondary lung malignancies, IRE failed to meet the expected efficacy and the trial was terminated prematurely after inclusion of 23 patients, in which 61% showed progressive disease [63]. The disappointing results may be explained by high differences in electric conductivity between normal lung parenchyma and tumor tissue. Of note, needle tract seeding happened in 13% of cases.

5. Safety and complications of percutaneous ablation

Percutaneous ablation of lung tumors is generally considered safe. A list of potential complications is presented in **Table 2**. In a nationwide analysis of 3344 patients who underwent percutaneous lung ablation in the United States [16], in-hospital mortality was 1.3%, and patients with more comorbidities (Charlson comorbidity index score $\geq$ 4) was associated with significantly higher mortality. The most common complication was pneumothorax (38.4%), followed by pneumonia (5.7%) and effusion (4.0%). In a Japanese review of 1000 RFA sessions [64], there was a 0.4% procedure-related mortality, of which three died of interstitial pneumonia and another died of hemothorax. Major complication rate was 9.8%, consisting of 2.3% aseptic pleuritis, 1.9% pneumonia, 1.6% lung abscess (**Figure 5**), 1.6% pneumothorax requiring pleural sclerosis, 0.4% bronchopleural fistula and 0.3% brachial nerve injury. Previous radiotherapy and age were significant risk factors for pneumonia, as were emphysema for lung abscess, and platelet count and tumor size for bleeding [64].

Pneumothorax occurs as a result of pleural puncture by the ablation catheter leading to air leak. Hence, unlike standard lung biopsy technique, in which the shortest path to tumor is preferred, some operators advocated a longer distance between pleura puncture site and tumor is more desirable for ablation. An indirect approach that leaves an unablated tract of at least 2 cm of normal lung is preferable [29], because

Complications		Treatment/remarks
Pneumothorax	3.5–54% (Up to 10% delayed pneumothorax)	Only 6–29% require chest tube insertion
Pleural effusion/aseptic pleuritis	2.3–19%	Only a minority require drainage
Bleeding	1.6–18%	Rarely require emergency arterial embolization or surgery
Pneumonia	1.8%	Antibiotics
Lung abscess	1.6%	Antibiotics, drainage
Bronchopleural fistula	0.4–0.6%	Prolonged chest tube drainage, chemical pleurodesis, endobronchial valves/ embolization
Needle tract seeding	0.3–0.7%	Associated with biopsy prior to RFA
Thermal injury to nearby structures	0.3–0.5% (brachial plexus) 1.3% (phrenic nerve) 0.1% (diaphragm)	Phrenic nerve injury can lead to significant reduction in vital capacity and referred pain to shoulder
Pneumonitis	0.4%	Pulse steroid
Pulmonary artery pseudoaneurysm	0.2%	Transcatheter coil embolization
Systemic air embolism	Very rare	Hyperbaric oxygen

Table 2.
Complications following thermal ablation in the lung.

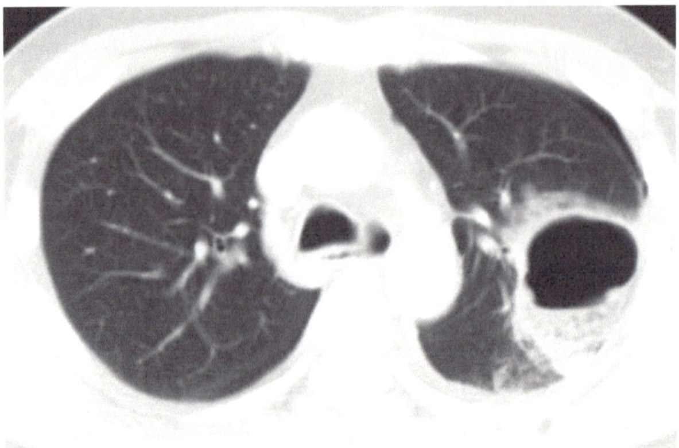

Figure 5.
A small pneumothorax and a large cavity with soft tissue content at 2 weeks after microwave ablation of a left upper lobe lung tumor. If the patient had fever and air-fluid level was seen in the cavity, a suspicion for lung abscess should be raised, and the abscess should be drained with contents sent for culture and intravenous antibiotics should be commenced.

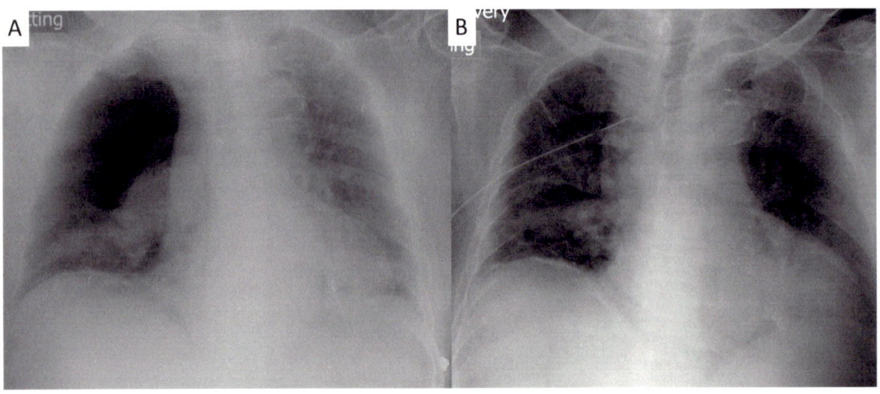

Figure 6.
(A) A large right pneumothorax immediately after CT-guided radiofrequency ablation of a right lower lobe lung cancer. (B) Shows the lung re-expands after right chest drain insertion in the same patient.

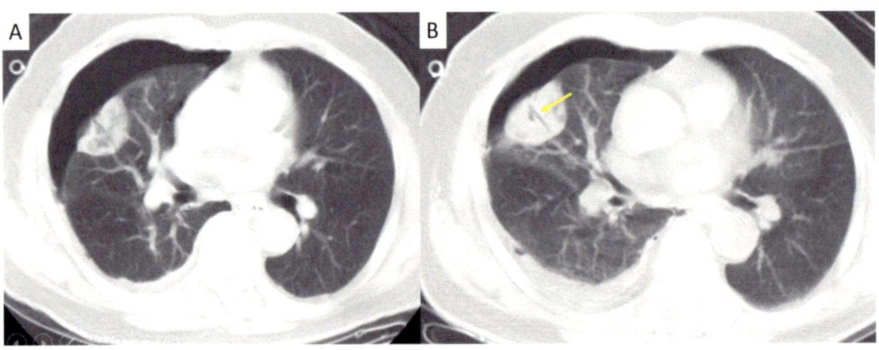

Figure 7.
(A) A patient with right lower lobe lung cancer was treated with CT-guided microwave ablation, but complicated by persistent air leak for 2 weeks despite chest drain insertion. CT scan showed a moderate right pneumothorax and an area of ground glass opacity in the anterior right lower lobe representing the ablation zone. (B) CT scan performed at 3 weeks after ablation demonstrated a bronchopleural fistula (yellow arrow) joining a lobar bronchus to the pleural space through the ablated needle tract.

unablated pleura contracts less and heals quicker. Emphysema is the most significant risk factor for pneumothorax in multiple studies [65, 66]. Other risk factors include male gender, no previous lung surgery, high number of tumors ablated, advanced age, and traversal of major fissure by electrode [67]. The rate of pneumothorax ranges from 3.5–54%, but only 6–29% required chest tube placement [68] (**Figure 6**). Delayed pneumothorax could occur in up to 10% of cases [69, 70]. Around 0.4–0.6% of all patients develop bronchopleural fistula [64, 71] leading to intractable pneumothorax not resolving with chest drainage (**Figure 7**). Treatment strategies include repeated chemical pleurodesis, placement of endobronchial valves (**Figure 8**), and bronchoscopic embolization of relevant fistulae [68].

Aseptic pleuritis and pleural effusion is postulated to be due to ablation zone reaching pleura leading of pleural inflammation, and is associated with higher

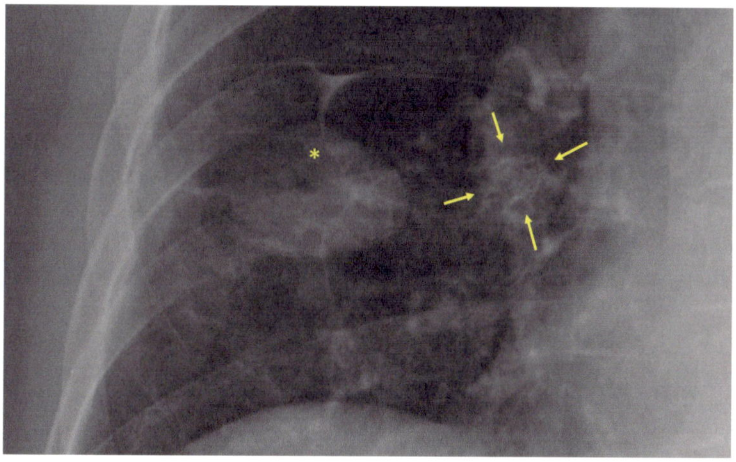

Figure 8.
Resolution of pneumothorax after implantation of an endobronchial valve (faint metallic shadow surrounded by yellow arrows) for bronchopleural fistula. This is the same patient as **Figure 7** *And the ablation zone is marked by (*) on this chest x-ray.*

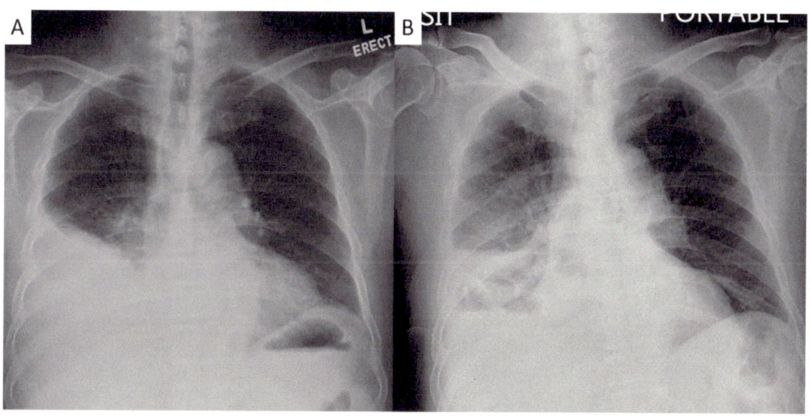

Figure 9.
(A) Moderate right pleural effusion that has accumulated for 3 days following CT-guided microwave ablation of a right lower lobe lung tumor. The patient had low grade fever and complained of shortness of breath. (B) partial drainage of the effusion by a medium bore chest drain. The pleural fluid was exudative but sterile, and the patient was discharged home after a course of antibiotics and complete drainage of the effusion.

pleural temperatures [72]. Repeated punctures and previous systemic chemotherapy were significant risk factors [64]. Aseptic pleuritis gives rise to pleuritic pain, but most resolve spontaneously. Only a minority of pleural effusion required drainage (**Figure 9**).

The incidence of hemoptysis after percutaneous RFA is 3–9% [68], while the incidence of all forms of hemorrhage is approximately double that rate. Risk factors for intraparenchymal hemorrhage include basal and middle lung zone lesions, needle track traversing lung parenchyma by more than 2.5 cm, electrode traversing pulmonary vessels and the use of multi-tined electrodes [73]. Although most hemorrhages are self-limiting, rarely ablation injury to intercostal artery may occur leading to massive bleeding [68].

6. Bronchoscopic ablation techniques

Most of the thermal ablative techniques in literature involved percutaneous placement of electrodes. Since 2010, a Japanese group pioneered a bronchoscopy-guided cooled RFA technique for lung tumors in humans [74, 75], followed by a Chinese group using electromagnetic navigation bronchoscopy (ENB) guidance [76]. Compared to percutaneous approach, a major advantage of bronchoscopic ablation is lack of pleural puncture, and hence fewer pleural-based complications. The Japanese group reported no pneumothorax, bronchopleural fistula nor pleural effusion in 28 cases of bronchoscopic RFA [75], while the rate of pneumothorax for percutaneous ablation ranges from 3.5–54% as mentioned above. Bronchoscopic ablation also eliminates the risk of needle tract seeding. Another edge of bronchoscopic ablation is its ability to reach certain regions of lung which are otherwise difficult or dangerous for percutaneous access, for instance areas near mediastinal pleura, diaphragm, lung apex, or areas shielded by scapula.

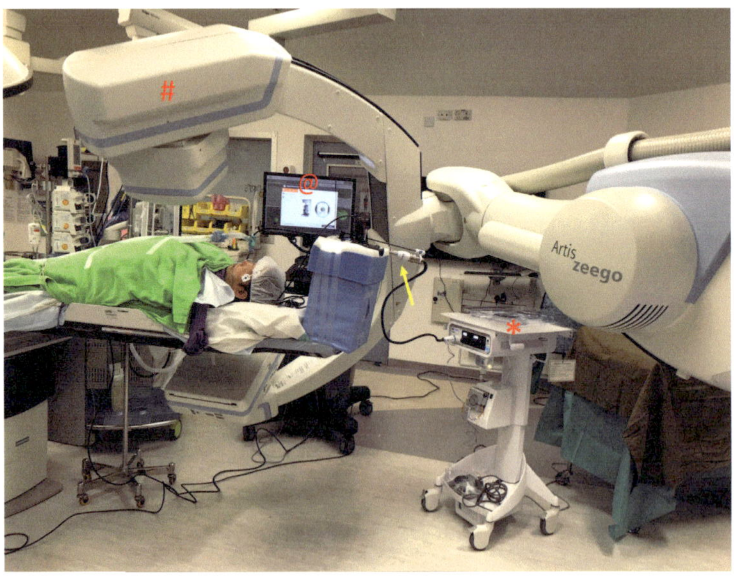

Figure 10.
The set-up for microwave ablation of lung nodules under electromagnetic navigation bronchoscopy (ENB) is shown. Within the hybrid theater, the patient lies supine and is intubated with single lumen endotracheal tube. With the help of navigation software like SuperDimension™ (@), and fine adjustment of position with cone-beam CT (#), the target lung lesion is localized with a ENB bronchoscope. The microwave ablation catheter is inserted through the bronchoscope into the lung tumor, which is then connected to the microwave generator (*). The yellow arrow is pointing to the external part of microwave ablation catheter.

With evidence of safety and technical success of bronchoscopic ablation in animal models [77], and the above-mentioned advantages in mind, the author's institute is one of the first to perform ENB-guided microwave ablation on patients in the hybrid operating room (**Figure 10**). Navigation precision has been much improved following the advent of ENB with the help of navigation systems like SuperDimension™ (Covidien, Plymouth, MN, USA) (**Figures 11** and **12**), supplemented by position confirmation by fluoroscopy and cone beam CT. The microwave catheter (Emprint™ Ablation Catheter with Thermosphere™ technology, Covidien, Plymouth, MN, USA) is inserted within the lung tumor via bronchoscopy and ablated for up to 10 minutes per burn (**Figure 13**). Since early

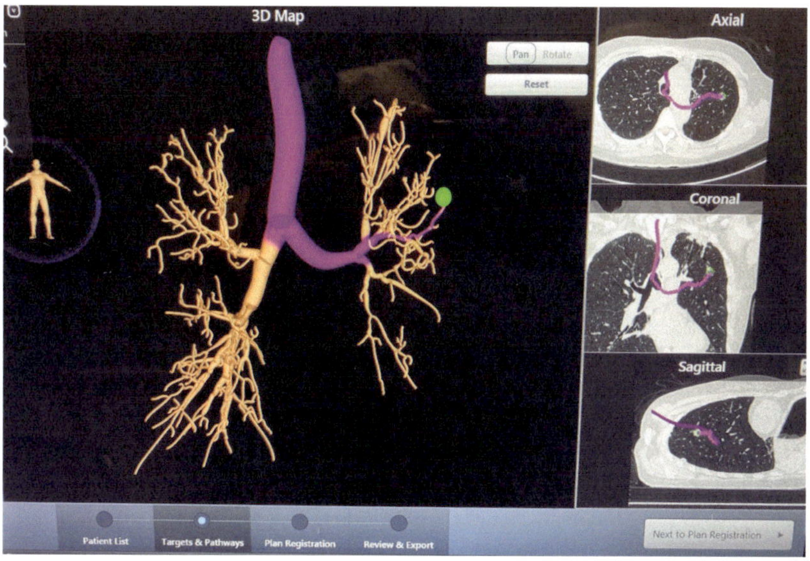

Figure 11.
The planned navigation pathway (pink) from trachea to the target lung lesion in left upper lobe with the help of navigation software like SuperDimension™.

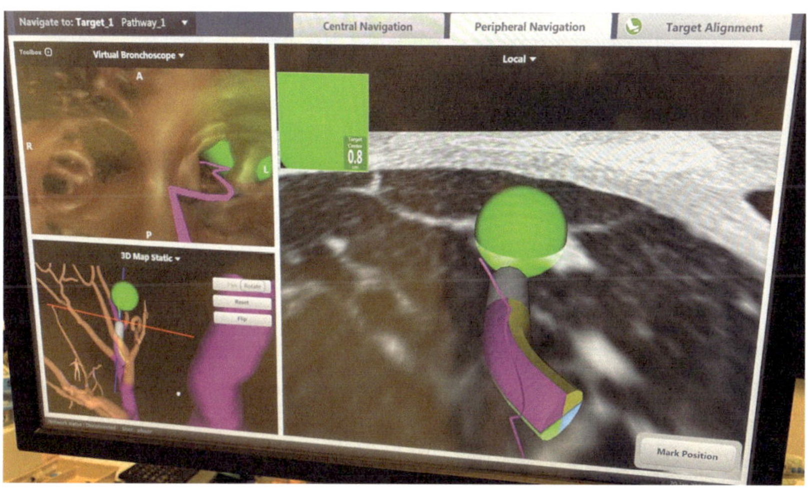

Figure 12.
The SuperDimension™ software allows multiple views to guide navigation to a target lung lesion (green ball). The upper left panel shows the navigation pathway (pink) in virtual bronchoscopy view, while the lower left panel shows it in 3D map view. On the right side panel, the Centre of the target lung lesion is shown to be 0.8 cm from the tip of the locatable guide.

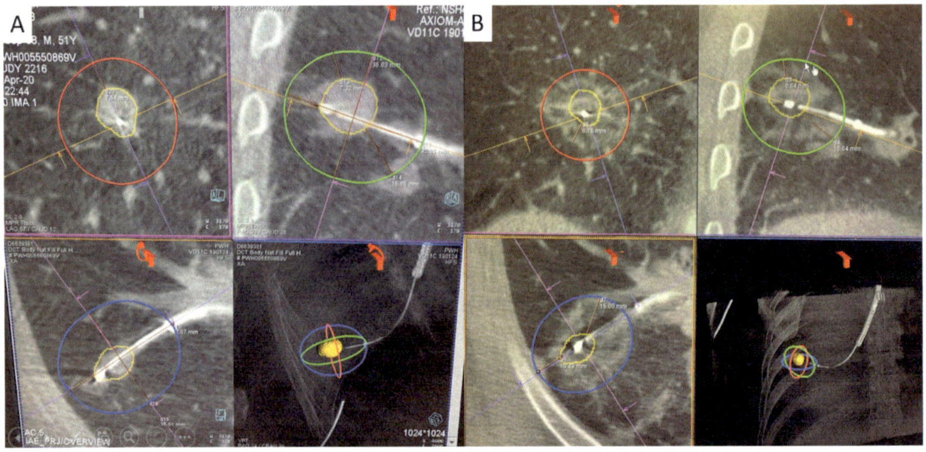

Figure 13.
(A) The target lung lesion (yellow tracing) in 3 axes on CT before bronchoscopic microwave ablation. The green, red and blue ovals mark the expected ablation zone margins. (B) The post-ablation appearance of the same lung nodule. The lung tumor has been encompassed in the ablation zone, represented by ground-glass opacities.

2019, we have performed 45 cases with 100% technical success rate. Similar to percutaneous approach, the median length of stay was 1 day only. Only 2 patients (4.4%) developed pneumothorax requiring chest drainage. Post-ablation reaction and fever occurred in 8.9%, minor hemoptysis or hemorrhage in 4.4%, and pleural effusion in 2.2%. As of the time of writing, there was no progressive disease at a mean follow up of 290 days. We believe that bronchoscopic ablation represents the future for lung cancer ablation as it offers a truly wound-less option with likely fewer complications.

7. Conclusions

Image-guided ablative therapy is an important armamentarium in the treatment of lung cancers, either for early stage lung cancers in patients who are medically inoperable or refuse surgery, or for palliation of late stage lung cancers. Radiofrequency ablation is the most studied modality with a large body of evidence supporting its safety and efficacy, with comparable outcomes to sublobar resections and stereotactic radiation therapy in select patients. Nonetheless, microwave ablation is quickly catching up in popularity due to its superior properties over RFA. Traditionally, lung ablation was performed percutaneously, but the latest development of bronchoscopic ablation techniques are promising and may drive the future of lung cancer ablation research.

Conflict of interest

Dr. Joyce WY Chan and Dr. Rainbow WH Lau declare no conflict of interest.

Professor Calvin SH Ng is a consultant for Johnson and Johnson; Medtronic, USA.

Author details

Joyce W.Y. Chan, Rainbow W.H. Lau and Calvin S.H. Ng*
Division of Cardiothoracic Surgery, Department of Surgery, Prince of Wales Hospital, The Chinese University of Hong Kong, Hong Kong SAR

*Address all correspondence to: calvinng@surgery.cuhk.edu.hk

References

[1] Rami-PortaR, TsuboiM. Sublobar resection for lung cancer. European Respiratory Journal 2009; 33(2): 426-435. DOI: 10.1183/09031936.00099808.

[2] El-SherifA, GoodingWE, SantosR, et al. Outcomes of Sublobar Resection Versus Lobectomy for Stage I Non-Small Cell Lung Cancer: A 13-Year Analysis. Annals of Thoracic Surgery 2006; 82(2): 408-416. DOI: 10.1016/j.athoracsur.2006.02.029.

[3] BerfieldKS, WoodDE. Sublobar resection for stage IA non-small cell lung cancer. Journal of Thoracic Disease 2017; 9(Suppl 3): 208-210. DOI: 10.21037/jtd.2017.03.135.

[4] AbreuCECV, FerreiraPPR, deMoraesFY, NevesWFP, GadiaR, CarvalhoH de A. Radioterapia estereotáxica extracraniana em câncer de pulmão: Atualização. Jornal Brasileiro de Pneumologia 2015; 41(4): 376-387. DOI: 10.1590/S1806-37132015000000034.

[5] Anon. Long-term Results of Stereotactic Body Radiation Therapy in Medically Inoperable Stage I Non-Small Cell Lung Cancer - PubMed.

[6] DupuyDE, ZagoriaRJ, AkerleyW, Mayo-SmithWW, KavanaghPV., SafranH. Technical innovation: Percutaneous radiofrequency ablation of malignancies in the lung. American Journal of Roentgenology 2000; 174(1): 57-59. DOI: 10.2214/ajr.174.1.1740057.

[7] AlexanderE, DupuyD. Lung cancer ablation: Technologies and techniques. Seminars in Interventional Radiology 2013; 30(2): 141-150. DOI: 10.1055/s-0033-1342955.

[8] DupuyDE, Mayo-SmithWW, AbbottGF, DiPetrilloT. Clinical applications of radio-frequency tumor ablation in the thorax. Radiographics 2002; 22(SPEC. ISS). DOI: 10.1148/radiographics.22.suppl_1.g02oc03s259.

[9] DupuyDE, FernandoHC, HillmanS, et al. Radiofrequency ablation of stage IA non-small cell lung cancer in medically inoperable patients: Results from the American College of Surgeons Oncology Group Z4033 (Alliance) trial. Cancer 2015; 121(19): 3491-3498. DOI: 10.1002/cncr.29507.

[10] SimonCJ, DupuyDE, DiPetrilloTA, et al. Pulmonary radiofrequency ablation: Long-term safety and efficacy in 153 patients. Radiology 2007; 243(1): 268-275. DOI: 10.1148/radiol.2431060088.

[11] LeeJM, JinGY, GoldbergSN, et al. Percutaneous Radiofrequency Ablation for Inoperable Non-Small Cell Lung Cancer and Metastases: Preliminary Report. Radiology 2004; 230(1): 125-134. DOI: 10.1148/radiol.2301020934.

[12] SolomonSB, ThorntonRH, DupuyDE, DowneyRJ. Protection of the Mediastinum and Chest Wall with an Artificial Pneumothorax during Lung Ablations. Journal of Vascular and Interventional Radiology 2008; 19(4): 610-615. DOI: 10.1016/j.jvir.2008.01.004.

[13] YasuiK, KanazawaS, SanoY, et al. Thoracic tumors treated with CT-guided radiofrequency ablation: Initial experience. Radiology 2004; 231(3): 850-857. DOI: 10.1148/radiol.2313030347.

[14] KimC. Understanding the nuances of microwave ablation for more accurate post-treatment assessment. Future Oncology 2018; 14(17): 1755-1764. DOI: 10.2217/fon-2017-0736.

[15] BraceCL, HinshawJL, LaesekePF, SampsonLA, LeeFT. Pulmonary thermal ablation: Comparison of radiofrequency

and microwave devices by using gross pathologic and CT findings in a swine model. Radiology 2009; 251(3): 705-711. DOI: 10.1148/radiol.2513081564.

[16] WelchBT, BrinjikjiW, SchmitGD, et al. A national analysis of the complications, cost, and mortality of percutaneous lung ablation. Journal of Vascular and Interventional Radiology 2015; 26(6): 787-791. DOI: 10.1016/j.jvir.2015.02.019.

[17] ChheangS, AbtinF, GuteirrezA, GenshaftS, SuhR. Imaging features following thermal ablation of lung malignancies. Seminars in Interventional Radiology 2013; 30(2): 157-168. DOI: 10.1055/s-0033-1342957.

[18] SuhRD, WallaceAB, SheehanRE, HeinzeSB, GoldinJG. Unresectable Pulmonary Malignancies: CT-guided Percutaneous Radiofrequency Ablation - Preliminary Results. Radiology 2003; 229(3): 821-829. DOI: 10.1148/radiol.2293021756.

[19] AbtinFG, EradatJ, GutierrezAJ, LeeC, FishbeinMC, SuhRD. Radiofrequency ablation of lung tumors: Imaging features of the postablation zone. Radiographics 2012; 32(4): 947-969. DOI: 10.1148/rg.324105181.

[20] OrganLW. Electrophysiologic principles of radiofrequency lesion making. Applied Neurophysiology 1976; 32(2): 69-76. DOI: 10.1159/000102478.

[21] LencioniR, CrocettiL, CioniR, et al. Response to radiofrequency ablation of pulmonary tumours: a prospective, intention-to-treat, multicentre clinical trial (the RAPTURE study). The Lancet Oncology 2008; 9(7): 621-628. DOI: 10.1016/S1470-2045(08)70155-4.

[22] AmbrogiMC, FanucchiO, CioniR, et al. Long-term results of radiofrequency ablation treatment of stage i non-small cell lung cancer: A prospective intention-to-treat study. Journal of Thoracic Oncology 2011; 6(12): 2044-2051. DOI: 10.1097/JTO.0b013e31822d538d.

[23] DeBaèreT, PalussièreJ, AupérinA, et al. Midterm local efficacy and survival after radiofrequency ablation of lung tumors with minimum follow-up of 1 year: Prospective evaluation. Radiology 2006; 240(2): 587-596. DOI: 10.1148/radiol.2402050807.

[24] KimSR, HanHJ, ParkSJ, et al. Comparison between surgery and radiofrequency ablation for stage i non-small cell lung cancer. European Journal of Radiology 2012; 81(2): 395-399. DOI: 10.1016/j.ejrad.2010.12.091.

[25] UhligJ, LudwigJM, GoldbergSB, ChiangA, BlasbergJD, KimHS. Survival rates after thermal ablation versus stereotactic radiation therapy for stage 1 non–small cell lung cancer: A national cancer database study. Radiology 2018; 289(3): 862-870. DOI: 10.1148/radiol.2018180979.

[26] BiN, SheddenK, ZhengX, KongFMS. Comparison of the Effectiveness of Radiofrequency Ablation With Stereotactic Body Radiation Therapy in Inoperable Stage I Non-Small Cell Lung Cancer: A Systemic Review and Pooled Analysis. In International Journal of Radiation Oncology Biology Physics, vol 95. Elsevier Inc., 2016; 1378-1390. DOI: 10.1016/j.ijrobp.2016.04.016.

[27] SimonCJ, DupuyDE, Mayo-SmithWW. Microwave ablation: Principles and applications. In Radiographics, vol 25. Radiographics, 2005. DOI: 10.1148/rg.25si055501.

[28] LubnerMG, BraceCL, HinshawJL, LeeFT. Microwave tumor ablation: Mechanism of action, clinical results, and devices. Journal of Vascular and Interventional Radiology 2010; 21(SUPPL. 8): S192. DOI: 10.1016/j.jvir.2010.04.007.

[29] Louis HinshawJ, LubnerMG, ZiemlewiczTJ, LeeFT, BraceCL. Percutaneous tumor ablation tools: Microwave, radiofrequency, or cryoablation-what should you use and why? Radiographics 2014; 34(5): 1344-1362. DOI: 10.1148/rg.345140054.

[30] WardRC, HealeyTT, DupuyDE. Microwave ablation devices for interventional oncology. Expert Review of Medical Devices 2013; 10(2): 225-238. DOI: 10.1586/erd.12.77.

[31] WolfFJ, GrandDJ, MachanJT, DiPetrilloTA, Mayo-SmithWW, DupuyDE. Microwave ablation of lung malignancies: Effectiveness, CT findings, and safety in 50 patients. Radiology 2008; 247(3): 871-879. DOI: 10.1148/radiol.2473070996.

[32] BelfioreG, RonzaF, BelfioreMP, et al. Patients' survival in lung malignancies treated by microwave ablation: Our experience on 56 patients. European Journal of Radiology 2013; 82(1): 177-181. DOI: 10.1016/j.ejrad.2012.08.024.

[33] KoWC, LeeYF, ChenYC, et al. CT-guided percutaneous microwave ablation of pulmonary malignant tumors. Journal of Thoracic Disease 2016; 8(Suppl 9): S659–S665. DOI: 10.21037/jtd.2016.09.44.

[34] HealeyTT, MarchBT, BairdG, DupuyDE. Microwave Ablation for Lung Neoplasms: A Retrospective Analysis of Long-Term Results. Journal of Vascular and Interventional Radiology 2017; 28(2): 206-211. DOI: 10.1016/j.jvir.2016.10.030.

[35] PusceddduC, MelisL, SotgiaB, GuerzoniD, PorcuA, FancelluA. Usefulness of percutaneous microwave ablation for large non-small cell lung cancer: A preliminary report. Oncology Letters 2019; 18(1): 659-666. DOI: 10.3892/ol.2019.10375.

[36] VoglTJ, WorstTS, NaguibNNN, AckermannH, Gruber-RouhT, Nour-EldinNEA. Factors influencing local tumor control in patients with neoplastic pulmonary nodules treated with microwave ablation: A risk-factor analysis. American Journal of Roentgenology 2013; 200(3): 665-672. DOI: 10.2214/AJR.12.8721.

[37] YaoW, LuM, FanW, et al. Comparison between microwave ablation and lobectomy for stage I non-small cell lung cancer: a propensity score analysis. International Journal of Hyperthermia 2018; 34(8): 1329-1336. DOI: 10.1080/02656736.2018.1434901.

[38] WatsonRA, TolI, GunawardanaS, TsakokMT. Is microwave ablation an alternative to stereotactic ablative body radiotherapy in patients with inoperable early-stage primary lung cancer? Interactive Cardiovascular and Thoracic Surgery 2019; 29(4): 539-543. DOI: 10.1093/icvts/ivz123.

[39] MacchiM, BelfioreMP, FloridiC, et al. Radiofrequency versus microwave ablation for treatment of the lung tumours: LUMIRA (lung microwave radiofrequency) randomized trial. Medical Oncology 2017; 34(5). DOI: 10.1007/s12032-017-0946-x.

[40] ErinjeriJP, ClarkTWI. Cryoablation: Mechanism of action and devices. Journal of Vascular and Interventional Radiology 2010; 21(SUPPL. 8): S187. DOI: 10.1016/j.jvir.2009.12.403.

[41] GageAA, BaustJ. Mechanisms of Tissue Injury in Cryosurgery. Cryobiology 1998; 37(3): 171-186. DOI: 10.1006/cryo.1998.2115.

[42] IzumiY, OyamaT, IkedaE, KawamuraM, KobayashiK. The acute effects of transthoracic cryoablation on normal lung evaluated in a porcine model. Annals of Thoracic Surgery 2005; 79(1): 318-322. DOI: 10.1016/j.athoracsur.2003.09.082.

[43] HinshawJL, LittrupPJ, DurickN, et al. Optimizing the protocol for

pulmonary cryoablation: A comparison of a dual- and triple-freeze protocol. CardioVascular and Interventional Radiology 2010; 33(6): 1180-1185. DOI: 10.1007/s00270-010-9868-0.

[44] DasSK, HuangYY, LiB, YuXX, XiaoRH, YangHF. Comparing cryoablation and microwave ablation for the treatment of patients with stage IIIB/IV non-small cell lung cancer. Oncology Letters 2020; 19(1): 1031-1041. DOI: 10.3892/ol.2019.11149.

[45] MaiwandMO. The role of cryosurgery in palliation of tracheo-bronchial carcinoma. European Journal of Cardio-thoracic Surgery 1999; 15(6): 764-768. DOI: 10.1016/S1010-7940(99)00121-9.

[46] InoueM, NakatsukaS, YashiroH, et al. Percutaneous cryoablation of lung tumors: Feasibility and safety. Journal of Vascular and Interventional Radiology 2012; 23(3): 295-302. DOI: 10.1016/j.jvir.2011.11.019.

[47] YamauchiY, IzumiY, HashimotoK, et al. Percutaneous cryoablation for the treatment of medically inoperable Stage I non-small cell lung cancer. PLoS ONE 2012; 7(3). DOI: 10.1371/journal.pone.0033223.

[48] ZemlyakA, MooreWH, BilfingerTV. Comparison of Survival after Sublobar Resections and Ablative Therapies for Stage I Non-Small Cell Lung Cancer. Journal of the American College of Surgeons 2010; 211(1): 68-72. DOI: 10.1016/j.jamcollsurg.2010.03.020.

[49] YashiroH, NakatsukaS, InoueM, et al. Factors affecting local progression after percutaneous cryoablation of lung tumors. Journal of Vascular and Interventional Radiology 2013; 24(6): 813-821. DOI: 10.1016/j.jvir.2012.12.026.

[50] MooreW, TalatiR, BhattacharjiP, BilfingerT. Five-year survival after cryoablation of stage I non-small cell lung cancer in medically inoperable patients. Journal of Vascular and Interventional Radiology 2015; 26(3): 312-319. DOI: 10.1016/j.jvir.2014.12.006.

[51] DeBaereT, TselikasL, WoodrumD, et al. Evaluating cryoablation of metastatic lung tumors in patients-safety and efficacy the ECLIPSE trial-interim analysis at 1 year. Journal of Thoracic Oncology 2015; 10(10): 1468-1474. DOI: 10.1097/JTO.0000000000000632.

[52] CallstromMR, WoodrumDA, NicholsFC, et al. Multicenter Study of Metastatic Lung Tumors Targeted by Interventional Cryoablation Evaluation (SOLSTICE). In Journal of Thoracic Oncology, vol 15. Elsevier Inc, 2020; 1200-1209. DOI: 10.1016/j.jtho.2020.02.022.

[53] NiuL, ChenJ, YaoF, et al. Percutaneous cryoablation for stage IV lung cancer: A retrospective analysis. Cryobiology 2013; 67(2): 151-155. DOI: 10.1016/j.cryobiol.2013.06.005.

[54] NiuL, XuK, MuF. Cryosurgery for lung cancer. Journal of Thoracic Disease 2012; 4(4): 408-419. DOI: 10.3978/j.issn.2072-1439.2012.07.13.

[55] VoglTJ, StraubR, LehnertT, et al. Perkutane thermoablation von lungenmetastasen - Erfahrungen mit dem einsatz der LITT, der radiofrequenzablation (RFA) und literaturübersicht. RoFo Fortschritte auf dem Gebiet der Rontgenstrahlen und der Bildgebenden Verfahren 2004; 176(11): 1658-1666. DOI: 10.1055/s-2004-813465.

[56] ZhaoQ, TianG, ChenF, ZhongL, JiangT. CT-guided percutaneous laser ablation of metastatic lung cancer: Three cases report and literature review. Oncotarget 2017; 8(2): 2187-2196. DOI: 10.18632/oncotarget.13901.

[57] RosenbergC, PuisR, HegenscheidK, et al. Laser Ablation of Metastatic

Lesions of the Lung: Long-Term Outcome. American Journal of Roentgenology 2009; 192(3): 785-792. DOI: 10.2214/AJR.08.1425.

[58] MaorE, IvorraA, LeorJ, RubinskyB. The effect of irreversible electroporation on blood vessels. Technology in Cancer Research and Treatment 2007; 6(4): 307-312. DOI: 10.1177/153303460700600407.

[59] ThomsonKR, CheungW, EllisSJ, et al. Investigation of the safety of irreversible electroporation in humans. Journal of Vascular and Interventional Radiology 2011; 22(5): 611-621. DOI: 10.1016/j.jvir.2010.12.014.

[60] SongZ, XuX, LiuM, et al. Efficacy and mechanism of steep pulse irreversible electroporation technology on xenograft model of nude mice: a preclinical study. World journal of surgical oncology 2018; 16(1): 84. DOI: 10.1186/s12957-018-1386-6.

[61] VroomenLGPH, PetreEN, CornelisFH, SolomonSB, SrimathveeravalliG. Irreversible electroporation and thermal ablation of tumors in the liver, lung, kidney and bone: What are the differences? Diagnostic and Interventional Imaging 2017; 98(9): 609-617. DOI: 10.1016/j.diii.2017.07.007.

[62] UsmanM, MooreW, TalatiR, WatkinsK, BilfingerTV. Irreversible electroporation of lung neoplasm: A case series. Medical Science Monitor 2012; 18(6). DOI: 10.12659/MSM.882888.

[63] RickeJ, JürgensJHW, DeschampsF, et al. Irreversible Electroporation (IRE) Fails to Demonstrate Efficacy in a Prospective Multicenter Phase II Trial on Lung Malignancies: The ALICE Trial. CardioVascular and Interventional Radiology 2015; 38(2): 401-408. DOI: 10.1007/s00270-014-1049-0.

[64] KashimaM, YamakadoK, TakakiH, et al. Complications After 1000 Lung Radiofrequency Ablation Sessions in 420 Patients: A Single Center's Experiences. American Journal of Roentgenology 2011; 197(4): W576–W580. DOI: 10.2214/AJR.11.6408.

[65] YamagamiT, KatoT, HirotaT, YoshimatsuR, MatsumotoT, NishimuraT. Pneumothorax as a complication of percutaneous radiofrequency ablation for lung neoplasms. Journal of Vascular and Interventional Radiology 2006; 17(10): 1625-1629. DOI: 10.1097/01.RVI.0000236607.05698.4A.

[66] OkumaT, MatsuokaT, YamamotoA, et al. Frequency and risk factors of various complications after computed tomography-guided radiofrequency ablation of lung tumors. CardioVascular and Interventional Radiology 2008; 31(1): 122-130. DOI: 10.1007/s00270-007-9225-0.

[67] KennedySA, MilovanovicL, DaoD, FarrokhyarF, MidiaM. Risk factors for pneumothorax complicating radiofrequency ablation for lung malignancy: A systematic review and meta-analysis. Journal of Vascular and Interventional Radiology 2014; 25(11): 1671-1681.e1. DOI: 10.1016/j.jvir.2014.07.025.

[68] HirakiT, GobaraH, FujiwaraH, et al. Lung cancer ablation: Complications. Seminars in Interventional Radiology 2013; 30(2): 169-175. DOI: 10.1055/s-0033-1342958.

[69] ClasenS, KettenbachJ, KosanB, et al. Delayed development of pneumothorax after pulmonary radiofrequency ablation. CardioVascular and Interventional Radiology 2009; 32(3): 484-490. DOI: 10.1007/s00270-008-9489-z.

[70] YoshimatsuR, YamagamiT, TerayamaK, MatsumotoT, MiuraH,

NishimuraT. Delayed and recurrent pneumothorax after radiofrequency ablation of lung tumors. Chest 2009; 135(4): 1002-1009. DOI: 10.1378/chest.08-1499.

[71] SakuraiJ, HirakiT, MukaiT, et al. Intractable Pneumothorax Due to Bronchopleural Fistula after Radiofrequency Ablation of Lung Tumors. Journal of Vascular and Interventional Radiology 2007; 18(1): 141-145. DOI: 10.1016/j.jvir.2006.10.011.

[72] TajiriN, HirakiT, MimuraH, et al. Measurement of pleural temperature during radiofrequency ablation of lung tumors to investigate its relationship to occurrence of pneumothorax or pleural effusion. CardioVascular and Interventional Radiology 2008; 31(3): 581-586. DOI: 10.1007/s00270-007-9283-3.

[73] Nour-EldinNEA, NaguibNNN, MacKM, AbskharonJE, VoglTJ. Pulmonary hemorrhage complicating radiofrequency ablation, from mild hemoptysis to life-threatening pattern. European Radiology 2011; 21(1): 197-204. DOI: 10.1007/s00330-010-1889-1.

[74] TanabeT, KoizumiT, TsushimaK, et al. Comparative study of three different catheters for ct imaging-bronchoscopy-guided radiofrequency ablation as a potential and novel interventional therapy for lung cancer. Chest 2010; 137(4): 890-897. DOI: 10.1378/chest.09-1065.

[75] KoizumiT, TsushimaK, TanabeT, et al. Bronchoscopy-Guided Cooled Radiofrequency Ablation as a Novel Intervention Therapy for Peripheral Lung Cancer. Respiration 2015; 90(1): 47-55. DOI: 10.1159/000430825.

[76] XieF, ZhengX, XiaoB, HanB, HerthFJF, SunJ. Navigation Bronchoscopy-Guided Radiofrequency Ablation for Nonsurgical Peripheral Pulmonary Tumors. Respiration 2017; 94(3): 293-298. DOI: 10.1159/000477764.

[77] YuanHBin, WangXY, SunJY, et al. Flexible bronchoscopy-guided microwave ablation in peripheral porcine lung: A new minimally-invasive ablation. Translational Lung Cancer Research 2019; 8(6): 787-796. DOI: 10.21037/tlcr.2019.10.12.

Section 4

Systemic Therapy Personalization

Chapter 7

Precision Medicine in Lung Cancer: Challenges and Opportunities in Diagnostic and Therapeutic Purposes

Beatrice Aramini, Valentina Masciale, Federico Banchelli, Roberto D'Amico, Massimo Dominici and Khawaja Husnain Haider

Abstract

Lung cancer is one of the leading causes of cancer death among both men and women, making up almost 25% of all cancer deaths. Precision medicine shows promise for improving many aspects of health and healthcare, including tests, drugs, and other technologies that support innovation, with the possibility of new partnerships with scientists in a wide range of specialties. Non–small-cell lung cancer (NSCLC) has become a prominent example of the success of precision medicine in treating solid tumor malignancies. The first step in this process involves new blood-based diagnostics, which can now noninvasively provide clinically useful information. However, the identification of novel biomarkers that could be used in early diagnosis is urgently needed, especially for guiding initial therapy and predicting relapse or drug resistance following the administration of novel targeted therapies.

Keywords: precision medicine, target therapy, liquid biopsy, CTC, CSCs, miRNA, NGS, NSCLC

1. Introduction

1.1 Lung cancer and the meaning of "precision medicine"

The scientific community tends to conflate the meanings of "precision medicine" and "personalized medicine" [1, 2]. In fact, the National Research Council defines "personalized medicine" with an old meaning quite similar to that of "precision medicine." However, whereas personalized medicine mainly focuses on medical actions for a single person, precision medicine explores various factors affecting that person's condition, such as diseases, the environment, etc. [3].

Precision medicine is able to provide specific genetic maps for patients with elevated cancer risks, potentially revealing gene mutations and thus calculating the likelihood of family members' developing a certain type of cancer.

Recently, the use of precision medicine has been expanded to attempt treatment of several solid tumors, including those of breast, brain, and lung cancer [4, 5]. In general, the aim of precision medicine is to find the right treatment for a specific patient at the right dose and time, which is particularly important in cancer therapy.

Finding a precise treatment for a patient could eradicate the potential problem of the variability of treatment response, including resistance. In fact, one of the main problems with cancer treatments is a nonresponse to drug therapy and the consequent metastatization of the disease.

Precision medicine is being used to treat certain cancers to help discover what tests and treatments are best. In addition, doctors could employ precision medicine to identify those at high risk for cancer, to prevent certain types of cancer, for early cancer detection, to make specific cancer diagnoses, to select the best treatment options, and to evaluate treatment efficacy [6].

The history of focused therapies to combat lung cancer began with the approval of the small molecule tyrosine kinase inhibitors (TKIs) of epidermal growth factor receptor (EGFR) [7]. This marked the beginning of the era of targeted therapies for lung cancer. On a related note, in 2004 and 2007, the first discoveries of adenocarcinoma of the lung were identified as *EGFR* mutations and *ALK*-rearrangements. These new findings paved the way for new targeted therapies – namely, tyrosine kinase inhibitors (TKIs) [8]. The responses to these inhibitors and the subsequent discoveries from numerous clinical trials (NCT00322452, NCT00932893) [9, 10], led to incorporating them into daily clinical activities. This demonstrated that TKIs are more effective than traditional treatments, such as chemotherapy. In contrast, patients with non-EGFR mutant lung cancers do not respond to EGFR TKIs, and, for this reason, chemotherapy a more effective treatment for them [9]. To complicate cancer's frequent resistance to chemotherapy, consequent threat of recurrence, and the related costs of targeted therapies, no drugs have been very effective in its treatment. Thus, the latter must be considered when introducing targeted therapies into clinical practice [11]. However, scientists have proceeded to define and characterize other oncogenic driver mutations in lung adenocarcinoma, such as KRAS. This mutation was first described in 1980 [12, 13], with a presence of 25–30% in lung adenocarcinoma and high aggression, which is even more dangerous without specific targeted therapies. Interestingly, the first recent study with promising clinical data came from a Phase I trial, in which the KRAS G12C inhibitor AMG 510 shrank lung cancer tumors harboring KRAS G12C mutations [14, 15]. This highlighted the importance of identifying new drivers' mutations therapies in lung cancer for decreasing mortality and recurrence. Other mutations have been identified in lung cancer, including ERBB2 (3%), BRAF (2%), PIK3CA (1%), MAP2K1 (1%), and NRAS (1%), [16], although these are defined as *niche* mutations. Beyond the fact that these niche mutations are infrequent, they are no less dangerous, with a high level of mortality. On this subject, a recent study by Aramini et al. examined three cohorts of mutations selected from patients with lung adenocarcinoma [17]. These mutations were 1) BRAF, c-MET, DDR2, HER2, MAP2K1, NRAS, PIK3CA, and RET; 2) K-RAS; and 3) EGFR. In this pilot study, the researchers demonstrated that niche mutations exhibited an increased risk of death when compared with EGFR mutations and a similar risk of death when compared with KRAS mutations. This aspect is key in highlighting the importance of focusing attention not only on general mutations but also on niche mutations to develop more effective cures in larger populations. In fact, a clinical trial is currently being conducted to better define the less common oncogenic driver mutations (e.g., NCT01336634).

In lung adenocarcinoma patients, the importance of testing eventual genetic mutations introduced new diagnostic perspectives. These have enhanced the treatment recommendations of the International Association for the Study of Lung Cancer (IASLC) and National Comprehensive Cancer Network (NCCN) for patients with EGFR mutation and ALK positivity. Moreover, new mutations have been studied for diagnostic purposes, including ROS, RET, MET, BRAF, and HER2, although these are infrequent mutations [18–20]. These studies have laid crucial groundwork for creating more focused treatments tailored to each patient [18–20].

Precise molecular tests led to the correlation of EGFR mutations and sensitivity to gefitinib and erlotinib in lung adenocarcinoma, especially in non-smokers or low-smokers. The EGFR tyrosine kinase inhibitors (TKIs) are considered the baseline treatment for this cancer, although a high percentage of patients develop resistance to therapy and experience a disease recurrence within nine months [18]. However, scientists discovered new mutations, developing a more focused panel of patients' genetic characteristics. These researchers discovered that 50% of patients developing tumor dissemination showed a secondary EGFR mutation, such as T790M, which has been used for developing new target therapies, including AZD9291 and CO-1686 [21].

ALK, ROS, and RET, defined as receptor tyrosine kinase gene rearrangements, present at a frequency between 1 and 8% in lung adenocarcinoma, although patients harboring ALK fusion or ROS1 mutations have positively responded to crizotinib and to TKIs. However, these patients frequently develop recurrence, probably due to an acquired resistance and from mechanisms which must be further investigated [22, 23].

The target of mutations is particularly difficult, especially the study of the mitogen activation pathway (MAPK). This has been of recent interest for its implications regarding lung adenocarcinoma development and the subsequent results of therapeutics. Specifically, the MAPK activation mechanism has been found frequently along certain KRAS amino acids. Currently, KRAS is considered an aggressive mutation for its impact on overall survival (OS) in early-stage NSCLC. Finding specific RAS inhibitors may open the door to new target treatments that improve long-term survival and responses to therapies, even in patients with KRAS mutations. New treatments have been set against the downstream effectors of activated KRAS, such as MEK1/MEK2, PI3K, and AKT [24]. In addition, recent phase II data analyzing the inhibition of MEK1/MEK2 by selumetinib and docetaxel showed promising results in KRAS-muted patients [25].

Additional work on downstream effectors in the KRAS mutant pathway is crucial. Currently, several clinical trials employing the inhibition of PI3KCA, MEK, and PTEN are in progress [26].

Recently precision medicine is used not only in clinical practice to drive oncological decision but also in patients with rare tumors, likely due to their frequency in these patients' family histories. This aspect is important for making medical decisions, as well as for screening.

The most frequent tests used at this time are biomarker tests, chromosome tests, gene tests, and biochemical tests, all of which are derived from blood, saliva, a tissue biopsy, or body fluids. These tests are named as follows: DNA mutational analysis, genomic testing, proteomics, biomarker testing, tumor profiling, cytogenetics, next generation sequencing, or molecular testing [27, 28].

1.2 NSCLC biomarkers

The use of drugs against NSCLC in locally advanced or advanced stages may help identify targeted drugs, which are more useful and better tolerated, as well as more responsive against lung cancer. The latter remains a serious problem in the world, accounting for over 1.7 million deaths in 2018 [29], showing that therapies are still largely ineffective. In particular, EGFR and ALK are considered biomarkers that predict positive responses to specific drugs. However, not all patients with lung cancer show these mutations, and this is why not all patients respond to gefitinib, erlotinib, or afatinib, which are currently considered the most effective against EGFR mutations [30, 31].

In addition, the ALK-positive gene is rare, occurring in approximately 5% of patients with NSCLC and eliciting production of a growth-promoting enzyme [32]. Patients who are ALK-positive are usually treated with crizotinib, a tyrosine kinase inhibitor that blocks the input of the growth signals to the nucleus of the cancer cell. Immunotherapy is the last defense against cancer, and it has been developed in the last decades, including cancer vaccines, oncolytic viruses, and administration of antibodies or recombinant proteins that co-stimulate or block the immune checkpoint pathways [33]. However, there is a pressing need to identify new targets specific to a larger cohort of patients with better outcomes than those of current chemotherapeutic treatments. This need has induced the scientific community to deeply analyze other mechanisms or approaches.

Although targeted drugs and chemotherapeutic agents may be useful for weeks or months against tumors in terms of disease control, the majority of tumor relapses occur after several months of treatment.

1.3 A new kind of drug treatment: Immune checkpoint inhibitors

A new class of drugs was recently developed by Allison et al. and named *checkpoint inhibitors* [34, 35]. This group has the specific role of enhancing patients' immunity, thus increasing their chances of fighting cancer. The first one created was nivolumab, followed by pembrolizumab, which targets a receptor called programmed cell death-1 (PD-1).

However, not all patients have shown high levels of PD-1 expression in their cancer cells, revealing the major limitation of these therapies. In fact, the prognostic role of PD-L1 in solid tumors such as lung cancer, melanoma, etc. is still debated [36]. In patients with an overexpression of PD-L1, the use of antibodies able to target PD-1 and PD-L1 is one of the main points to consider for the setting of more effective therapies [37]. However, for the low immunohistochemistry accuracy based on PD-L1, the use of this biomarker as a possible predictor for satisfying immunotherapeutic results against cancer is under examination [38]. The main shortfalls of this marker are, first, the different cut-off values of positivity in different solid tumors; second, the sensitivity, which is very variable as demonstrated in several studies; and third, the potential involvement and impact of the tumor microenvironment associated with the use of other genes markers which, combined together, may be more helpful for a better-focused PD-1/PD-L1 blocking immunotherapy [39].

In particular, pembrolizumab—a humanized antibody used in cancer immunotherapy as a programmed cell death 1 (PD-1) inhibitor—seems to improve survival significantly more than standard chemotherapy in NSCLC patients with an expression of PD-1 ligand ≥50% in cancer cells [40, 41]. In addition, in nonsquamous NSCLC patients the PD-L1 positively expression of at least 1% represents a good responder against antitumor action. This aspect highlighted the importance of the presence of at least 1% PD-L1 expression for the treatment of NSCLC patients, which seem to represent two-thirds of all NSCLC population [42, 43]. In contrast, for small cell lung cancer (SCLC) which represents 15% of all types of lung cancers, there are actually few choices of cancer treatments and no molecularly targeted drug has been approved. In particular, the potential role of PD-1/PD-L1 inhibitors in SCLC has not been yet considered [44]. Recently, the first study analyzing the PD-L1 expression in SCLC has been conducted at Kyoto University Hospital, where the researchers analyzed the immunohistochemical expression of this marker in paraffin blocks from 39 patients affected by SCLC [45]. Although previous studies have been conducted—most likely for the use of different types of antibodies—the expression was arbitrary, and this represented an impediment in the elucidation of the possible expression and role of PD-L1 in SCLC [46]. For the first time, the team from Kyoto University thought to use the standard PD-L1 antibody already tested in NSCLC with the same cut-off level (1%) as in NSCLC [45]. This approach was important to elucidate the presence of this marker, even in SCLC, although the correlation with the clinical aspects has not been yet defined.

In summary, all the aspects described would suggest that the use of PD-L1 as an exclusive biomarker in cancer may not represent a completely satisfying choice in terms of accuracy and efficacy. On the other side, at the moment, scientists cannot ignore the good responses against cancer that patients with at least 1% of positivity for PD-L1 show through the most-used checkpoint inhibitors [47]. In summary, further studies set on the combination among PD-1/PD-L1 pathways, the tumor microenvironment and other genes markers may open the way for new discoveries that are tailored to the individual patient and more effective against cancer.

2. Precision medicine and solid tumors

The development of new techniques and approaches to discovering signaling pathways to better understand tumor growth has opened to precision medicine for solid tumors [48].

In particular, the major field is to create future treatments tailored to each patient to improve their results against cancer. However, this aspect has not yet been focalized for the numerous difficulties related to the new cancer cells targets. Through current clinical trials, pharmaceutical companies are developing studies based on specific markers to find multiple options for the best treatment [49].

Recent advances regarding the biology behind these tumors have shown promising results. In several centers, patients are analyzed by RNA expression testing and protein analyses [50, 51]. These genetic analyses have already been taken into consideration, especially for hereditary tumors. Certain companies, such as Myriad Genetics Inc., have developed in the last decades several molecular diagnostic kits to test patients at risk of developing hereditary tumors [52–54]. Thus far, this aspect has been extensively analyzed for prostate cancer and breast cancer [55, 56]. It has been examined for the genes mutations that are more frequent in these diseases, as well as the development of prognostic scores related to cancer recurrence [57].

At the moment, the possibility of developing a molecular profile is limited for the presence of mutations and other genetic variations. However, scientists are planning to develop a molecular profile based on RNA expression, as described for familiar genetic diseases or by immunity profiles. There is an urgent need to develop new approaches and targeted treatments to better stratify cancer patients, to prevent recurrence, and to more effectively treat these patients.

Several clinical trials are running regarding the possibility of targeting oncologic patients. Some of these trials involve specific tumors, such as BATTLE I and II [58], and some are non-tumor specific. These studies have been designed as observational, randomized, and non-randomized [59–62].

Non-randomized trials are studying molecular profiles in the Clinical Laboratory Improvement Amendments (CLIA) certified laboratories, which were founded in 2013 in collaboration with pharmaceutical societies to identify a specific genes patent for each patient. In particular, pharmaceutical companies have been conducting independent trials of drugs in patients with specific genetic profiles [63].

However, these profiles may not be the same for patients with several solid tumors, but at this time, this aspect is not well known. The National Cancer Institute (NCI) is preparing a study with the involvement of agents from different companies [64]. The baseline for these studies, called NCI-MATCH studies, will be the analysis by a consortium of NCI-selected CLIA-certified laboratories of the genomic profiles of several cancer patients. This process will use a new approach called next generation sequencing (NGS) for a number of selected genes.

Another interesting study, the SHIVA study, randomizes patients with specific genetic abnormalities matching generic types of cancer and patients' specific genes. It examines the possible results from standard treatments in terms of cytotoxicity and disease progression [65].

These types of combined studies involving several companies and certified laboratories may be very important to further discoveries, but the difficulty of coordinating multiple companies constitutes an effective impediment. Basic research is suggested to more deeply analyze the mechanisms and mutations involved in development and tumor progression [66, 67]. A representative panel during time of the major achievements for lung cancer therapy (**Figure 1**).

Regarding the mutations, those in the scientific community do not believe that studying a single mutation or a small panel of genes would be enough to influence future decisions or treatments for oncological patients. For this reason, the new advanced technologies require a larger panel of genes or intra- and inter-tumor heterogeneity at the protein, genetic, and epigenetic levels [68, 69]. Specifically, the genetic analysis of RNA and proteins in primary or metastatic diseases in patients with renal carcinomas have shown a large heterogeneity of cells and genes inside the tumors. This is one of the main obstacles in the battle against cancer [68, 69]. On the other hand, in colorectal and lung cancer, the panel of genes that seem to be involved is limited [70, 71]. One must be considered, such as in the case of lung cancer. Such a tumor could develop several mutations during its progression, and these would be persistent in evolving. For this reason, future patients' tumor profiles

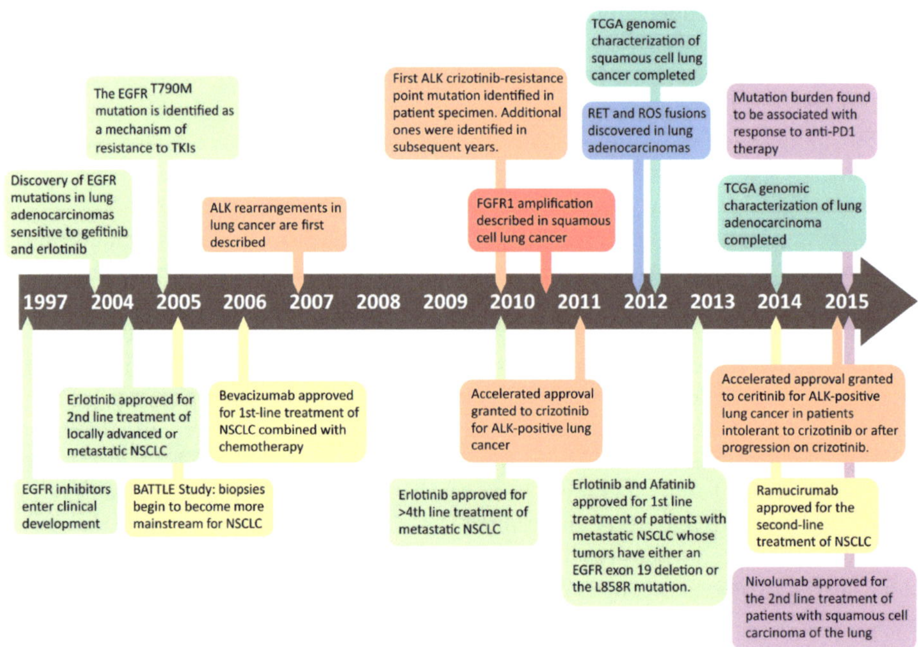

Figure 1.
Timeline of major discoveries and related therapeutic approaches in non-small cells lung cancer.

would need to be frequently updated to guarantee the best treatment options. One problem would be the impossibility of obtaining sufficient material from biopsies. In addition, it would be difficult to ask to these patients to perform several biopsies in order to have a more focused treatment. Thus, in order to minimize invasive procedures, scientists have attempted to develop the best approach with the least aggressiveness toward the patient. For example, the analysis of circulating free DNA (cfDNA)by liquid biopsy, widely discussed at this time, and CTCs may be considered of great value if these approaches are able to replace multiple biopsies. For the moment, the results of these techniques seem to be promising, but further investigation is needed regarding each type of solid tumor, as well as each patient [72–74].

Even the serum proteins are of interest; however, the difficulty in identifying a specific protein has made this approach very difficult to use for tumor patients. For example, PSA levels for prostate cancer patients, as well as CEA measurements, are commonly used markers, but several clinical trials and basic research are necessary to identify more markers for future cancer diagnoses [75–77].

In summary, important progress has been made in terms of molecular profiles and developing advanced genetic technologies. However, the coming years will be crucial in determining whether these new aspects will revolutionize treatments and improve prognoses in cancer patients.

3. Recent discoveries in *precision*-diagnostic and *precision*-therapeutic approaches to lung cancer

New genetic discoveries through high-throughput techniques could allow the establishment of a new era in which precision medicine could be routinely used for cancer treatment, as well as in its diagnosis and therapy [78]. Since the earlies 2000s, innovative sequencing systems called next-generation sequencing methods (NGS, Next Generation Sequencing), or massive parallel sequencing (MPS, Massive Parallel Sequencing), have been used to define high-efficiency nucleotide sequences in the simultaneous, independent analysis of millions of bp of DNA. In particular, the association of genomic data and the identification of new biomarkers may modify cancer treatments in the near future. This would require extensive knowledge of the mutational analysis of a panel of cancer genes, along with determination of copy-number variations and any other structural rearrangements. As with lung cancer, which has a high rate of recurrence after surgery independent from stages, it would be useful in treating other solid tumors to have some predictor of relapse based on genetic tests identifying the individual risks of various cancers and their consequent relapses. This chapter will discuss technical considerations for developing genomic precision diagnostic tools for clinicians to support their further use in oncological care and research trials, as represented schematically in **Figure 2**.

3.1 Single-gene assays versus next-generation sequencing

Until now, the most commonly used methods have included DNA or RNA amplification using polymerase chain reaction (PCR), followed by classical Sanger sequencing or pyrosequencing, analysis of fragments by electrophoresis after digestion with restriction enzymes, or fluorescent in situ hybridization with specific probes (FISH) [79]. Single gene analysis often has significant advantages over large-scale genomic sequencing due to the lower cost and reduced complexity in test development, execution, and interpretation. In molecular oncology, for example, there is frequent identification of BCR-ABL1 translocation by FISH in patients

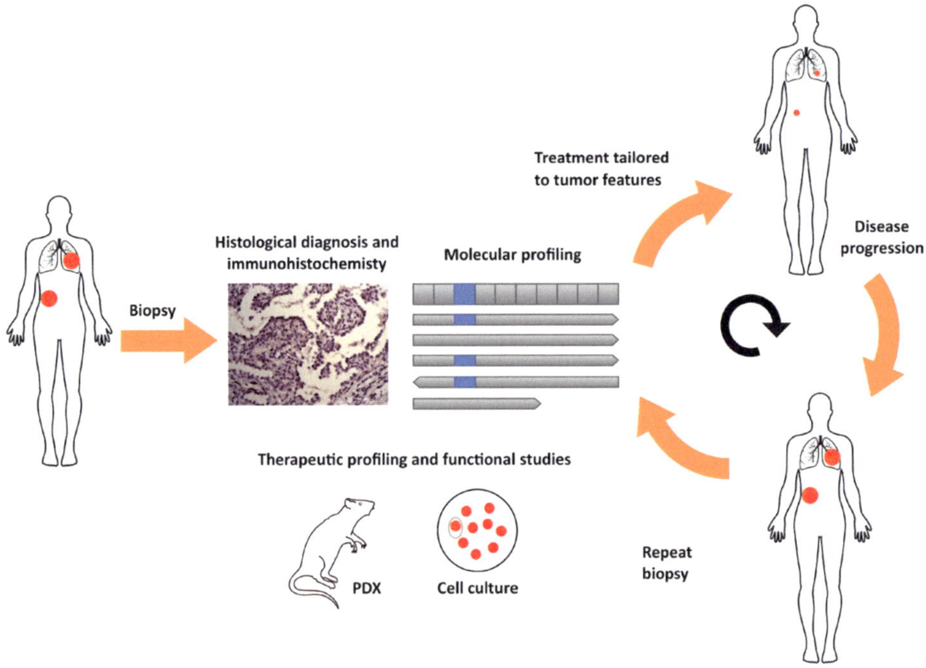

Figure 2.
Future perspectives in molecular profiling and diagnostic approaches in lung cancer.

with chronic myeloid leukemia. Single gene analysis is a useful approach when the genetic alterations are well known. On the other hand, high-throughput screening, such as NGS, is more sensitive than many monogenic methodologies, such as Sanger sequencing. As a consequence of the discovery of more relevant genes in a clinical context, NGS has become an increasingly attractive approach. Molecular testing of advanced non-small cell lung cancer (NSCLC) provides a good example of the rapidly growing need for the molecular profile of several genes, especially cancer. Initially, the only knowledge about the genetics of lung cancer was the deletion of exon19 in the EGFR gene and the mutation of the L858R gene, which could lead to the first targeted therapy with tyrosine kinase inhibitor (TKI) [80–88]. However, within a few years, effective targeted therapies approved by the U.S. Food and Drug Administration (FDA) have been developed and are now effective in treating lung cancer with other EGFR and BRAF mutations [83, 84], as well as ALK and ROS1 rearrangements [84–88]. Other solid tumors have been associated with target therapies involving other molecular alterations, such as exon 14 MET skip mutations [89–91], RET rearrangements [92–94], and ERBB2 (HER2) mutations [95], which have led to a new setting for therapeutic recommendations from the National Comprehensive Cancer Network (NCCN) [96].

3.2 Gene panels versus unbiased genomic and transcriptomic analyses

Given their high speed of execution, NGS techniques have been used for the identification of disease genes by whole genome sequencing (WGS) or whole exome sequencing (WES), as well as target gene panels [97]. The potential advantage of these techniques is the possibility of detecting essentially any genomic alteration, including novel or rare alterations. However, certain critical points must be considered. To begin, WGS is far too expensive and generates a huge amount of raw data requiring complex bioinformatics analyses to extract useful information.

As a consequence, analysis may be performed only on selected cases. In NSCLC, for instance, whole-genome studies have demonstrated a median of 888 and 15,659 mutations in NSCLC samples from, respectively, nonsmokers and smokers [98]. The major part of these variants lacks any relevant pathogenic significance. Nevertheless, the comparison between tumor and normal DNA is mandatory, distinguishing somatic mutations, due to cancer, from germline polymorphisms, which will be inherited by patients' offspring. However, WES is an unbiased approach that has also found utility in certain laboratories as a tool for unraveling cancers. WES limits sequencing to the ~1.5% of the genome that lies in the exons of genes. Nevertheless, this approach also generates a large number of potential variants, the vast majority of which even in this case currently do not have annotated clinical implications. Exome sequencing would also fail to detect pathogenic variants, such as structural rearrangements with intronic breakpoints. DNA quality requirements are lower than those of WGS, so the drawbacks of this approach include the fact that the depth of sequencing obtained through WES is much lower than that obtained from targeted panels. For diagnostic purposes, it has been argued that a high sensitivity is needed to reduce the number of false negatives. Although a genetic variant of uncertain significance can be detected, it would be better to be cautious even if there were no clinical treatment for the alteration. Another crucial element that may be investigated with WGS is the copy number alteration (CNA), which is a parameter that takes into account the number of repeated alterations in the DNA. These hallmarks in cancer often lead to the activation of oncogenes and inactivation of tumor suppressor [99]. The WES is primarily used to discover all of the variations in the DNA sequence, but the RNA-Seq is specifically used for the measurement of gene expression, gene fusion detection, and identification of splicing events, since it is based on direct sequencing of cDNA. One of the most important applications of the RNA-Seq is for cancer. For example, a large-scale RNA-Seq has been useful for the detection of several cancer driver genes in adenocarcinoma of the lungs [100, 101]. That study compared the transcriptome of lung cancers between smokers and nonsmokers and found a significant difference in the number of point mutations between the two groups. In summary, the amount of smoking (packs/year) was positively correlated with the number of somatic point mutations in the cancer genome. As for the study described, a complete molecular analysis conducted on the transcriptome or the entire genome or exosome through higher coverage of the genomic regions allowed the detection of lower-level molecular alterations. Moreover, the principle difference between targeted genetic panels and unbiased, extensive genomic and transcriptomic analysis is not necessary in the last case to know a priori the molecular alterations to be detected.

3.3 Applications of molecular oncology

3.3.1 Diagnosis

For different tumors, molecular diagnostic tests, as for example, BCR-ABL1 in chronic myeloid leukemia or other data, may be very helpful in influencing the decisions of oncologists or pathologists. That is, they could develop more detailed diagnoses, as well as more appropriate approaches, although molecular analyses would need to be correlated with clinicopathological patients' characteristics.

In particular, certain mutations detected in malignant tumors have also been found in healthy individuals [102–104]. However, the new technologies related to advanced molecular analysis are now able to distinguish between cancer mutations and normal tissue mutations. One of the most important aspects of this precision medicine tailored to the patient is the possibility of stratifying the prognosis. Several studies are examining this aspect in several solid tumors [105–108].

3.3.2 Therapy

Several clinical trials are currently being conducted regarding specific target alterations in different cancer types. The Molecular Analysis for Therapy Choice (MATCH; http://www.cancer.gov/aboutcancer/treatment/clinical-trials/nci-supported/nci-match) trial and the Targeted Agent and Profiling Utilization Registry (TAPUR) trial were designed to identify particular molecular targets able to determine a specific therapy against cancer. The main difficulty arises from the fact that each tumor shows a specific mutation that may be different in each patient. This genetic heterogeneity has led to targeting specific drivers in each tumor. Furthermore, the identification through the NGS technique introduced new possibilities for finding specific oncogenic drivers that could maximize the possibility of receiving the benefit of a very focused, tailored therapy. The use of NGS is intended to guide treatment decisions. In fact, this technique can identify oncogenic alterations, which may be target inhibitors or monoclonal antibodies. For example, the BRAF V600E mutation can be cured by BRAF inhibitors and MEK inhibitors approved by the FDA. For instance, patients with colorectal cancer and KRAS and NRAS mutations showed a therapeutic resistance to EGFR antibody therapy [109, 110].

The integration of genomic results into reports and the clinical decision supported by NGS are a powerful tool that enables the simultaneous interrogation of many regions of the human genome [111]. However, as the volume of data from NGS testing grows, so does the challenge of distinguishing the findings that are clinically meaningful and prioritizing their clinical utility. Given the large number of genetic variants that occur in cancer genomes and the many low-frequency or nonrecurring mutations detected using NGS, a systematic approach to prioritizing variants is necessary to effectively implement NGS-based precision diagnostics in routine clinical contexts [112]. Molecular pathologists, in collaboration with their oncology colleagues, have been tasked with evaluating this abundance of data, distilling it to what is clinically relevant, and communicating this information in the most cogent, manageable manner possible. Several components are required to properly integrate genomic results into clinical reports, among which is the understanding of the clinical evolution of the genomic variant in patients.

4. Future perspectives on lung cancer treatments

The role of cfDNA has been extensively analyzed in terms of the definition of new-targeted therapies, and the interpretation of this role in driving immunotherapy has just begun [113]. The mutation in a cancer patient can be studied from cfDNA by NGS [114]. Only one study has found conflicting results from the blood tumor mutation burden (TMB) [115]. It has been found that a high blood sample, TMB, is correlated with the reaction to inhibitors of programmed cell death (PD)1 and its ligand (PD-L1) [115, 116], as in NSCLC with atezolizumab in POPLAR and OAK trials [117]. The TMB is more correlated with advanced disease, and it expresses a high value of circulating tumor DNA (ctDNA) concentrations [118]. Different studies have shown that there is a correlation between ctDNA kinetics and clinical course in terms of possibility of predicting the prognosis [119]. In particular, it has been demonstrated that the variation of circulating the tumor DNA burden is able to distinguish a real and unreal tumor progression. Another interesting application of cfDNA, which scientists are studying, is the possibility of detecting the minimal residual disease (MRD) for the setting of immunotherapy or the possibility of finding the drug resistance as JAK1/2 or B2M mutations [120]. With regard to the early stages' NSCLC, the prospect of setting screening tests is very challenging. The National Lung Screening Trial [121] and the NELSON trial have shown that to test asymptomatic men with high risks factors by chest CT reduced the deaths in men to 26% and in women to 41% [122]. However, the problem of false positives is still one of the most difficult factors to eliminate [123]. These trials showed that the combination of the high sensitivity of CT scans and liquid biopsy may have an important effect in driving clinical decisions, as well as therapeutic approaches. One limitation is the fact that ctDNA quantities may be low or absent in the early stages of disease [124]. Another important value of cfDNA assay may be the opportunity to identify recurrent mutations. This aspect is important in terms of prognosis and developing new targeted treatments. For example, the Cancer SEEK assay can combine the genomic analysis of 16 genes in ctDNA and eight biomarkers detectable for eight non metastatic diseases [125–127]. Nevertheless, certain limitations remain regarding sensitivity to early-stage detection. For instance, lung cancer does not currently have a specific circulating protein marker. The most promising test at the moment is the multi-region exome sequencing of a tumor, but this technique is limited by the costs and the excessive time required, which make this approach currently unavailable to the patients. However, the most discussed approaches developed for circulating tumor cells (CTC) isolation are based on the following: 1) antigen expression and 2) biophysical characteristics [128–130].

In summary, the microfluidic technologies have probably been the most common approach to CTC isolation since 2007, with the "CTC-ship" [131]. However, several limitations are ongoing, and further studies must better stratify this approach not only in the early stages of NSCLC but also for other solid tumors. The world of exosomes is complex because of their vast numbers and various roles. In particular, they were found to contain microRNA (miRNA) that could be exchanged via horizontal intercellular transfer with the possibility of activating an oncogene or a tumor suppressor gene. In 60–75% NSCLC, miRNAs play crucial roles. Moreover, recent studies have provided evidence that exosomes may mediate interactions among different types of cells to enhance cell–cell communication within the tumor microenvironment. In particular, exosome signaling may provide new insights into how cancer stem cells (CSCs) confer drug resistance between drug-resistant and drug-sensitive cells [132]. In fact, CSCs exhibit self-renewal, proliferation, tumor initiation, and propagation, and the "stemness" of cancer cells seems to be supported by the release of exosomes [133–135]. Cancer stem cells are thought to secrete microvesicles and exosomes that interact with neighboring stromal cells. For instance, experimental evidence has shown that breast cancer stem cells secrete exosomes with characteristics of cancer cell-derived exosomes [135, 136]. Exosomes released by cancer stem cells mediate tumor growth in different cancer types. For example, in a renal cancer model, microvesicles released from human renal cancer stem cells were described to stimulate angiogenesis and the formation of a pre-metastatic niche in the lungs [137]. Elsewhere, a study on glioma stem cells reported that glioma-associated stem cells increased the biological aggressiveness of glioma-initiating cells through the release of exosomes. However, both exosomes and cancer stem cells targeted against tumors must be thoroughly analyzed in the future. This is important because there is no clear identification of a specific target against NSCLC [138, 139] or tumors in general, and it is difficult to characterize cancer stem cells and necessary to optimize the roles and definitions of specific exosomes for each type of cancer. Such research would be a milestone in developing new therapies and new approaches to screening oncologic patients.

Author details

Beatrice Aramini[1*], Valentina Masciale[1], Federico Banchelli[2], Roberto D'Amico[2], Massimo Dominici[3] and Khawaja Husnain Haider[4]

1 Division of Thoracic Surgery, University of Modena and Reggio Emilia, Modena, Italy

2 Center of Statistic, Department of Medical and Surgical Sciences, University of Modena and Reggio Emilia, Modena, Italy

3 Division of Oncology, Department of Medical and Surgical Sciences, University of Modena and Reggio Emilia, Modena, Italy

4 Department of Basic Sciences, Sulaiman AlRajhi Medical School, Sulaiman Alrajhi University, Kingdom of Saudi Arabia

*Address all correspondence to: beatrice.aramini@unimore.it

References

[1] Marson FAL, Bertuzzo CS, Ribeiro JD. (2017) Personalized or Precision Medicine? The Example of Cystic Fibrosis. Front Pharmacol.;8:390. Published 2017 Jun 20. doi:10.3389/fphar.2017.00390

[2] Ho D, Quake SR, McCabe ERB, Chng WJ, Chow EK, et al. (2020) Enabling Technologies for Personalized and Precision Medicine. Trends Biotechnol. 38(5):497-518. doi: 10.1016/j.tibtech.2019.12.021.

[3] Goetz LH, Schork NJ. (2018) Personalized medicine: motivation, challenges, and progress. Fertil Steril. 109(6):952-963. doi:10.1016/j.fertnstert.2018.05.006.

[4] Malone ER, Oliva M, Sabatini PJB, Stockley TL, Siu LL. (2020) Molecular profiling for precision cancer therapies. Genome Med. 12(1):8. doi:10.1186/s13073-019-0703-1.

[5] Davis AA, McKee AE, Warren AK, and Villaflor VM. (2018) Complexity of Delivering Precision Medicine: Opportunities and Challenges. American Society of Clinical Oncology Educational Book 38, 998-1007.

[6] Morgensztern D, Campo MJ, Dahlberg SE, Doebele RC, Garon E. et al. (2014) Molecularly targeted therapies in non-small-cell lung cancer annual update 2014. J Thorac Oncol. 2015;10(1 Suppl 1):S1-S63. doi:10.1097/JTO.0000000000000405.

[7] Mambetsariev I, Wang Y, Chen C, Nadaf S, Pharaon R, et al. (2020) Precision medicine and actionable alterations in lung cancer: A single institution experience. PLoS One. 15(2):e0228188. doi: 10.1371/journal.pone.0228188.

[8] Politi K, Herbst RS. Lung cancer in the era of precision medicine. (2015) Clin Cancer Res. 21(10):2213-2220. doi:10.1158/1078-0432.CCR-14-2748.

[9] Mok TS, Wu YL, Thongprasert S, Yang CH, Chu DT, Saijo N, et al. (2009) Gefitinib or carboplatin-paclitaxel in pulmonary adenocarcinoma. N Engl J Med361:947-57. doi: 10.1056/NEJMoa0810699.

[10] Shaw AT, Kim DW, Nakagawa K, Seto T, Crino L, et al. (2013) Crizotinib versus chemotherapy in advanced ALK-positive lung cancer. N Engl J Med. 368:2385-94. doi: 10.1056/NEJMoa1214886.

[11] Djalalov S, Beca J, Hoch JS, Krahn M, Tsao MS, et al. (2014) Cost effectiveness of EML4-ALK fusion testing and first-line crizotinib treatment for patients with advanced ALK-positive non-small-cell lung cancer. J Clin Oncol. 32:1012-9. doi: 10.1200/JCO.2013.53.1186.

[12] Santos E, Martin-Zanca D, Reddy EP, Pierotti MA, Della Porta G, et al. (1984) Malignant activation of a K-ras oncogene in lung carcinoma but not in normal tissue of the same patient. Science. 223:661-4. doi: 10.1126/science.6695174.

[13] Rodenhuis S, van de Wetering ML, Mooi WJ, Evers SG, van Zandwijk N, et al. (1987) Mutational activation of the K-ras oncogene. A possible pathogenetic factor in adenocarcinoma of the lung. N Engl J Med. 317:929-35. doi: 10.1056/NEJM198710083171504.

[14] Yang H, Liang SQ, Schmid RA, Peng RW. (2019) New Horizons in KRAS-Mutant Lung Cancer: Dawn After Darkness. Front Oncol. 9:953. doi:10.3389/fonc.2019.00953.

[15] Hallin J, Engstrom LD, Hargis L, Calinisan A, Aranda R, et al. (2020) The KRASG12C Inhibitor MRTX849

Provides Insight toward Therapeutic Susceptibility of KRAS-Mutant Cancers in Mouse Models and Patients. Cancer Discov. 10(1):54-71. doi: 10.1158/2159-8290.CD-19-1167.

[16] Pao W, Girard N. New driver mutations in non-small-cell lung cancer. (2011) Lancet Oncol. 12:175-80. doi: 10.1016/S1470-2045(10)70087-5.

[17] Aramini B, Banchelli F, Bettelli S, Manfredini S, D'Amico R. et al. (2020) Overall survival in patients with lung adenocarcinoma harboring "niche" mutations: an observational study. Oncotarget.11(5):550-559. Published 2020 Feb 4. doi:10.18632/oncotarget.27472.

[18] Lindeman NI, Cagle PT, Beasley MB, Chitale DA, Dacic S. et al. (2013) Molecular testing guideline for selection of lung cancer patients for EGFR and ALK tyrosine kinase inhibitors: guideline from the College of American Pathologists, International Association for the Study of Lung Cancer, and Association for Molecular Pathology [published correction appears in J Thorac Oncol. 8(10):1343]. J Thorac Oncol. 2013;8(7):823-859. doi:10.1097/JTO.0b013e318290868f.

[19] Cardarella S, Johnson BE. (2013) The impact of genomic changes on treatment of lung cancer. Am J Respir Crit Care Med. 188(7):770-775. doi:10.1164/rccm.201305-0843PP.

[20] Pennell NA, Arcila ME, Gandara DR, and West H. (2019) Biomarker Testing for Patients With Advanced Non–Small Cell Lung Cancer: Real-World Issues and Tough Choices. American Society of Clinical Oncology Educational Book 39, 531-542.

[21] Ma C, Wei S, Song Y. (2011) T790M and acquired resistance of EGFR TKI: a literature review of clinical reports. J Thorac Dis. 3(1):10-18. doi:10.3978/j.issn.2072-1439.2010.12.02

[22] Shaw AT, Kim DW, Nakagawa K, Seto T, Crinó L. et al. (2013) Crizotinib versus chemotherapy in advanced ALK-positive lung cancer. The New England journal of medicine. 368:2385-2394. doi: 10.1056/NEJMoa1214886.

[23] Kwak EL, Bang YJ, Camidge DR, Shaw AT, Solomon Bet al. (2010) Anaplastic lymphoma kinase inhibition in non-small-cell lung cancer. The New England journal of medicine. 363:1693-1703. doi: 10.1056/NEJMoa1006448.

[24] Ghimessy, A., Radeczky, P., Laszlo, V. Hegedus B, Renyi-Vamos F et al. (2020) Current therapy of KRAS-mutant lung cancer. Cancer Metastasis Rev . https://doi.org/10.1007/s10555-020-09903-9.

[25] Janne PA, Shaw AT, Pereira JR, Jeannin G, Vansteenkiste J. et al. (2013) Selumetinib plus docetaxel for KRAS-mutant advanced non-small-cell lung cancer: a randomised, multicentre, placebo-controlled, phase 2 study. The lancet oncology 14:38-47. doi: 10.1016/S1470-2045(12)70489-8.

[26] Temraz S, Mukherji D, Shamseddine A. (2015) Dual Inhibition of MEK and PI3K Pathway in KRAS and BRAF Mutated Colorectal Cancers. Int J Mol Sci. 2015;16(9):22976-22988. doi:10.3390/ijms160922976.

[27] Tainsky MA. Genomic and proteomic biomarkers for cancer: a multitude of opportunities. (2009) Biochim Biophys Acta. 1796(2):176-193. doi:10.1016/j.bbcan.2009.04.004.

[28] Chen ZQ, Huang LS, Zhu B. (2018) Assessment of Seven Clinical Tumor Markers in Diagnosis of Non-Small-Cell Lung Cancer. Dis Markers. 9845123. Published 2018 Dec 11. doi:10.1155/2018/9845123.

[29] Bray F, Ferlay J, Soerjomataram I, Siegel RL, Torre LA et al. Global cancer statistics 2018: GLOBOCAN estimates

of incidence and mortality worldwide for 36 cancers in 185 countries. A CANCER J CLIN 2018;68:394-424. doi: 10.3322/caac.21492.

[30] Chang LC, Lim CK, Chang LY, Chen KY, Shih JY, et al. (2019) Non-small cell lung cancer harbouring non-resistant uncommon EGFR mutations: Mutation patterns, effectiveness of epidermal growth factor receptor-tyrosine kinase inhibitors and prognostic factors. Eur J Cancer. 119:77-86. doi: 10.1016/j.ejca.2019.06.025.

[31] Crosbie PA, Shah R, Summers Y, Dive C, Blackhall F. (2013) Prognostic and predictive biomarkers in early stage NSCLC: CTCs and serum/plasma markers. Transl Lung Cancer Res. 2(5):382-397. doi:10.3978/j.issn.2218-6751.2013.09.02.

[32] Golding B, Luu A, Jones R, Viloria-Petit AM. (2018) The function and therapeutic targeting of anaplastic lymphoma kinase (ALK) in non-small cell lung cancer (NSCLC). Mol Cancer.;17(1):52. doi:10.1186/s12943-018-0810-4.

[33] Voena C, Menotti M, Mastini C, Di Giacomo F et al. Efficacy of a Cancer Vaccine against ALK-Rearranged Lung Tumors. (2015) Cancer Immunol Res. 3(12):1333-1343. doi:10.1158/2326-6066.CIR-15-0089.

[34] Sharma P, Allison JP. (2015) Immune checkpoint targeting in cancer therapy: toward combination strategies with curative potential. Cell.161(2):205-214. doi:10.1016/j.cell.2015.03.030.

[35] Farkona S, Diamandis EP, Blasutig IM. (2016) Cancer immunotherapy: the beginning of the end of cancer? BMC Med.;14:73. doi:10.1186/s12916-016-0623-5.

[36] Cottrell TR, Taube JM. (2018) PD-L1 and Emerging Biomarkers in Immune Checkpoint Blockade Therapy. CancerJ.;24(1):41-46. doi:10.1097/PPO.0000000000000301.

[37] Yi M, Jiao D, Xu H, Liu Q, Zhao W. et al. (2018) Biomarkers for predicting efficacy of PD-1/PD-L1 inhibitors. Mol Cancer.;17(1):129. Published 2018 Aug 23. doi:10.1186/s12943-018-0864-3.

[38] Chakravarti N, Prieto VG. (2015) Predictive factors of activity of anti-programmed death-1/programmed death ligand-1 drugs: immunohistochemistry analysis. Transl Lung Cancer Res. 4(6):743-751. doi:10.3978/j.issn.2218-6751.2015.12.10.

[39] Li H, Xu Y, Wan B, Song Y, Zha P. et al. (2019) The clinicopathological and prognostic significance of PD-L1 expression assessed by immunohistochemistry in lung cancer: a meta-analysis of 50 studies with 11,383 patients. Transl Lung Cancer Res.;8(4):429-449. doi:10.21037/tlcr.2019.08.04

[40] Dang TO, Ogunniyi A, Barbee MS, Drilon A. (2016) Pembrolizumab for the treatment of PD-L1 positive advanced or metastatic non-small cell lung cancer. Expert Rev Anticancer Ther. 16(1):13-20. doi:10.1586/14737140.2016.1123626.

[41] Incorvaia L, Fanale D, Badalamenti G, Barraco N, Bono M. et al. (2019) Programmed Death Ligand 1 (PD-L1) as a Predictive Biomarker for Pembrolizumab Therapy in Patients with Advanced Non-Small-Cell Lung Cancer (NSCLC). Adv Ther.;36(10):2600-2617. doi:10.1007/s12325-019-01057-7.

[42] Santini FC, Hellmann MD. (2018) PD-1/PD-L1 Axis in Lung Cancer. Cancer J.;24(1):15-19. doi:10.1097/PPO.0000000000000300.

[43] Davis, A.A., Patel, V.G. (2019) The role of PD-L1 expression as a predictive biomarker: an analysis of

all US Food and Drug Administration (FDA) approvals of immune checkpoint inhibitors. J. Immunotherapy Cancer 7, 278. https://doi.org/10.1186/s40425-019-0768-9.

[44] Onoi K, Chihara Y, Uchino J, Shimamoto T, Morimoto Y. et al. (2020) Immune Checkpoint Inhibitors for Lung Cancer Treatment: A Review. J Clin Med.;9(5):1362. Published 2020 May 6. doi:10.3390/jcm9051362.

[45] Nakajima N, Yoshizawa A, Moriyoshi K, Sonobe M, Menju T. et al. (2019) P40 expression in small cell lung cancer: The presence of p40-positive cells does not always indicate squamous differentiation. Thorac Cancer.;10(5):1188-1192. doi:10.1111/1759-7714.13062.

[46] McLaughlin J, Han G, Schalper KA, Carvajal-Hausdorf D, Pelekanou V. et al. (2016) Quantitative Assessment of the Heterogeneity of PD-L1 Expression in Non-Small-Cell Lung Cancer [published correction appears in JAMA Oncol. Jan;2(1):146]. JAMA Oncol. 2016;2(1):46-54. doi:10.1001/jamaoncol.2015.3638.

[47] Ancevski Hunter K, Socinski MA, Villaruz LC. (2018) PD-L1 Testing in Guiding Patient Selection for PD-1/PD-L1 Inhibitor Therapy in Lung Cancer. Mol Diagn Ther.;22(1):1-10. doi:10.1007/s40291-017-0308-6.

[48] Jürgensmeier JM, Eder JP, Herbst RS. (2014) New strategies in personalized medicine for solid tumors: molecular markers and clinical trial designs. Clin Cancer Res. 20(17):4425-4435. doi:10.1158/1078-0432.CCR-13-0753.

[49] Fogel DB. (2018) Factors associated with clinical trials that fail and opportunities for improving the likelihood of success: A review. Contemp Clin Trials Commun. 11:156-164. doi:10.1016/j.conctc.2018.08.001.

[50] Von Hoff DD, Stephenson JJ, Jr, Rosen P, Loesch DM, Borad MJ et al. Pilot study using molecular profiling of patients' tumors to find potential targets and select treatments for their refractory cancers. J Clin Oncol. 2010;28:4877-4883. doi: 10.1200/JCO.2009.26.5983.

[51] Meric-Bernstam F, Farhangfar C, Mendelsohn J, Mills GB. (2013) Building a personalized medicine infrastructure at a major cancer center. J Clin Oncol. 31:1849-1857. doi: 10.1200/JCO.2012.45.3043.

[52] Wang Y, Wang Y, Wang Y, Zhang Y. (2020) Identification of prognostic signature of non–small cell lung cancer based on TCGA methylation data. Scientific Reports 10:8575. doi: 10.1038/s41598-020-65479-y.

[53] Wistuba II, Behrens C, Lombardi F, Wagner S, Fujimoto J, et al. (2013) Validation of a Proliferation-Based Expression Signature as Prognostic Marker in Early Stage Lung Adenocarcinoma. Clin Cancer Res 19(22); 6261-71. doi: 10.1158/1078-0432.CCR-13-0596.

[54] Bueno R, Hughes E, Wagner S, Gutin AS, Lanchbury JS et al. (2015) Validation of a Molecular and Pathological Model for Five-Year Mortality Risk in Patients with Early Stage Lung Adenocarcinoma. J. Thorac Oncol. 10: 67-73. doi: 10.1097/JTO.0000000000000365.

[55] Cuzick J, Swanson GP, Fisher G, Brothman AR, Berney DM et al. (2011) Prognostic value of an RNA expression signature derived from cell cycle proliferation genes for recurrence and death from prostate cancer: A retrospective study in two cohorts. Lancet Oncol. 12:245-55. doi: 10.1016/S1470-2045(10)70295-3.

[56] Wirapati P, Sotiriou C, Kunkel S, Farmer P, Pradervand Set al. (2008)

Meta-analysis of gene expression profiles in breast cancer: toward a unified understanding of breast cancer subtyping and prognosis signatures. Breast Cancer Res 10, R65. doi: 10.1186/bcr2124.

[57] Aramini B, Casali C, Stefani A, Bettelli S, Wagner S et al. (2016) Prediction of distant recurrence in resected stage I and II lung adenocarcinoma. Lung Cancer 101 82-87. doi: 10.1016/j.lungcan.2016.09.005.

[58] Kim ES, Herbst RS, Wistuba II, Lee JJ, Blumenschein GR et al. (2011) The BATTLE trial: personalizing therapy for lung cancer. Cancer Discov. 1:44-53. doi: 10.1158/2159-8274.CD-10-0010.

[59] Tran B, Dancey JE, Kamel-Reid S, McPherson JD, Bedard PL et al. Cancer genomics: technology, discovery, and translation. J Clin Oncol. 2012;30:647-660. doi: 10.1200/JCO.2011.39.2316.

[60] Le Tourneau C, Kamal M, Tredan O, Delord JP, Campone M et al. (2012) Designs and challenges for personalized medicine studies in oncology: focus on the SHIVA trial. Target Oncol. 7:253-265. doi: 10.1007/s11523-012-0237-6.

[61] Tsimberidou AM, Iskander NG, Hong DS, Wheler JJ, Falchook GS et al. (2012) Personalized medicine in a phase I clinical trials program: the MD Anderson Cancer Center initiative. Clin Cancer Res. 18:6373-6383. doi: 10.1158/1078-0432.CCR-12-1627.

[62] Arnedos M, Andre F, Farace F, Lacroix L, Besse B et al. (2012) The challenge to bring personalized cancer medicine from clinical trials into routine clinical practice: the case of the Institut Gustave Roussy. Mol Oncol. 6:204-210. doi: 10.1016/j.molonc.2012.02.008.

[63] ClinicalTrials.gov. Novartis Pharmaceuticals, NCT01831726, NCT 01833169, NCT 01885195, NCT 01981187, NCT 02002689. ClinicalTrials.gov.

[64] Conley BA. Precision Cancer Medicine; Exceptional Responders; NCI-MATCH. http://deainfo.nci.nih.gov/advisory/ctac/1113/PrecisionCancerMedicine.pdf.

[65] Belin L, Kamal M, Mauborgne C, Plancher C, Mulot F, et al. (2017) Randomized phase II trial comparing molecularly targeted therapy based on tumor molecular profiling versus conventional therapy in patients with refractory cancer: cross-over analysis from the SHIVA trial. Ann Oncol. 28(3):590-596. doi: 10.1093/annonc/mdw666.

[66] Burrell RA, McGranahan N, Bartek J, Swanton C. (2013) The causes and consequences of genetic heterogeneity in cancer evolution. Nature.501:338-345. doi: 10.1038/nature12625.

[67] Awada A, Aftimos PG. (2013) Targeted therapies of solid cancers: new options, new challenges. Curr Opin Oncol.25:296-304. doi: 10.1097/CCO.0b013e32835ff318.

[68] Gerlinger M, Rowan AJ, Horswell S, Math M, Larkin J et al. (2012) Intratumor heterogeneity and branched evolution revealed by multiregion sequencing. N Engl J Med. 366:883-892. doi: 10.1056/NEJMoa1113205.

[69] Yachida S, Jones S, Bozic I, Antal T, Leary R et al. (2010) Distant metastasis occurs late during the genetic evolution of pancreatic cancer. Nature. 467:1114-1117. doi: 10.1038/nature09515.

[70] Vakiani E, Janakiraman M, Shen R, Sinha R, Zeng Z et al. (2012) Comparative genomic analysis of primary versus metastatic colorectal carcinomas. J Clin Oncol. 30:2956-2962. doi: 10.1200/JCO.2011.38.2994.

[71] Jakobsen JN, Sorensen JB. (2012) Intratumor heterogeneity and chemotherapy-induced changes in EGFR status in non-small cell lung cancer. Cancer Chemother Pharmacol. 69:289-299. doi: 10.1007/s00280-011-1791-9.

[72] Narayan A, Carriero NJ, Gettinger SN, Kluytenaar J, Kozak KR et al. (2012) Ultrasensitive measurement of hotspot mutations in tumor DNA in blood using error-suppressed multiplexed deep sequencing. Cancer Res. 72:3492-3498. doi: 10.1158/0008-5472.CAN-11-4037.

[73] Perkins G, Yap TA, Pope L, Cassidy AM, Dukes JP et al. (2012) Multi-purpose utility of circulating plasma DNA testing in patients with advanced cancers. PLoS One. 7:e47020. doi: 10.1371/journal.pone.0047020.

[74] Yu M, Stott S, Toner M, Maheswaran S, Haber DA . Circulating tumor cells: approaches to isolation and characterization. (2011) J Cell Biol. 2011;192:373-382. doi: 10.1083/jcb.201010021.

[75] Ebeling FG, Stieber P, Untch M, Nagel D, Konecny GE et al. (2002) Serum CEA and CA 15-3 as prognostic factors in primary breast cancer. Br J Cancer. 86:1217-1222. doi: 10.1038/sj.bjc.6600248.

[76] Okamoto T, Nakamura T, Ikeda J, Maruyama R, Shoji F, et al. (2005) Serum carcinoembryonic antigen as a predictive marker for sensitivity to gefitinib in advanced non-small cell lung cancer. Eur J Cancer 41:1286-1290. doi: 10.1016/j.ejca.2005.03.011.

[77] Jürgensmeier JM, Schmoll HJ, Robertson JD, Brooks L, Taboada M et al. (2013) Prognostic and predictive value of VEGF, sVEGFR-2 and CEA in mCRC studies comparing cediranib, bevacizumab and chemotherapy. Br J Cancer108:1316-1323. doi: 10.1038/bjc.2013.79.

[78] Politi K, Herbst RS. (2015) Lung cancer in the era of precision medicine. Clin Cancer Res. 21(10):2213-2220. doi:10.1158/1078-0432.CCR-14-2748.

[79] Yeung CC, Egan D, & Radich JP. (2016) Molecular monitoring of chronic myeloid leukemia: present and future. Expert review of molecular diagnostics, 16(10), 1083-1091. doi: 10.1080/14737159.2016.1227243.

[80] Principale- Gregg JP, Li T, & Yoneda KY. (2019). Molecular testing strategies in non-small cell lung cancer: optimizing the diagnostic journey. Translational lung cancer research, 8(3), 286-301. doi: 10.21037/tlcr.2019.04.14.

[81] Lindeman NI, Cagle PT, Aisner DL, Arcila ME, Beasley MB et al. (2018) Updated molecular testing guideline for the selection of lung cancer patients for treatment with targeted tyrosine kinase inhibitors: guideline from the College of American Pathologists, the International Association for the Study of Lung Cancer, and the Association for Molecular Pathology. Arch Pathol Lab Med 142:321-46.

[82] Cooper W, Fox S, O'Toole S, Morey A, Frances G et al. (2014) National Working Group Meeting on ALK diagnostics in lung cancer. Asia Pac J Clin Oncol. 10(suppl):211-217. doi: 10.1111/ajco.12190. doi: 10.1111/ajco.12190.

[83] Dietel M, Bubendorf L, Dingemans AM, Dooms C, Elmberger G et al. (2016) Diagnostic procedures for non-small-cell lung cancer (NSCLC): recommendations of the European Expert Group. Thorax. 71(2):177-184. doi: 10.1136/thoraxjnl-2014-206677.

[84] Duffy MJ, Sturgeon CM, Soletormos G, Barak V, Molina R et al. (2015) Validation of new cancer biomarkers: a position statement from the European group on tumor markers.

Clin Chem. 61(6):809-820. doi: 10.1373/clinchem.2015.239863.

[85] Garcia-Campelo R, Bernabe R, Cobo M, Corral J, Coves J et al. (2015) SEOM clinical guidelines for the treatment of non-small cell lung cancer (NSCLC) 2015. Clin Transl Oncol.;17(12):1020-1029. doi: 10.1007/s12094-015-1455-z.

[86] Gridelli C, Balducci L, Ciardiello F, Di Maio M, Felip E et al. (2015) Treatment of elderly patients with non-small-cell lung cancer: results of an International Expert Panel Meeting of the Italian Association of Thoracic Oncology. Clin Lung Cancer. 16(5):325-333. doi: 10.1016/j.cllc.2015.02.006.

[87] Joseph L, Cankovic M, Caughron S, Chandra P, Emmadi R et al. (2016) The spectrum of clinical utilities in molecular pathology testing procedures for inherited conditions and cancer: a report of the Association for Molecular Pathology. J Mol Diagn. 18(5):605-619. doi: 10.1016/j.jmoldx.2016.05.007.

[88] Kerr KM, Bubendorf L, Edelman MJ, Marchetti A, Mok T et al. (2014) Second ESMO consensus conference on lung cancer: pathology and molecular biomarkers for non-smallcell lung cancer. Ann Oncol. 25(9):1681-1690. doi: 10.1093/annonc/mdu145.

[89] Monso E, Montuenga LM, Sanchez de Cos J, Villena C; Lung Cancer CIBERES-RTICC-SEPAR-Plataforma Biobanco Pulmonar. Biological marker analysis as part of the CIBERES-RTIC Cancer-SEPAR Strategic Project on Lung Cancer. Arch Bronconeumol. 2015;51(9):462-467. doi: 10.1016/j.arbres.2014.11.010

[90] Popper HH, Gruber-Mosenbacher U, Hutarew G, Luka Brcic L, Malgorzata Szolkowska M et al. (2016) Recommendations of the Austrian Working Group on Pulmonary Pathology and Oncology for predictive molecular and immunohistochemical testing in non-small cell lung cancer. Memo. 9(4):191-200. doi: 10.21037/tlcr.2020.04.07.

[91] Sepulveda AR, Hamilton SR, Allegra CJ, Grody W, Cushman-Vokoun AM et al. (2017) Molecular biomarkers for the evaluation of colorectal cancer: guideline from the American Society for Clinical Pathology, College of American Pathologists, Association for Molecular Pathology, and the American Society of Clinical Oncology. J Clin Oncol. 35(13):1453-1486. doi: 10.1200/JCO.2016.71.9807.

[92] van der Heijden EH, Casal RF, Trisolini R, Steinfort DP, Hwangbo B, et al. (2014) Guideline for the acquisition and preparation of conventional and endobronchial ultrasoundguided transbronchial needle aspiration specimens for the diagnosis and molecular testing of patients with known or suspected lung cancer. Respiration. 88(6):500-517. doi: 10.1159/000368857.

[93] Villar Alvarez F, Muguruza Trueba I, Belda Sanchis J, Rodríguez Suárez PM, de Cos Escuín JS et al. (2016) Executive summary of the SEPAR recommendations for the diagnosis and treatment of nonsmall cell lung cancer. Arch Bronconeumol. 52(7):378-388. doi: 10.1016/j.arbr.2016.02.020

[94] von Laffert M, Schirmacher P, Warth A, Büttner R, Huber RM et al. (2017) ALK-testing in non-small cell lung cancer (NSCLC): immunohistochemistry (IHC) and/or fluorescence in-situ hybridisation (FISH)?: statement of the Germany Society for Pathology (DGP) and the Working Group Thoracic Oncology (AIO) of the German Cancer Society e.V. (Stellungnahme der Deutschen Gesellschaft fur Pathologie und der AG Thorakale Onkologie der

Arbeitsgemeinschaft Onkologie/ Deutsche Krebsgesellschaft e.V.). Lung Cancer103:1-5. doi: 10.1016/j.lungcan.2016.11.008.

[95] Scottish Intercollegiate Guidelines Network (SIGN). Management of lung cancer. Edinburgh: SIGN; 2014. SIGN publication no. 137. http://www.sign.ac.uk. Accessed June 12, 2017.

[96] Yale University School of Medicine. GuideLines Into DEcision Support (GLIDES). http://medicine.yale.edu/cmi/glides/index.aspx. Accessed June 21, 2017.

[97] van El CG, Cornel MC, Borry P, Hastings RJ, Fellmann F, et al., & ESHG Public and Professional Policy Committee (2013). Whole-genome sequencing in health care. Recommendations of the European Society of Human Genetics. European journal of human genetics : EJHG, 21 Suppl 1(Suppl 1), S1–S5. doi: 10.1038/ejhg.2013.46.

[98] Nakagawa H, & Fujita M. (2018). Whole genome sequencing analysis for cancer genomics and precision medicine. Cancer science, 109(3), 513-522. doi: 10.1111/cas.13505.

[99] O'Brien TD, Jia P, Xia J, Saxena U, Jin H, et al. (2015) Inconsistency and features of single nucleotide variants detected in whole exome sequencing versus transcriptome sequencing: A case study in lung cancer. Methods. 2015 Jul 15;83:118-27. doi: 10.1016/j.ymeth.2015.04.016.

[100] Seo JS, Ju YS, Lee WC, Shin JY, Lee JK, et al. (2012) The transcriptional landscape and mutational profile of lung adenocarcinoma. Genome Res. 22:2109-2119. doi: 10.1101/gr.145144.112.

[101] Horak P, Fröhling S, & Glimm H. (2016). Integrating next-generation sequencing into clinical oncology: strategies, promises and pitfalls. ESMO open, 1(5), e000094. doi: 10.1136/esmoopen-2016-000094.

[102] Jeromin S, Haferlach T, Weissmann S, Meggendorfer M, Eder C et al. (2015) Refractory anemia with ring sideroblasts and marked thrombocytosis cases harbor mutations in SF3B1 or other spliceosome genes accompanied by JAK2V617F and ASXL1 mutations. Haematologica. 100:e125-127. doi: 10.3324/haematol.2014.119032.

[103] Malcovati L, Karimi M, Papaemmanuil E, Ambaglio I, Jädersten M et al. (2015) SF3B1 mutation identifies a distinct subset of myelodysplastic syndrome with ring sideroblasts. Blood. 126:233-241. doi: 10.1182/blood-2015-03-633537.

[104] Ding L, Ley TJ , Larson DE, Miller CA, Koboldt DC, et al. (2012) Clonal evolution in relapsed acute myeloid leukaemia revealed by whole-genome sequencing. Nature. 481:506-510. doi: 10.1038/nature10738.

[105] Garg M, Nagata Y, Deepika Kanojia D, Mayakonda A, Yoshida K et al. (2015) Profiling of somatic mutations in acute myeloid leukemia with FLT3-ITD at diagnosis and relapse. Blood. 126:2491-2501. doi: 10.1182/blood-2015-05-646240.

[106] Jan M, Snyder TM, Corces-Zimmerman MR, Vyas P, Weissman IL, et al. (2012) Clonal evolution of preleukemic hematopoietic stem cells precedes human acute myeloid leukemia. Science translational medicine. 4:149ra118. doi: 10.1126/scitranslmed.3004315.

[107] Shlush LI, Zandi S, Mitchell A, Chen WC, Brandwein JM, et al. (2014) Identification of pre-leukaemic haematopoietic stem cells in acute leukaemia. Nature 506:328-333. doi: 10.1038/nature13038.

[108] Klco JM, Miller CA, Griffith M, Petti A, Spencer DH et al. (2015) Association Between Mutation Clearance After Induction Therapy and Outcomes in Acute Myeloid Leukemia. Jama. 314:811-822. doi: 10.1001/jama.2015.9643.

[109] Alexandrov LB, Nik-Zainal S, Wedge DC, Aparicio SA, Behjati S et al. (2013) Signatures of mutational processes in human cancer. Nature. 500:415-421. doi: 10.1038/nature12477.

[110] Greenman C, Stephens P, Smith R, Dalgliesh GL, Hunter C, et al. (2007) Patterns of somatic mutation in human cancer genomes. Nature. 446:153-158. doi: 10.1038/nature05610.

[111] Conway JR, Warner JL, Rubinstein WS, and Miller RS (2019). Next-Generation Sequencing and the Clinical Oncology Workflow: Data Challenges, Proposed Solutions, and a Call to Action. JCO Precision Oncology 3, 1-10. doi: 10.1200/PO.19.00232.

[112] Shyr, D., & Liu, Q. (2013). Next generation sequencing in cancer research and clinical application. Biological procedures online, 15(1), 4. doi: 10.1186/1480-9222-15-4.

[113] Fabrizio D, Lieber D, Malboeuf C, Silterra J , White E. et al. (2018) Abstract 5706: a blood-based next-generation sequencing assay to determine tumor mutational burden (bTMB) is associated with benefit to an anti-PD-L1 inhibitor, atezolizumab. Cancer Res 78: 13 Suppl., 5706-5717. doi: 10.1158/1538-7445.AM2018-5706.

[114] Koeppel F, Blanchard S, Jovelet C, Genin B, Marcaillou C et al. (2017) Whole exome sequencing for determination of tumor mutation load in liquid biopsy from advanced cancer patients. PLoS One 12: e0188174. doi:10.1371/journal.pone.0188174.

[115] Khagi Y, Goodman AM, Daniels GA, Patel SP, Sacco AG et al. (2017) Hypermutated circulating tumor DNA: correlation with response to checkpoint inhibitor-based immunotherapy. Clin Cancer Res 23: 5729-5736. doi:10.1158/1078-0432.CCR-17-1439.

[116] Chan TA, Yarchoan M, Jaffee E, Swanton C, Quezada SA et al. (2019) Development of tumor mutation burden as an immunotherapy biomarker: utility for the oncology clinic. Ann Oncol. 30(1):44-56. doi:10.1093/annonc/mdy495.

[117] Chalabi M, Cardona A, Nagarkar DR, Dhawahir Scala A, Gandara DR, et al. (2020) imCORE working group of early career investigators. Efficacy of chemotherapy and atezolizumab in patients with non-small-cell lung cancer receiving antibiotics and proton pump inhibitors: pooled post hoc analyses of the OAK and POPLAR trials. Ann Oncol.31(4):525-531. doi: 10.1016/j.annonc.2020.01.006.

[118] Yang N, Li Y, Liu Z Du D, Cao Xet al. (2018). The characteristics of ctDNA reveal the high complexity in matching the corresponding tumor tissues. BMC Cancer 18, 319. doi: 10.1186/s12885-018-4199-7.

[119] Guibert N, Mazieres J, Delaunay M, Casanova A, Farella M et al. (2017) Monitoring of KRAS-mutated ctDNA to discriminate pseudo-progression from true progression during anti-PD-1 treatment of lung adenocarcinoma. Oncotarget 8: 38056-38060. doi: 10.18632/oncotarget.16935.

[120] Cabel L, Proudhon C, Romano E, Girard N, Lantz O et al. (2018) Clinical potential of circulating tumour DNA in patients receiving anticancer immunotherapy. Nat Rev Clin Oncol 15: 639-650. doi: 10.1038/s41571-018-0074-3.

[121] Aberle DR, Adams AM, Berg CD, Black WC, Clapp JD et al. (2011) Reduced lung-cancer mortality with low-dose computed tomographic screening. National Lung Screening Trial Research Team, Aberle DR, Adams AM, et al. N Engl J Med 365: 395-409. doi: 10.1056/NEJMoa1102873.

[122] De Koning H, Van Der Aalst C, Ten Haaf K, M. Oudkerk (2018) PL02.05 Effects of volume CT lung cancer screening: mortality results of the NELSON randomised-controlled population-based trial. J Thorac Oncol ; 13: Suppl., S185. dOI:https://doi.org/10.1016/j.jtho.2018.08.012.

[123] Guibert N, Mazieres J, Delaunay M, Casanova A, Farella M et al. (2017) Monitoring of KRAS-mutated ctDNA to discriminate pseudo-progression from true progression during anti-PD-1 treatment of lung adenocarcinoma. Oncotarget 8: 38056-38060. doi:10.18632/oncotarget.16935.

[124] Cohen JD, Li L, Wang Y, Thoburn C, Afsari B, et al. (2018) Detection and localization of surgically resectable cancers with a multi-analyte blood test. Science 359: 926-930. doi:10.1126/science.aar3247.

[125] Jamal-Hanjani M, Wilson GA, McGranahan N, Birkbak NJ, Watkins TBK et al. (2017) Tracking the evolution of non-small-cell lung cancer. N Engl J Med 376: 2109-2121. doi:10.1056/NEJMoa1616288.

[126] Abbosh C, Birkbak NJ, Wilson GA, Jamal-Hanjani M, Constantin T et al. (2017) Phylogenetic ctDNA analysis depicts early-stage lung cancer evolution. Nature 545: 446-451. doi:10.1038/nature22364.

[127] Ulrich BC, Guibert N. (2017) Towards a comprehensive framework for cell-free DNA analysis: lessons from TRACERx. Ann Transl Med 5: 428. doi:10.21037/atm.2017.08.12.

[128] Oxnard GR, Paweletz CP, Kuang Y, Mach SL, O'Connell A, et al. (2014) Noninvasive detection of response and resistance in EGFR-mutant lung cancer using quantitative next-generation genotyping of cell-free plasma DNA. Clin Cancer Res 20: 1698-1705. doi:10.1158/1078-0432.CCR-13-2482

[129] Sacher AG, Alden RS, Oxnard GR. (2016) Early intervention in lung cancers with rapid plasma genotyping for EGFR and KRAS mutations-reply. JAMA Oncol. 2: 1096-1097. doi:10.1001/jamaoncol.2016.1963

[130] Yanagita M, Redig AJ, Paweletz CP, Dahlberg SE, O'Connell A, et al. (2016) A prospective evaluation of circulating tumor cells and cell-free DNA in EGFR-mutant non-small cell lung cancer patients treated with erlotinib on a phase II trial. Clin Cancer Res 22: 6010-6020. doi:10.1158/1078-0432.CCR-16-0909.

[131] Nagrath S, Sequist LV, Maheswaran S, Bell DW, Irimia D et al. (2007) Isolation of rare circulating tumour cells in cancer patients by microchip technology. Nature 450: 1235-1239. doi:10.1038/nature06385.

[132] Yang Z, Zhao N, Cui J, Wu H, Xiong J, et al. (2020) Exosomes derived from cancer stem cells of gemcitabine-resistant pancreatic cancer cells enhance drug resistance by delivering miR-210. Cell Oncol (Dordr). 43(1):123-136. doi: 10.1007/s13402-019-00476-6.

[133] Adorno-Cruz V, Kibria G, Liu X, Doherty M, Junk DJ, et al. (2015) Cancer stem cells: targeting the roots of cancer, seeds of metastasis, and sources of therapy resistance. Cancer Res. 15;75(6):924-929. doi: 10.1158/0008-5472.CAN-14-3225.

[134] Gernapudi R, Yao Y, Zhang Y, Wolfson B, Roy S, et al. (2015) Targeting exosomes from preadipocytes inhibits preadipocyte to cancer stem

cell signaling in early-stage breast cancer. Breast Cancer Res Treat. 2015 Apr;150(3):685-95. doi: 10.1007/s10549-015-3326-2.

[135] Aramini B, Masciale V, Haider KH. (2020) Defining lung cancer stem cells exosomal payload of miRNAs in clinical perspective. World J Stem Cells.;12(6):406-421. doi:10.4252/wjsc.v12.i6.406.

[136] Kumar D, Gupta D, Shankar S, Srivastava RK. (2015) Biomolecular characterization of exosomes released from cancer stem cells: Possible implications for biomarker and treatment of cancer. Oncotarget. 20;6(5):3280-91. doi: 10.18632/oncotarget.2462.

[137] Grange C, Tapparo M, Collino F, Vitillo L, Damasco C, et al. (2011) Microvesicles released from human renal cancer stem cells stimulate angiogenesis and formation of lung premetastatic niche. Cancer Res. 71(15):5346-56. doi: 10.1158/0008-5472.CAN-11-0241.

[138] Masciale V, Grisendi G, Banchelli F, D'Amico R, Maiorana A et al. (2019) Isolation and Identification of Cancer Stem-Like Cells in Adenocarcinoma and Squamous Cell Carcinoma of the Lung: A Pilot Study. Front Oncol. 9:1394. Published 2019 Dec 18. doi:10.3389/fonc.2019.01394.

[139] Masciale V, Grisendi G, Banchelli F, D'Amico R, Maiorana A et al. (2020) CD44+/EPCAM+ cells detect a subpopulation of ALDHhigh cells in human non-small cell lung cancer: A chance for targeting cancer stem cells? Oncotarget 11(17):1545-1555. Published 2020 Apr 28. doi:10.18632/oncotarget.27568.

Chapter 8

Challenges in the Treatment of Oligometastatic Non-small Cell Lung Cancer

Martina Vrankar

Abstract

Since 1995, when the concept of oligometastatic non-small cell lung cancer was first described, no high-level evidence has been introduced for management of those patients subset. Data from retrospective reports and analysis and from every-day clinical practice revealed that some of the non-small cell lung cancer patients with a few metastases could benefit significantly with local radical treatment approach of primary and metastatic lesions. Recent advances in modern local treatment approaches with minimally invasive surgery and stereotactic radiotherapy, as well as introduction of immunotherapy, open new field of interest for personalized treatment of limited metastatic non-small cell lung cancer. In this report, we are summarizing limited data of case reports, retrospective studies and few randomized studies of patients with oligometastatic non-small cell lung cancer and discuss challenges of treatment in the era of molecular targeted therapy and immunotherapy.

Keywords: oligometastases, non-small cell lung cancer, ablative treatment, stereotactic body radiation therapy, immunotherapy, molecular targeted therapy

1. Introduction

Lung cancer is the leading cause of cancer mortality worldwide, with over 1.7 million deaths and over 2 million newly diagnosed cases annually [1]. More than a half of all new diagnosed patients with non-small cell lung cancer (NSCLC) presents in stage IV disease with a median overall survival (OS) of 10–12 months. Stage IV NSCLC is generally considered incurable disease with a 5-year survival ranged from 0 to 10% [2]. However, the sub segment of patients in stage IV was recognized years ago with different clinical presentation and prolonged survival that overcomes expected for metastatic disease [3]. Oligometastatic disease was first described in 1995 as a state of limited systemic metastatic burden in which treatment of oligometastases with radical local therapies could be curative in selected patients [3, 4]. For decades, no high-level evidence has been introduced for management of these patients subset. Moreover, no uniform definition and staging requirements for usage the term oligometastatic NSCLC have been accepted until recently. Clinical data indicate that the number of patients with oligometastatic disease that undergo ablative local treatment is increasing at a great rate [5]. With the extension of imaging diagnostic methods like 2-deoxy-2-[fluorine-18]fluoro-D-glucose positron emission tomography/computed tomography (^{18}F-FDG PET/CT) and magnetic resonance imaging (MRI), oligometastatic NSCLC patients who benefit most from radical treatment could be selected precisely [6]. On the other hand, development in technical improvement of modern local treatment approaches and advances in new systemic treatment options for NSCLC patients offer new hope for improvement of outcomes in oligometastatic NSCLC. In this chapter, we present most relevant scientific evidence regarding oligometastatic NSCLC and discuss future perspectives in treatment of these patients in the era of molecular targeted treatment and immunotherapy.

2. Definition

Even the oligometastatic disease was first described in 1995, no uniform and clear definition has been accepted for years [3]. Most past clinical trial protocols have used an upper limit of metastases between one and eight as inclusion criteria; however, 90% of included patients actually had one metastasis [5, 7].

The concept of oligometastatic NSCLC include different clinical scenarios of limited number of metastatic lesions that are feasible to local ablative treatment. Regarding the time of presentation, in synchronous oligometastatic disease metastatic lesions are detected at the time of diagnosis of the primary tumor. In metachronous oligometastatic disease new metastatic lesions not present at the time of the primary diagnosis develop [8, 9]. Other related terms are currently used, like oligorecurrence, in which limited number of metastatic lesions develop in otherwise controlled primary tumor site followed radical treatment. Oligoprogression describes metastatic disease with controlled primary tumor and most metastases due to systemic therapy followed by progression of one or few metastatic lesions. Oligoressistance follows systemic therapy of patients with widespread metastases who have a near complete response but limited number of persistent lesions remains. First attempt to unify the oligometastatic state was inclusion oligometastatic disease in the 8th edition of the Tumor, Node, Metastasis (TNM) published by the International Association for the Study of Lung Cancer (IASLC). In the assessment for M descriptor, 225 (22%) of the 1025 metastatic patients were reported with a single metastasis in a single organ that had significantly better prognosis than those with multiple metastases in one or several organs [10]. Accordingly, single metastatic lesion in a single distant organ was assigned to the new M1b category [2, 10].

Recently, a pan-European multidisciplinary consensus statement on the definition and staging of synchronous oligometastatic NSCLC was formulated [11]. As it was concluded, the definition is relevant when a radical treatment is technically feasible with acceptable toxicity, with all sites being amenable to local treatment modality that may result in long-term disease control. A maximum of 5 metastases and 3 organs is proposed for definition of oligometastatic NSCLC. The presence of diffuse serosal metastases (meningeal, pericardial, pleural, and mesenteric) or bone marrow involvement excludes cases from the definition, as these cannot be treated with radical intent. For pulmonary metastases, the eight TNM classification should be followed. Metastasis in the same lobe (T3) or in the same lung (T4) should not be counted as a metastatic site, but it can influence the possibility of treatment with radical intent. Mediastinal lymph nodes must be considered as regional disease, but their involvements are of importance in the decision of feasibility for radical treatment of locoregional disease. The recommendations for staging include ^{18}F-FDG PET/CT and brain imaging, preferably magnetic resonance imaging (MRI), that are mandatory. Besides mediastinal lymph node staging with ^{18}F-FDG PET/CT, pathological confirmation is required if this influences the treatment decision. In addition, pathological confirmation at least of one metastasis is required unless the risk outweighs the benefit.

3. Incidence

Oligometastatic disease used to be reported sporadically [12]; however, with the improvement in diagnostic imaging, mainly ^{18}F-FDG PET/CT and MRI, oligometastases appear relatively frequent. While available data on incidence of oligometastatic NSCLC at diagnosis remains limited, even when published mostly in retrospective reports, the diversity of inclusion criteria about the maximum number of metastatic lesions accepted for study, makes it more difficult to compare. However, it has been estimated that aproximatelly 20–50% patients with metastatic NSCLC at diagnosis present with oligometastatic disease [10, 13, 14]. As mentioned before, in the IASLC TNM classification of lung cancer, 22% of all metastatic patients had a single metastatic lesion [10]. The most frequent site of a single lesion was bone, followed by brain, adrenals and liver. In an analysis of 725 NSCLC patients with metastatic disease at diagnosis, 186 (26%) were recognized with oligometastatic disease defined as ≤5 lesions [13]. Of those, 51% of the patients had a single metastatic lesion and in 81% of patients, metastases were limited to one organ site. As in previous analysis, the most common site of a single lesion appearance was brain, bone and adrenal glands. In the group of oligorecurrent NSCLC patients after treatment of the primary site, 50–60% were reported to present with only one to three metastatic sites [4, 15]. The majority of patients who have been treated with surgery, at recurrence presented with metastases in the brain, contralateral lung or adrenal gland. The pattern of oligoprogression in advanced or metastatic NSCLC patients after first-line chemotherapy has been barely reported. In a study of Rusthoven et al., local progression only, was the predominant pattern of failure in 64% of patients after systemic therapy, mostly platinum-based chemotherapy, suggesting that consolidation local therapy after first-line systemic treatment could potentially alter the patterns of failure and prolong time to progression in a substantial proportion of those patients [14]. With the introduction of new systemic treatment possibilities that prolong survival, like tyrosine kinase inhibitors (TKI) in patients with epidermal growth factor receptor (EGFR) mutation/anaplastic lymphoma kinase (ALK) rearrangement, oligoprogression has been reported more often. Molecular targeted therapy with TKI enable higher response rates and better progression-free survival (PFS), however, progression inevitably develops in most cases after 1 to 2 years of molecular targeted treatment due to acquired resistance [16]. Data from literature reveals that the proportion of patients progressing with an oligoprogressive pattern of disease ranges from 15 to 47% during EGFR TKI treatment [17–19]. Few series also suggest that as many as 25% of patient treated with TKI progress with single metastases and 50% with four or less lesions [17, 20]. For those patients with oligoprogressive or oligoresistance disease, local ablative therapy and continuation of molecular targeted therapy could result in more than 6 months of additional clinical benefits [20].

4. Prognostic factors

Oligometastatic disease is highly divers in prognosis, ranged from rapid progression with demise during treatment to long-term survivals. It is assumed that about 25% of oligometastatic patients will have prolonged disease-free interval [7, 12, 21]. Therefore, the identification of oligometastatic patients that will benefit most from aggressive local treatment is of the crucial importance.

As already mentioned, results from IASLC 8th TNM classification validation study revealed significantly longer OS in patients with a single extrathoracic metastasis than in those with multiple metastases [10]. In the individual patients data meta-analysis of Ashworth et al. 757 oligometastatic NSCLC patients were included from 1985 to 2012 and managed with ablative treatments to all sites of disease, however, half of the patients had only a single metastasis [7]. Surgery was the most commonly used treatment for the primary tumor (83.9%) and metastases (62.3%). Factors predictive for OS were synchronous versus metachronous metastases ($P < .001$), N-stage ($P = .002$), and adenocarcinoma histology ($P = .036$). In recursive partitioning analysis, three risk groups were identified: low-risk, metachronous metastases (5-year OS, 47.8%); intermediate risk, synchronous metastases and N0 disease (5-year OS, 36.2%); and high risk, synchronous metastases and N1/N2 disease (5-year OS, 13.8%). In the analysis of Parikh et al., 186 patients with five or fewer distant metastatic lesions at diagnosis were included, of whom 52% patients had a single metastatic lesion [13]. On multivariable analysis, Eastern Cooperate Oncology Group (ECOG PS) performance status, nodal status N2–3, squamous pathology, and metastases to multiple organs were associated with a greater hazard of death (all $P < .01$). However, the number of metastatic lesions and radiologic size of the primary tumor were not associated with OS. Definitive local therapy to the primary tumor was associated with prolonged survival. Data from twenty-four studies that included altogether 1935 patients with oligometastatic NSCLC were analyzed in a meta-analysis by Li et al. [22]. Among patients with oligometastatic disease, defined as 5 or fewer lesions, they identified several factors associated with improved survival, including aggressive treatment to the primary lung tumor, female gender, lower nodal stage, adenocarcinoma histology and thoracic stage. Other retrospective publications reported importance of aggressive local treatment [23, 24]; moreover, the major predictors of OS were the extent of intra-thoracic disease including nodal status and possibilities for resection or radical radiotherapy [25–27]. In the trial by Gomez et al. besides treatment type (local treatment versus no local treatment) presence of driver mutations were associated with improved PFS [28, 29]. Aside of the number of metastases, mediastinal node involvement, time until onset of metastases, histology, PS, T stage, treatment of the primary and metastatic lesions, diagnosis-specific graded prognostic assessment (DS-GPA classification, and Lung-molGPA) is well known for patients with brain metastasis.

Additionally, a specific genetic or epigenetic alterations ("initiation," "progression," and "virulence" genes) have been described so far that together with failures in immunosurveillance impact patients'clinical outcomes. The oligometastatic tumors are believed to have more indolent biology [3]. Initial investigations of the mechanisms running occurrence of oligometastases identified a central role of microRNAs (miRNAs). Lussier and colleagues evaluated miRNA profiles in an analysis of patients with five metastases manageable for RT. They found that overexpression of the miR-200 family was correlated with polymetastatic progression [30]. Moreover, they observed a specific microRNA expression that identified the patients most likely to remain oligometastatic after metastases directed treatment and therefore associated with a better prognosis.

5. Treatment

Since oligometastatic NSCLC is considered as intermediate state between localized lung cancer and widespread metastatic disease, the therapeutic approaches used for treatment of these patients besides standard systemic therapy include aggressive local therapy.

Several early case and retrospective reports showed that a subset of NSCLC patients with mostly solitary metastasis that were radically treated to all known metastatic sites, could achieve long-term survival [31–33]. Following years, more retrospective reports of oligometastatic patients treated with radical intent were published that demonstrating better-than-expected prolonged survival with median OS between 13.5 to 26 months and 5-year survival between 10 to 36% [13, 23–25, 34–37]. In an individual patient data meta-analysis on 757 oligometastatic NSCLC treated between 1985 and 2012 with surgical metastasectomy, stereotactic radiotherapy/radiosurgery, or radical external-beam radiotherapy for metastases and with curative treatment of the primary lung cancer, median OS was 26 months, 1-year OS 70.2%, and 5-year OS 29.4% [7].

While the last decade use of effective local treatment with minimally invasive surgery or advanced radiation technics for oligometastatic lesions in NSCLC patients has risen, the evidence from prospective studies has been lacking. The first prospective single-arm phase II trial of oligometastatic NSCLC patient with up to five metastases at primary diagnosis amendable for radical local treatment was published in 2012 [27]. Forty patients were enrolled with brain, bone and adrenal gland metastases. Of all included, 87% had a single metastatic lesion and 95% of all received chemotherapy as part of their primary treatment. Median OS was 13.5 months and two- and three- year survival rates were 23.3% and 17.5%, respectively. In 2016, Gomez et al. published the results of a prospective multicentre randomized phase 2 trial that enrolled 74 oligometastatic NSCLC patients with the maximum of 3 metastatic lesion [28]. All patients received standard first-line systemic therapy including platinum-based chemotherapy or TKI in patients with EGFR mutations or ALK rearrangements. Patients were randomly assigned to either local consolidative therapy consisting of resection or (chemo) radiotherapy or to maintenance treatment alone. The study was terminated early after randomization of 49 patients as part of the annual analyses due to substantial efficacy improvement in the local consolidative group compared with the maintenance group. At a median follow-up time of 12.39 months, the median PFS in the consolidative group was significantly longer with 11.9 months versus 3.9 months in the maintenance group. Importantly, time to appearance of a new lesion was longer in the consolidative group arm (11.9 months vs. 5.7 months) suggesting that local consolidative treatment may have altered the natural course of the disease, either by limiting the potential for subsequent dissemination or by altering systemic anticancer immune response. In 2018, the updated survival data at a median follow-up of 38.8 month, confirmed the PFS benefit in consolidative group with 14.2 months compared to 4.4 months in the maintenance group and median OS of 41.2 months in the consolidative arm versus 17.0 months in the maintenance arm [29].

In a phase II randomized clinical trial conducted by Iyengar et al., a total of 29 patients with oligometastatic NSCLC were included [38]. Inclusion criteria allowed up to six sites of extra cranial lesions (including primary) and exclude patients receiving first-line molecular targeted therapy with EGFR/ALK TKI. Fourteen patients were assign to the stereotactic body radiation therapy (SBRT)-plus-maintenance chemotherapy arm, and 15 patients to the maintenance chemotherapy–alone arm. In the SBRT group, all residual disease sites were treated with SBRT. A total of 31 lesions were treated in 14 patients with intrathoracic sites the most common locations of SBRT treatment. Likewise, the trial was stopped to accrual early after an interim analysis found a significant improvement in PFS in the SBRT-plus-maintenance chemotherapy arm with 9.7 months vs. 3.5 months in the maintenance chemotherapy–alone arm (P = .01).

A third completed randomized phase II trial, SABR (stereotactic ablative radiotherapy)-COMET international trial included patients with a controlled primary malignancy of different solid cancers and 1–5 metastatic lesions manageable for SABR treated between 2012 and 2016 [39]. Ninety-nine patients, of those 18% NSCLC patients, were randomly assigned in a 1:2 ratio between standard-of-care treatments and standard-of-care treatments plus SABR. Median OS was 28 months in the control group versus 41 months in the SABR group. Adverse events of grade 2 or worse were significantly higher in SABR group (29% vs. 9%) with three deaths after SABR. Recently, results of extended follow-up were published [40]. With the median follow-up of 51 months, median OS was 28 months in the control arm versus 50 months in the SABR group. Five-year OS rates were 17.7% versus 42.3%, respectively. There were no new grade 2–5 adverse events.

All three randomized studies have contributed increasingly in the evidence that radical local treatment approach added to standard therapy may yield prolonged survival in selected oligometastatic NSCLC. However, last decade most studies have still been retrospective in nature and biased with respect to definition of oligometastatic disease. Systematic review by Schanne et al. included 54 studies that were published between 1987 and 2018 with altogether 1994 patients with oligometastatic NSCLC [5]. Even with a wide range of oligometastatic definitions, 90% of patients were treated for a single metastasis. 60% of patients were diagnosed with adenocarcinoma and 55% of the metastases were located in the brain, 17% in the lung, 11% in the adrenal gland and 17% in other organs. Systemic therapy was used in 68% of patients in a variety of settings, mostly adjuvant/maintenance or neoadjuvant but also combined with RT. Molecular targeted therapy was used in 5% of cases; however, immunotherapy was not used treatment modality in any of analyzed studies. Surgical resection was the most common local treatment modality used in 76% of patients for primary tumor and in 65% of patients for distant metastases. RT was used as neoadjuvant/adjuvant or definitive treatment of primary tumor in 9% and 22%, respectively. Adjuvant RT after surgical resection for metastatic lesions was used in 27% of patients, mostly after resection of brain metastases. Radiation as primary treatment modality was more common for treatment of metastases than for primary tumors (69% vs. 35%). Median OS in the analyzed studies was 19.6 months (6.2–52.9 months) with an observed plateau and possible long-term survival of 20%. Importantly, this analysis also gives us insight in time trends of management oligometastatic NSCLC patients for the last three decades. Relating to time analysis, in the studies published after 2011 radiotherapy has almost surpassed surgical approaches. Local treatment changed in favor to wider use of radiotherapy for primary tumors from 23 to 41%. Moreover, wider adoption of SBRT instead of conventionally fractionated RT with an increase from 0 to 23% for primary tumors and from 15 to 60% for distant metastases was reported. Additionally, the number of patients receiving no systemic therapies was reduced from 45% before 2011 to 24% afterwards. Notably, a trend for improved median OS over time was observed: patients from reports published after 2011 revealed better OS compared to the earlier period: 28.1 months versus 17.2 months, respectively. Comparing the effect of different type of local treatment, when only studies after 2011 were included, no significant effect on median OS was detected neither for primary tumor nor for metastases.

Despite the lack of evidence for optimal treatment of patients with oligometastatic NSCLC, the concept of delivering local radical treatment in patients with oligometastatic NSCLC was incorporated in NSCLC guidelines. The European Society for Medical Oncology (ESMO) Clinical Practice Guidelines due to the limited available evidence propose preferred inclusion in clinical trials [41, 42]. The National Comprehensive Cancer Network (NCCN) guidelines state that patients with NSCLC with limited metastases can receive local radical treatment [43].

6. Challenges in the era of molecular targeted and immunotherapy

The management of oligometastatic NSCLC has changed significantly over the past decades. While surgery, radiotherapy, stereotactic radiotherapy and systemic therapy are the cornerstones of current treatment strategies, treatment modalities have varied over time with respect to the advantages of local treatment techniques as introduction of new systemic treatment possibilities. According to the literature, surgery has been mostly used in oligometastatic NSCLC patients for resection of brain, contralateral lung and adrenal gland metastases [5, 23, 35, 44] Considering the significant morbidity associated with surgical resection of multiple sites of metastatic disease, SBRT has become an alternative treatment approach for achieving local ablation. The highest level of evidence for incorporation of local treatment in oligometastatic NSCLC patients based on small randomize phase II clinical trials, which regularly reported higher PFS and OS with the use of SBRT compared with no SBRT [28, 29, 38–40]. However, the efficacy of SBRT in potentially curable patients with the stage I NSCLC is already confirmed [45]. The broader adoption of SBRT in clinical practice reflects its non-invasive nature, ability to simultaneous treatment of multiple sites in a short time, feasibility of concurrent local and systemic treatment, utility to treatment in the outpatient setting and relatively low toxicity profile [46, 47]. Moreover, SBRT to the progressing lesions may delay the need to start or change systemic therapy that might reflect in prolonged PFS, OS and quality of life for the patients [48–50]. In a systematic review by Tsao et al., reported median OS ranged from 13.5 to 55 months and PFS from 4.4 to 14.7 months. [50] SBRT has currently become a treatment option for tumors in almost any body site, with many publications documenting its efficacy for lung, liver, adrenal, and bone/spine metastases, achieving high as much as 70–90% of local control [51].

Systemic therapy is the backbone treatment for metastatic NSCLC patients; though it is not well defined in management for oligometastatic NSCLC [41–43]. Despite potentially successful local treatment, the majority of oligometastatic NSCLC patients will develop distant progression due to undetectable micrometastases at the time of diagnosis. Therefore, all recent prospective trials combined local treatment with addition of systemic therapy standardly used at the time of the study. However, the therapeutic sequence of systemic therapy might be important for oligometastatic disease, as usually only the patients who do not progress with induction systemic treatment were capable for aggressive local treatment. We are currently not able to reliably predict the course of oligometastatic disease at the time of diagnosis, therefore upfront local therapy colud represent an overtreatment due to rapid progression to multimetastatic disease. Although studies with oligometastatic NSCLC have included patients treated with systemic therapy, mostly chemotherapy and minority molecular targeted therapies, current clinical practice and guidelines for treatment of metastatic NSCLC include molecular targeted agents, immunotherapy or combination of immunotherapy and chemotherapy in first-line setting [52–64]. The introduction of new agents as molecular targeted and immunotherapy has resulted in the improved survival in patients with metastatic and locally advanced NSCLC. As a result, the first line systemic therapies used in most retrospective and prospective studies of oligometastatic NSCLC do not reflect those currently used. With onset of new systemic therapies in the management of NSCLC patients, great interest has risen in exploring the safety and efficacy of combined SBRT with new agents to improve the therapeutic outcomes in metastatic NSCLC as well as in oligometastatic disease.

6.1 Molecular targeted therapy in oligometastatic NSCLC

Patients with actionable tumor mutations have high response rates and long PFS times when treated with molecular targeted therapy [54–62]. However, progression inevitably occurs due to either insufficient CNS passage of the drug in some cases of CNS progression, or to acquired resistance with biological change in the tumor cells. The concept of oligoprogression supports the idea of disease progression due to the development of TKI-resistant clones with subsequent distant progression [65]. Different scenarios of progression in patients with actionable tumor mutations including oligoressistance, oligoreccurence or oligoprogression requiring consideration for local treatment. In the analysis of Guo et al. the majority of progressive disease on osimertinib was reported within residual lesions in initially involved sites, thus consolidative SBRT may prolong time to progression in a selected subgroup of patients [66]. In a retrospective study of Xu et al., 145 patients with oligometastatic EGFR-mutant NSCLC diagnosed from 2010 to 2016 were enrolled [67]. According to consolidative local treatment with surgery or radiotherapy, patients were grouped in three category, 51 in the all-local therapy group (consolidative to all residual disease, including primary tumor, lymph nodes, and metastatic sites), 55 in the part-local therapy group (consolidative to either primary tumor or oligometastatic sites), and 39 in the non-local therapy group (not receive any local therapy). Radiotherapy included standard-fractionation radiotherapy (60 Gy in 2-Gy fractions), aggressive palliation radiotherapy (45 Gy in 3-Gy fractions, a biologically equivalent dose of approximately 60 Gy) or stereotactic radiosurgery (SRS), with curative intent when possible. The median PFS in all-local, part-local, and non-local groups were 20.6, 15.6, and 13.9 months, respectively ($p < 0.001$). The median OS in all-local, part-local, and non-local groups were 40.9, 34.1, and 30.8 months, respectively ($p < 0.001$). The difference was significant between the all-local group and part-local or non-local group. The median OS was significantly better with consolidative local therapy for primary tumor (40.5 versus 31.5 months, $p < 0.001$), brain metastases (38.2 versus 29.2 months, $p < 0.002$), and adrenal metastases (37.1 versus 29.2 months, $p < 0.032$). Radiation toxicity was acceptable, included grade ≥ 3 pneumonitis (7.7%) and esophagitis (16.9%). No grade 5 toxicity was reported. A retrospective multi-institutional analysis by Magnuson et al. explored the optimal management of patients with EGFR-mutant NSCLC who developed brain metastases and have not received EGFR TKI [68]. A total of 351 patients from six institutions were included. Patients were treated with SRS followed by EGFR-TKI, WBRT followed by EGFR-TKI, or EGFR-TKI followed by SRS or WBRT at intracranial progression. The median OS for the SRS, WBRT, and EGFR-TKI cohorts was 46, 30 and 25 months, respectively ($P < .001$). On multivariable analysis, SRS versus EGFR-TKI, WBRT versus EGFR-TKI, age, performance status, EGFR exon 19 mutation, and absence of extracranial metastases were associated with improved OS. SRS followed by EGFR-TKI resulted in the longest OS and allowed patients to avoid the potential neurocognitive sequelae of WBRT.

In a retrospective analysis of Elamin et al. 129 patients with EGFR-mutant NSCLC who were treated with first-line TKI and 12 that were treated with TKI followed by local consolidation therapy were included [69]. Among the 12 patients treated with TKI plus local consolidative treatment, 8 patients had oligometastatic disease (defined as 3 metastases), and 4 patients had >3 metastases. Local consolidative treatment regimens were hypofractionated radiotherapy or SBRT for 11 patients and surgery for 1 patient. TKI followed by local consolidative treatment resulted in a significantly longer PFS (36 months) compared with TKI alone (14 months). Recently, Wang et al. presented an interim result of a randomized phase III, open-label clinical trial of first-line tyrosine kinase inhibitor with or without upfront local RT in patients with EGFR oligometastatic NSCLC [70]. From January 2016 to January 2019, 133 participants were enrolled, including 65 in the TKI arm who received standard of care TKI alone and 68 in the SBRT arm who received SBRT and TKI. At a median follow-up of 19.6 months, the median PFS for TKI alone was 12.5 months, and for TKI and SBRT was 20.20 months, respectively ($P < .001$). The median OS in the TKI alone arm was 17.40 months, and for TKI and SBRT arm was 25.50 months, respectively ($P < .001$).

Concerning the safety profile for combining EGFR or ALK TKI inhibitors and high dose RT, treatment was well tolerated and none of the available studies reported a significant increase in side effects [66–69]. To conclude, SBRT in combination with molecular targeted agents in actionable mutations NSCLC patients seem rationale for improving long-lasting disease control in synchronous oligometastatic oncogene addicted NSCLC patients; however no prospective data are available to confirm this.

6.2 Combining immunotherapy and radiotherapy

Immunotherapy with immune checkpoint inhibitors has revolutionized the management of stage IV NSCLC. In recent years, the blockade of programmed cell death 1 (PD-1) / programmed cell death ligand 1 (PD-L1) axis which served as a mechanism for tumor evasion of host tumor antigen-specific T-cell immunity, has demonstrated evident benefit in PFS and OS in metastatic and locally advanced NSCLC [61–64, 71, 72]. The indications for PD-1/PD-L1 blockade with immune checkpoint inhibitors (ICI) currently include most metastatic NSCLC patients without actionable tumor mutations, either as a single agent or combined with cytotoxic chemotherapy. The anti-PD-1/PD-L1 drugs approved at the moment for NSCLC are pembrolizumab, nivolumab, atezolizumab and durvalumab. Despite this paradigm shift, most patients present some kind of resistance to ICI, therefore arise the interest of researchers to combine multiple therapies. According to growing preclinical data describing mechanistic synergy between radiotherapy and immunotherapy, the most promising investigated combination is ICI with RT [73, 74]. Rational for combining radiotherapy and immunotherapy arises from the significant immune-stimulatory effects they both possess increasing the natural antitumor immune response through synergistic potentiation of an immunomodulatory effect [75, 76]. Increasing evidence indicates that cancer cells killed by radiation release tumor-associated antigens and immunoregulatory cytokines that serve as a kind of in situ vaccine against cancer [77, 78]. Cytokines also activate systemic tumor-specific immune response to eliminate tumor cells even outside the radiation field, so called abscopal effect [79]. This radiation-induced immune-mediated systemic antitumor phenomenon has high therapeutic potential, but is rare and relating to preclinical data more probable induced by high ablative doses, combined with checkpoint inhibitors [80, 81]. SBRT, through released neo-antigens and consequent maturation and proliferation of naive T-cells, and immunotherapy through activation and amplification of naive T-cells, may reciprocally potentiate each other amplification of T-cells-mediated tumoricidal effects [82–84]. Due to the lack of evidence, most "immunogenic" time sequencing of radio-immunotherapy and radiation dose-fractionation is not determined. Some data indicate that concurrent treatment or close sequencing of immunotherapy following radiotherapy may be the most effective [82]. However, according to data the radiation dose for the optimal antitumor immune response should be sub-tumoricidal. Several preclinical studies suggested that 8 to 10 Gy per fraction in 1–3 fractions represent optimal immunogenic dose [82–84].

Clinical interest for the combination of ICI and RT in NSCLC started to arise after the results of the KEYNOTE-001 study that enrolled progressive locally advanced or metastatic NSCLC [85]. A secondary analysis of the phase I trial revealed that of 97 included patients, 43% had been treated with RT prior to the administration of pembrolizumab. Those patients had significantly longer PFS (4.4 vs. 2.1 months) and OS (11.6 vs. 5.3 months) comparing patients with no RT. A single-arm phase 2 study of Bauml et al. included 45 patients with oligometastatic NSCLC with up to 4 metastatic sites [86]. Pembrolizumab was administered 4 to 12 weeks after prior comprehensive locally ablative therapy consisting of radiotherapy, chemoradiotherapy, surgery, or radiofrequency ablation, but most received ablative radiotherapy. Median PFS was 19.1 months, significantly greater than the historical median of 6.6 months (P = .005). OS at 12 months was 90.9% and at 24 months 77.5%. Even not conducted in oligometastatic NSCLC patients, the results of a multicetre, randomized phase 2 study (PEMBRO-RT) are interested. 92 patients were enrolled with advanced NSCLC after at least one regiment of chemotherapy with at least two metastases but upper limit was not specified [87]. Altogether, 76 patients were randomized to the pembrolizumab alone (control, 40 patients) or pembrolizumab after radiotherapy (3 fraction of 8 Gy) that was applied to a single metastatic site (experimental, 36 patients) to increase the likelihood of abscopal effect. The overall response rate at 12 weeks was 18% in the control arm vs. 36% in the experimental arm (P = .07). Median PFS was 1.9 months vs. 6.6 months (P = .19), and median OS was 7.6 months vs. 15.9 months (P = .16). Although a doubling of overall response rate was observed, the results did not meet the study's prespecified end point criteria for meaningful clinical benefit. Interestingly, subgroup analyses showed the largest benefit of radiotherapy in patients with PD-L1 – negative tumors. In a retrospective study of Samstein et al. 758 patients treated with ICI and RT were analyzed [88]. Median OS was 9 months in the entire cohort. Subanalysis regarding sequencing ICI and RT revealed increased OS in patients who received ICI and RT simultaneously. Median OS was 20 months for patients who started with ICI for at least 1 month before RT and continued throughout RT compared with 11 months for those that started ICI less than 30 days prior to RT and continued ICI throughout RT. In the cohort of patients who received concurrent therapy, hypofractionated radiotherapy (dose >4.00 Gy per fraction) and ICI greater than 30 days before RT was associated with improved OS.

Prospective data for management of patients with oligometastatic NSCLC in the era of immunooncology is scarce. Most of the available data on combining ICI and SBRT has been retrospective experiences on patients with metastatic NSCLC; however the benefit of combined treatment has been persistently demonstrated [89–91]. Importantly, the available data suggest that toxicity profile from the combination treatment has not increased in comparison to immunotherapy alone in the metastatic setting. A recent systematic review from prospective studies revealed grade ≥ 3 median toxicity rates of 14.5% with anti-PD-1/L1 plus SABR and 26% with anti-CTLA-4 plus SABR [92]. Concerning toxicity, no increased rates of immune-related adverse events using SBRT in the different organs or tissue types have been reported. However, reports from the studies that combined dual ICI therapy with SBRT in different cancers in prospective trials detected more toxicity.

In the future management of oligometastatic NSCLC patients, more questions should be answered. In the era of immunooncology, local treatment still presents the backbone of management with adding ICI to improve outcome of oligometastatic NSCLC patients. However, future prospective studies should give us answers to what sequence of local treatment and ICI is the most optimal combination, which radiation technique and fractionation would offer the best results, which patients should be selected for radical-intent treatment regarding biomarkers.

A great number of trials combining ICI and RT are ongoing. Regarding oligometastatic NSCLC, one is of particular interest, a randomized trial of consolidative immunotherapy with vs. without thoracic radiotherapy and/or SBRT after first-line systemic therapy for metastatic NSCLC comparing PFS as primary objective (NCT03867175).

7. Beyond progression: oligoprogression in NSCLC patients

An important growing subsegment of NSCLC patients is a group with oligoprogressive disease. With more effective systemic therapies that offer high response rates and long PFS times in patients with metastatic NSCLC, the oligoprogressive disease has become more and more common clinical scenario. Oligoprogressive disease, presented in oncogene driven NSCLC mostly occur due to the isolated emergence of well-described resistance mutations [65]. According to the literature, the occurrence of oligoprogression during TKI treatment seems to be quite frequent, reported in the range of 32–49% [17, 19, 20]. However, the optimal therapeutic approach in these patients is still unclear. Three main treatment options include changing systemic therapy, continuing the same systemic therapy beyond progression or using local therapy for eradicate the resistant clones while continuing the same systemic therapy [41]. The evidence supporting local treatment is limited to small retrospective reports. Weckhard et al. reported that 49% of ALK or EGFR positive metastatic NSCLC patients are treated with TKI presented with intracranial or extracranial oligoprogression suitable for local treatment [20]. Of 25 patients, 24 were treated with RT and one underwent surgery; however, 19 of 25 locally treated patients progressed again with PFS of 6.2 months. Yu et al. reported on 184 patients with EGFR mutation, of these 42 progressed with intracranial and 18 with extracranial oligometastases. These 18 were treated with local therapy, including surgery, radiofrequency ablation or RT with the median TTP of 10 months. Gan et al. reported on 33 ALK+NSCLC patients treated with crizotinib that had extracranial oligoprogression. Of these, 14 were suitable for local treatment with SBRT. Median overall time on crizotinib among those treated with SBRT versus those who progressed but were not suitable for SBRT was 28 and 10.1 months, respectively. Patients remaining on crizotinib for >12 months vs. ≤12 months had a 2 year OS of 72% vs. 12%, respectively ($p < 0.0001$) [93]. Xu et al. reported on 206 EGFR-mutant NSCLC patients included in the analysis of the survival benefit of adding local ablative therapy after oligoprogression during first-line TKI. With the median follow-up time of 42 months, the median PFS1, median PFS2 and median OS were 10.7 months, 18.3 months and 37.4 months, respectively. Survival rates of 1 year, 2 years and 3 years were 94.1%, 78.9%, and 54.7%, respectively. Altogether, the data suggest that local ablative treatment of progressive lesions in actionable mutations NSCLC patients can prolong treatment with first-line TKI without reported unacceptable excess toxicity. Moreover, despite the paucity and the heterogeneity of clinical data the use of local therapy in oligoprogressive oncogene driven NSCLC is already considered as standard clinical practice [94].

Currently, a few prospective randomized clinical trials are ongoing researching the benefit of local ablative treatment in oligoprogressive NSCLC. A Canadian trial, the STOP-NSCLC (NCT02756793) is a randomized phase II trial with estimated enrolment of 54 patients with oligoprogressive NSCLC during TKI or maintenance chemotherapy that evaluate either SBRT with continuation of current systemic agents or standard of care that may include continuation of current systemic agent, observation or switch to next-line treatment. Primary end-point will be PFS, while secondary end-points will be OS, local control, toxicity, quality of life and patterns of further progression. Similarly, European HALT study (NCT03256981) is a phase II/III, randomized study with question whether the use of SBRT to ≤3 sites of oligoprogressive disease in mutation positive advanced NSCLC patients with continuation of TKI improves PFS compared to continuation of TKI alone. The study aims to recruit 110 patients with oligoprogressive mutation positive advanced NSCLC following initial response to TKI. Third ongoing randomized trial is PROMISE-004 (NCT03808662) study with heterogeneous cohort including breast and NSCLC patients and estimated enrolment of 160 patients with either no targetable mutations upfront or targetable mutations after progression on first-line TKI. The purpose of the study is to evaluate the role of SBRT when metastatic lesions have just begun to grow with PFS as primary end-point.

In the context of immunotherapy in NSCLC patients, which includes the majority of lung cancer patients currently, tumor escape is not uncommon, but studies of oligoprogression are lacking. According to mechanism, oligoprogression might represent local immune tolerance due to stromal or tumor changes. Recently, in order to specify oligoprogression in NSCLC patients treated with immunotherapy, the results of a retrospective analysis of the failure pattern of 297 on ICI and 75 patients treated combined with chemotherapy and ICI were published [95]. Under ICI monotherapy in the first-line treatment, oligoprogression was more frequent (20% vs. 10%, $p < .05$), occurred later (median 11 vs. 5 months, $p < .01$) and affected fewer sites (mean 1.1 vs. 1.5, $p < .05$) compared to oligoprogression in patients treated with ICI monotherapy in later lines. Lymph nodes (42%, manly mediastinal) and the brain (39%) were mostly affected, followed by the lung (24%) and other organs. Compared to multifocal progression, oligoprogression occurred later (11 vs. 4 months, $p < .001$) and was associated with longer survival (26 vs. 13 months, $p < .001$) and higher tumor PD-L1 expression ($p < .001$). Chemoimmunotherapy showed a similar incidence of oligoprogression as ICI monotherapy (13% vs. 11% at 2 years). Local treatments were applied regularly for brain but only in 50% for extracranial lesions. However, oligoprogression in NSCLC patients is less common under ICI treatmnet than under TKI and its frequency descent with time. Few prospective trials evaluate the value of RT in oligoprogressive NSCLC treated with ICI, with one randomized phase II study designed to evaluate the effect of local consolidative RT to all sites of oligoprogressive disease in patients with metastatic NSCLC who have progressed through first-line systemic therapy containing an ICI (NCT04485026).

8. Conclusion

The number of patients with oligometastatic NSCLC has increased significantly over the last decade as well as the use of the locally ablative therapy to treat these patients. The evidence supporting this approach includes three randomized phase II clinical trials and substantial retrospective data; however, the inclusion criteria in these trials were mostly incomparable. Oligometastatic NSCLC has recently been defined by a consensus of multidisciplinary group of European thoracic oncology experts and this was the first step to unify future researching regarding diagnostic procedures and inclusion criteria. Recently, the therapeutic landscape of metastatic NSCLC has dramatically changed with the introduction of new systemic agents as molecular targeted and immunotherapy resulting in the prolonged survival and changing the field of oligometastatic framework significantly. A new concept that emerged with more effective systemic therapy is oligoprogression, frequently presents in patients treated with TKI. Additionally, combining radiotherapy and immunotherapy represent an increasing filed of interest due to synergistic potentiation of an immunomodulatory effect as a way to overcome the resistance of immunotherapy that exist in a substantial part of metastatic NSCLC patients. Especially for oligometastatic NSCLC patients, this integration might be meaningful due to a low tumor burden that seems to be one of the most important predictive factors for the benefit of SBRT-immunotherapy combination. In the future, further studies are needed to assess different treatment variables in order to optimize management of oligometastatic NSCLC in the way that the intent of treatment might not be just prolonged survival but cure.

Author details

Martina Vrankar
Institute of Oncology Ljubljana, Slovenia

*Address all correspondence to: mvrankar@onko-i.si

References

[1] Bray F, Ferlay J, Soerjomataram I, et al. Global cancer statistics 2018: GLOBOCAN estimates of incidence and mortality worldwide for 36 cancers in 185 countries. CA Cancer J Clin. 2018; 68: 394-424.

[2] Goldstraw P, Chansky K, Crowley J,et al. The IASLC Lung Cancer Staging Project: Proposal for Revision of the TNM Stage Groupings in the Forthcoming (Eight) Edition of the TNM Classification for Lung Cancer. J Thorac Oncol. 2016;11(1):39-51.

[3] Hellman S, Weichselbaum RR. Oligometastases. J Clin Oncol 1995; 13: 8-10.

[4] Torok JA, Gu L, Tandberg DJ, et al. Patterns of Distant Metastases After Surgical Management of Non-Small-cell Lung Cancer. Clin Lung Cancer. 2017; 18: e57-e70.

[5] Schanne DH, Heitmann J, Guckenberger M, et al. Evolution of treatment strategies for oligometastatic NSCLC patients – A systematic review of the literature. Cancer Treat Rev. 2019;80:101892

[6] Volpi S, Ali JM, Tasker A, et al. The role of positron emission tomography in the diagnosis, staging and response assessment on non-small cell lung cancer. Ann Transl Med. 2018;6(5):95

[7] Ashworth AB, Senan S, Palma DA, et al. An individual patient data metaanalysis of outcomes and prognostic factors after treatment of oligometastatic non-small cell lung cancer. Clin Lung Cancer 2014; 15: 346-355.

[8] Niibe Y, Hayakawa K. Oligometastases and oligo-recurrence: the new era of cancer therapy. Jpn J Clin Oncol 2010; 40: 107-111.

[9] Palma DA, Salama JK, Lo SS, et al. The oligometastatic state – separating truth from wishful thinking. Nat Rev Clin Oncol. 2014;11(9):549-57.

[10] Eberhardt WE, Mitchell A, Crowley J, et al. International Association for Study of Lung Cancer Staging and Prognostic Factors Committee, Advisory Board Members, and Participating Institutions. The IASLC Lung Cancer Staging Project: Proposals for the Revision of the M Descriptors in the Forthcoming Eighth Edition of the TNM Classification of Lung Cancer. J Thorac Oncol 2015; 10: 1515-1522.

[11] Dingemans AC, Hendriks LEL, Berghmans T, et al. Definition of Synchronous Oligometastatic Non-Small Cell Lung Cancer-A Consensus Report. J Thorac Oncol. 2019;14(12):2109-2119.

[12] Albain KS, Crowley JJ, LeBlanc M, et al. Survival determinants in extensive-stage non-small-cell lung cancer: the Southwest Oncology Group experience. J Clin Oncol. 1991;9(9):1618-26.

[13] Parikh RB, Cronin AM, Konozo DE, et al. Definitive primary therapy in patients presenting with oligometastatic non-small cell lung cancer. Int J Radiat Oncol Biol Phys. 2014;89(4):880-7.

[14] Rusthoven KE, Hammerman SF, Kavanagh BD, et al. Is there a role for consolidative stereotactic body radiation therapy following first-line systemic therapy for metastatic lung cancer? A patterns-of-failure analysis. Acta Oncol. 2009;48(4):578.83.

[15] Yano T, Okamoto T, Haro A, et al. Local treatment of oligometastatic recurrence in patients with resected non-small cell lung cancer. Lung Cancer. 2013;82(3):431-5.

[16] Camidge DR, Pao W, Sequist LV. Acquired resistance to TKIs in solid tumours: learning from lung cancer. Nat Rev Clin Oncol. 2014;11:473-481.

[17] Yoshida, K. Yoh, S. Niho S, et al. RECIST progression patterns during EGFR tyrosine kinase inhibitor treatment of advanced non-small cell lung cancer patients harboring an EGFRmutation. Lung Cancer. 2019;90:477-483.

[18] Doebele RC, Pilling AB, Aisner DL, et al. Mechanisms of resistance to crizotinib in patients with ALK gene rearranged non-small cell lung cancer. Clin Cancer Res. 2012;18(5):1472-82.

[19] Yu HA, Sima CS, Huang J, et al. Local therapy with continued EGFR tyrosine kinase inhibitor therapy as a treatment strategy in EGFR-mutant advanced lung cancers that have developed acquired resistance to EGFR tyrosine kinase inhibitors, J. Thorac. Oncol. 2013;8:346-351.

[20] Weickhardt AJ, Scheier B, Burke JM, et al. Local ablative therapy of oligoprogressive disease prolongs disease control by tyrosine kinase inhibitors in oncogene-addicted non-small-cell lung cancer. J Thorac Oncol. 2012;7(12):1807-1814.

[21] Hendriks LE, Derks JL, Postmus PE, et al. Single organ metastatic disease and local disease status, prognostic factors for overall survival in stage IV non-small cell lung cancer: Results from a population-based study. Eur J Cancer. 2015;51(17):2534-44.

[22] Li S, Zhu R, Li D, et al. Prognostic factors of oligometastatic non-small cell lung cancer: a meta-analysis. J Thorac Dis. 2018;10(6):3701-3713.

[23] Collaud S, Stahel R, Inci I, et al. Survival of patients treated surgically for synchronous single-organ metastatic NSCLC and advanced pathologic TN stage. Lung Cancer. 2012;78(3):234-8.

[24] Sheu T, Heymach JV, Swisher SG, et al. Propensity score-matched analysis of comprehensive local therapy for oligometastatic non-small-cell lung cancer that did not progress after front-line chemotherapy. Int J Radiat Oncol Biol Phys. 2014;90(4):850-7.

[25] Griffioen GH, Toguri D, Dahele M, et al. Radical treatment of synchronous oligometastatic non-small cell lung carcinoma (NSCLC): patient outcomes and prognostic factors. Lung Cancer. 2013;82(1):95-102.

[26] Lopez Guerra JL, Gomez D, Zhuang Y, et al. Prognostic impact of radiation therapy to the primary tumor in patients with non-small cell lung cancer and oligometastasis at diagnosis. Int J Radiat Oncol Biol Phys. 2012;84(1):e61-7.

[27] De Ruysscher D, Wanders R, van Baardwijk A, et al. Radical treatment of non-small-cell lung cancer patients with synchronous oligometastases: long-term results of a prospective phase II trial (Nct01282450). J Thorac Oncol. 2012;7(10);1547-55.

[28] Gomez DR, Blumenschein GR Jr, Lee JJ, et al. Local consolidative therapy versus maintenance therapy or observation for patients with oligometastatic non-small-cell lung cancer without progression after first-line systemic therapy: a multicentre, randomised, controlled, phase 2 study. The Lancet Oncol. 2016;17(12):1672-1682.

[29] Gomez DR, Tang C, Zhang J, et al. Local Consolidative Therapy Vs. Maintenance Therapy or Observation for Patients With Oligometastatic Non-Small-Cell Lung Cancer: Long-Term Results of a Multi-Institutional, Phase II, Randomized Study. J Clin Oncol. 2019;37(18):1558-1565.

[30] Lussier YA, Khodarev NN, Regan K, et al. Oligo- and polymetastatic progression in lung metastasis (es) patients is associated with specific microRNAs. PLoS One. 2012;7(12):e50141.

[31] Tanvetyanon T, Robinson LA, Schell MJ, et al. Outcomes of adrenalectomy for isolated synchronous versus metachronous adrenal metastases in non-small-cell lung cancer: a systematic review and pooled analysis. J Clin Oncol. 2008;26(7):1142-7.

[32] Porte H, Siat J, Guibert B, et al. Resection of adrenal metastases from non-small-cell lung cancer: a multicentre study. Ann Thorac Surg. 2001;71(3):981-5.

[33] Ambrogi V, Tonini G, Mineo TC. Prolonged survival after extracranial metastasectomy from synchronous resectable lung cancer. Ann Surg Oncol. 2001;8(8):663-6.

[34] Collen C, Christian N, Schallier D, et al. Phase II study of stereotactic body radiotherapy to primary tumor and metastatic locations in oligometastatic non-small-cell lung cancer patients. Ann Oncol. 2014;25(10):1954-1959.

[35] Congedo MT, Cesario A, Lococo F, et al. Surgery for oligometastatic non-small cell lung cancer: long-term results from a single center experience. J Thorac Cardiovasc Surg. 2012;144(2):444-52.

[36] Fleckenstein J, Petroff A, Schäfers HJ, et al. Long-term outcomes in radically treated synchronous vs. metachronous oligometastatic non-small-cell lung cancer. BMC Cancer. 2016;16:348.

[37] Inoue T, Katoh N, Aoyama H, et al. Clinical outcomes of stereotactic brain and/or body radiotherapy for patients with oligometastatic lesions. Jpn J Clin Oncol. 2010;40(8):788-94.

[38] Iyengar P, Wardak Z, Gerber DE, et al. Consolidative Radiotherapy for Limited Metastatic Non-Small-Cell Lung Cancer: A Phase 2 Randomized Clinical Trial. JAMA Oncol. 2018;4(1):e173501.

[39] Palma DA, Olson R, Harrow S, et al. Stereotactic ablative radiotherapy versus standard of care palliative treatment in patients with oligometastatic cancers (SABR-COMET): a randomised, phase 2, open-label trial. Lancet. 2019;393(10185):2051-2058.

[40] Palma DA, Olson R, Harrow S, et al. Stereotactic Ablative adiotherapy for the Comprehensive Treatment of Oligometastatic Cancers: Long-Term Results of the SABR-COMET Phase II Randomized Trial. J Clin Oncol. 2020;38(25):2830-2838.

[41] Planchard D, Popat S, Kerr K, et al. Metastatic non-small cell lung cancer: ESMO Clinical Practice Guidelines for diagnosis, treatment and follow-up. Updated version published 15 September 2020 by the ESMO Guidelines Committee. Originally published in 2018 – Ann Oncol (2018) 29(Suppl 4): iv192–iv237.

[42] Postmus PE, Kerr KM, Oudkerk M, et al. Early and Locally Advanced Non-Small-Cell Lung Cancer (NSCLC) Treatment Recommendations. Updated version published 04 May 2020 by the ESMO Guidelines Committee. Originally published in 2017 – Ann Oncol 2017;28(suppl 4):iv1-iv21.

[43] NCCN Guidelines. NSCLC version 7.2019. Available at: https://www.nccn.org/professionls/physician_gls/pdf/nscl.pdf (Accessed September 2020)

[44] Plönes T, Osei-Agyemang T, Krohn A, et al. Surgical Treatment of Extrapulmonary Oligometastatic Non-Small Cell Lung Cancer. Indian J Surg. 2015;77(Suppl 2):216-220.

[45] Videtic GMM, Donington J, Giuliani M, et al. Stereotactic body radiation therapy for early-stage non-small cell lung cancer: Executive Summary of an ASTRO Evidence-Based Guideline. Pract Radiat Oncol. 2017;7(5):295-301.

[46] Chmura SJ, Winter K, Salama JK, et al. Phase I trial of stereotactic body radiation therapy (SBRT) to multiple metastatic sites: a NRG oncology study. Int J Radiat Oncol Biol Phys. 2018;102(03):S68-S69.

[47] Klement RJ, Hoerner-Rieber J, Adebahr S, et al. Stereotactic body radiotherapy (SBRT) for multiple pulmonary oligometastases: Analysis of number and timing of repeat SBRT as impact factors on treatment safety and efficacy. Radiother Oncol. 2018;127(2):246-252.

[48] Cheung P. Stereotactic body radiotherapy for oligoprogressive cancer. Br J Radiol. 2016;89(1066):20160251.

[49] Merino Lara T, Helou J, Poon I, et al. Multisite stereotactic body radiotherapy for metastatic non-small-cell lung cancer: Delaying the need to start or change systemic therapy? Lung cancer. 2018;124:219-226.

[50] Tsao MN, Ven LI, Cheung P, et al. Stereotactic Body Radiation Therapy for Extracranial Oligometastatic Non-small-cell Lung Cancer: A Systematic Review. Clin Lung Cancer. 2020;21(2):95-105.e1

[51] Timmerman RD, Herman J, Cho LC. Emergence of stereotactic body radiation therapy and its impact on current and future clinical practice. J Clin Oncol. 2014;32(26):2847-54.

[52] Mok TS, Wu YL, Thongprasert S, et al. Gefitinib or carboplatin-paclitaxel in pulmonary adenocarcinoma. N Engl J Med. 2009;361(10):947-57.

[53] Han JY, Park K, Kim SW, et al. First-SIGNAL: first-line single-agent iressa versus gemcitabine and cisplatin trial in never-smokers with adenocarcinoma of the lung. J Clin Oncol. 2012;30(10):1122-8.

[54] Maemondo M, Inoue A, Kobayashi K, et al. Gefitinib or chemotherapy for non-small-cell lung cancer with mutated EGFR. N Engl J Med. 2010;362(25):2380-8.

[55] Rosell R, Carcereny E, Gervais R, et al. Erlotinib versus standard chemotherapy as first-line treatment for European patients with advanced EGFR mutation-positive non-small-cell lung cancer (EURTAC): a multicentre, open-label, randomised phase 3 trial. Lancet Oncol. 2012;13(3):239-46.

[56] Sequist LV, Yang JC, Yamamoto N, et al. Phase III study of afatinib or cisplatin plus pemetrexed in patients with metastatic lung adenocarcinoma with EGFR mutations. J Clin Oncol. 2013;31(27):3327-34.

[57] Camidge DR, Bang YJ, Kwak EL, et al. Activity and safety of crizotinib in patients with ALK-positive non-small-cell lung cancer: updated results from a phase 1 study. Lancet Oncol. 2012;13(10):1011-9.

[58] Shaw AT, Yeap BY, Solomon BJ, et al. Effect of crizotinib on overall survival in patients with advanced non-small-cell lung cancer harbouring ALK gene rearrangement: a retrospective analysis. Lancet Oncol. 2011;12(11):1004-12.

[59] Solomon BJ, Mok T, Kim DW, et al. First-line crizotinib versus chemotherapy in ALK-positive lung cancer. N Engl J Med. 2014;371(23):2167-77.

[60] Soria JC, Tan DSW, Chiari R, et al. First-line ceritinib versus platinum-based chemotherapy in advanced ALK-rearranged non-small-cell lung

cancer (ASCEND-4): a randomised, open-label, phase 3 study. Lancet. 2017;389(10072):917-929.

[61] Reck M, Rodriguez-Abreu D, Robinson AG, et al. Updated Analysis of KEYNOTE-024: Pembrolizumab Versus Platinum-Based Chemotherapy for Advanced Non-Small-Cell Lung Cancer With PD-L1 Tumor Proportion Score of 50% or Greater. J Clin Oncol. 2019;37(7):537-546.

[62] Gandhi L, Rodriguez-Abreu D, Gadgeel S, et al. Pembrolizumab plus Chemotherapy in Metastatic Non-Small-Cell Lung Cancer. N Engl J Med. 2018;378(22):2078-2092.

[63] Paz-Ares L, Luft A, Vicente D, et al. Pembrolizumab plus Chemotherapy for Squamous Non-Small-Cell Lung Cancer. N Engl J Med. 2018:379(21):2040-2051.

[64] Hellmann MD, Ciuleanu TE, Pluzanski A, et al. Nivolumab plus Ipilimumab in Lung Cancer with a High Tumor Mutational Burden. N Engl J Med. 2018;378(22):2093-2104.

[65] Basler L, Kroeze SG, Guckenberger M. SBRT for oligoprogressive oncogene addicted NSCLC. Lung Cancer. 2017; 106:50-57.

[66] Guo T, Ni J, Yang X, et al. Pattern of Recurrence Analysis in Metastatic EGFR-Mutant NSCLC Treated with Osimertinib: Implications for Consolidative Stereotactic Body Radiation Therapy. Int J Rad Oncol Biol Phys. 2020;107(1):62-71.

[67] Xu Q, Zhou F, Liu H, et al. Consolidative Local Ablative Therapy Improves the Survival of Patients With Synchronous Oligometastatic NSCLC Harboring EGFR Activating Mutation Treated With First-Line EGFR-TKIs. J Thorac Oncol. 2018;13(9):1383-1392.

[68] Magnuson WJ, Lester-Coll NH, Wu AJ, et al. Management of Brain Metastases in Tyrosine Kinase Inhibitor-Naïve Epidermal Growth Factor Receptor-Mutant Non-Small-Cell Lung Cancer: A Retrospective Multi-Institutional Analysis. J Clin Oncol. 2017;35(10):1070-1077.

[69] Elamin YY, Gomez DR, Antonoff MB, et al. Local Consolidation Therapy (LCT) After First Line Tyrosine Kinase Inhibitor (TKI) for Patients With EGFR Mutant Metastatic Mutant Non-small-cell Lung Cancer (NSCLC). Clin Lung Cancer. 2019;20(1):43-47.

[70] Wang X, Zeng M. First-line tyrosine kinase inhibitor with or without aggressive upfront local radiation therapy in patients with EGFRm oligometastatic non-small cell lung cancer: interim results of a randomized phase III, open-label clinical trial (SINDAS) (NCT02893332). J Clin Oncol. 2020;38(suppl 15):9508.

[71] Antonia SJ, Villegas A, Daniel D, et al. Durvalumab after Chemoradiotherapy in Stage III Non-Small-Cell Lung Cancer. N Engl J Med. 2017;377(20):1919-1929.

[72] Antonia SJ, Villegas A, Daniel D, et al. Overall Survival with Durvalumab after Chemoradiotherapy in Stage III NSCLC. N Engl J Med. 2018;379(24):2342-2350.

[73] Deng L, Liang H, Burnette B, et al. Irradiation and anti-PD-L1 treatment synergistically promote antitumor immunity in mice. J Clin Invest. 2014;124(2):687-95.

[74] Lugade AA, Moran JP, Gerber SA, et al. Local radiation therapy of B16 melanoma tumors increases the generation of tumor antigen-specific effector cells that traffic to the tumor. J Immunol. 2005;174(12):7516-23.

[75] Gupta A, Probst HC, Vuong V, et al. Radiotherapy promotes

tumor-specific effector CD8+ T cells via dendritic cell activation. J Immunol. 2012;189(2):558-66.

[76] Deng L, Liang H, Xu M, et al. STING-Dependent Cytosolic DNA Sensing Promotes Radiation-Induced Type I Interferon-Dependent Antitumor Immunity in Immunogenic Tumors. Immunity. 2014;41(5):843-52.

[77] Tang C, Wang X, Soh H, et al. Combining radiation and immunotherapy: a new systemic therapy for solid tumors? Cancer Immunol Res. 2014;2(9):831-8.

[78] Demaria S, Golden EB, Formenti SC. Role of Local Radiation Therapy in Cancer Immunotherapy. JAMA Oncol. 2015;1(9):1325-32.

[79] Abuodeh Y, Venkat P, Kim S. Systematic review of case reports on the abscopal effect. Curr Probl Cancer. 2016;**40**(1):25-37

[80] Weichselbaum RR, Liang H, Deng L, et al. Radiotherapy and immunotherapy: a beneficial liaison? Nat Rev Clin Oncol. 2017;14(6);365-379.

[81] Ngwa W, Irabor OC, Schoenfeld JD, et al. Using immunotherapy to boost the abscopal effect. Nat Rev Cancer. 2018;18(5):313-322.

[82] Buchwald ZS, Wynne J, Nasti TH, et al. Radiation, Immune Checkpoint Blockade and the Abscopal Effect: A Critical Review on Timing, Dose and Fractionation. Front Oncol. 2018;8:612.

[83] Twyman-Saint Victor C, Rech AJ, Maity A, et al. Radiation and dual checkpoint blockade activate non-redundant immune mechanisms in cancer. Nature. 2015;520(7547);373-7.

[84] Dovedi SJ, Adlard AL, Lipowska-Bhalla G, et al. Acquired resistance to fractionated radiotherapy can be overcome by concurrent PD-L1 blockade. Cancer Res. 2014;74(19):5458-68.

[85] Shaverdian N, Lisberg AE, Bornazyan K, et al. Previous radiotherapy and the clinical activity and toxicity of pembrolizumab in the treatment of non-small-cell lung cancer: a secondary analysis of the KEYNOTE-001 phase 1 trial. Lancet Oncol. 2017;18(7);895-903.

[86] Bauml JM, Mick R, Ciunci C, et al. Pembrolizumab After Completion of Locally Ablative Therapy for Oligometastatic Non-Small Cell Lung Cancer: A Phase 2 Trial. JAMA Oncol. 2019;5(9):1283-90.

[87] Theelen WSME, Peulen HMU, Lalezari F, et al. Effect of Pembrolizumab After Stereotactic Body Radiotherapy vs Pembrolizumab Alone on Tumor Response in Patients With Advanced Non-Small Cell Lung Cancer: Results of the PEMBRO-RT Phase 2 Randomized Clinical Trial. JAMA Oncol. 2019;5(9):1276-82.

[88] Samstein R, Rimner A, Barker CA, et al. Combined Immune Checkpoint Blockade and Radiation Therapy: Timing and Dose Fractionation Associated with Greatest Survival Duration Among Over 750 Treated Patients. Int J Radiat Oncol Biol Phys. 2017;99(2):S129-S130.

[89] Chen L, Douglass J, Kleinberg L, et al. Concurrent Immune Checkpoint Inhibitors and Stereotactic Radiosurgery for Brain Metastases in Non-Small Cell Lung Cancer, Melanoma, and Renal Cell Carcinoma. Int J Radiat Oncol Biol Phys. 2018;100(4):916-925.

[90] Verma V, Cushman TR, Selek U, et al. Safety of Combined Immunotherapy and Thoracic Radiation Therapy: Analysis of 3 Single-Institutional Phase I/II Trials. Int J Radiat Oncol Biol Phys. 2018;101(5):1141-1148.

[91] Schapira E, Hubbeling H, Yeap BY, et al. Improved Overall Survival and Locoregional Disease Control With Concurrent PD-1 Pathway Inhibitors and Stereotactic Radiosurgery for Lung Cancer Patients With Brain Metastases. Int J Radiat Oncol Biol Phys. 2018;101(3):624-629.

[92] Chicas-Sett R, Morales-Orue I, Castilla-Martinez J, et al. Stereotactic Ablative Radiotherapy Combined with Immune Checkpoint Inhibitors Reboots the Immune Response Assisted by Immunotherapy in Metastatic Lung Cancer: A Systematic Review. Int J Mol Sci. 2019;20(9):2173.

[93] Gan GN, Weickhardt AJ, Scheier B, et al. Stereotactic radiation therapy can safely and durably control sites of extra–central nervous system oligoprogressive disease in anaplastic lymphoma kinase-positive lung cancer patients receiving crizotinib. Ini J Radiat Oncol Biol Phys. 2014;88:892-898.

[94] Franceschini D, De Rose F, Cozzi S, et al. The use of radiation therapy for oligoprogressive/oligopersistant oncogene-driven non-small cell lung cancer: State of the art. Crit Rev Oncol Hematol. 2020;148:102894.

[95] Rheinheimer S, Heussel CP, Mayer P, et al. Oligoprogressive Non-Small-Cell Lung Cancer under Treatment with PD-(L)1 Inhibitors. Cancers (Basel). 2020;12(4):1046.

Chapter 9

Bone Metastases in Lung Cancer

Ana C. Belzarena

Abstract

Lung cancer patients frequently present with to bone metastases. Such lesions are responsible for increased morbidity, low quality of life, and increased costs to patients and the health care system. Pain is the most common symptom; however, these lesions also present as skeletal related events (SRE) which include pathological fractures, hypercalcemia, spinal cord and nerve compressions and cause the need for surgery and/or radiotherapy. Even though bone metastases are associated with poor prognosis, current treatment multimodalities continue to improve survival. Awareness and effective treatment of these lesions is paramount to maintain a good quality of life and function in lung cancer patients.

Keywords: bone metastases, lung cancer, diagnosis, treatment

1. Introduction

Lung cancer is the second most common cancer, for both genders. More than 235.000 new cases are expected to occur this year in the United States only. Additionally, this disease is also expected to cause more than 130.000 deaths yearly, being responsible for a fourth of the cancer fatalities in this country as well [1]. Lung cancer has different subtypes, the most frequent being Non-small cell lung cancer (NSCLC) which includes adenocarcinoma, squamous cell carcinoma and large cell carcinoma; those comprise 80% of the lung cancer cases [2].

This disease tends to have an asymptomatic presentation, leading to many of these patients presenting at a later stage with disease already spread to other sites [3]. Bone metastases occur when the tumor has spread from its original site, the lung, to bones. This event occurs via blood stream or lymphatic pathways [4]. Bone seeding is more frequent in the trunk bones due to a richer bone marrow, vast in blood vessels [5]. Prostate, breast and lung are the most common cancers to cause bone secondary disease [6]. Within the subtypes of lung cancer, adenocarcinoma is the subtype with the highest incidence of bone lesions [7]. Additionally, bone is the third most common site of spread for most cancers after lung and liver [8]. Likewise, bone metastases can be the initial presentation of an occult lung cancer. Occult primary malignancies occur in 4% of the cancer patients [9].

Obvious bone lesions are found in about 36% of these patients, while micro-metastasis in up to 60% of the lung cancer population [4]. An increased number of bone lesions is a reflection of more aggressive disease and as such is associated with decreased survival and a poor prognosis [10].

2. Clinical presentation

The axial bones are the most frequent location of bone lesions, the vertebral bodies being the most common followed by ribs, pelvis and calvarium (**Figure 1**) [7]. Less than 1% of bone lesions are present below the elbow or distal to the knee, but when those, also known as acral metastases, are present 44% are originated in the lung (**Figure 2**). Acral metastases are associated with a poor prognosis [11]. Bone metastases are known to cause pain and several other complications such as pathologic fractures, hypercalcemia, spinal cord and nerve compressions and cause the requirement for surgery and/or radiotherapy, all of these are known as skeletal related events (SRE) [4, 12]. Bone pain is present in about 80% of lung cancer patients at some point during their disease [4]. Approximately 10–30% of lung cancer patients will suffer a pathological fracture, fact that worsens survival times compared to patients without a fracture (**Figure 3**) [13, 14]. SREs are more likely to occur after a prior SRE has taken place [15]. More than half of these patients will suffer at least one SRE which will cause morbidity, will impair function and quality of life along with increased costs to the patient and health care system [16, 17]. On average patients suffer a SRE every 3 to 6 months, usually in periods of progression of their disease [4].

Hypercalcemia is a frequent SRE, present in one in eight patients, and oftentimes can be potentially life-threatening if untreated [18]. Hypercalcemia can occur associated with bone lesions or not; in the latter scenario it is due to an imbalance of

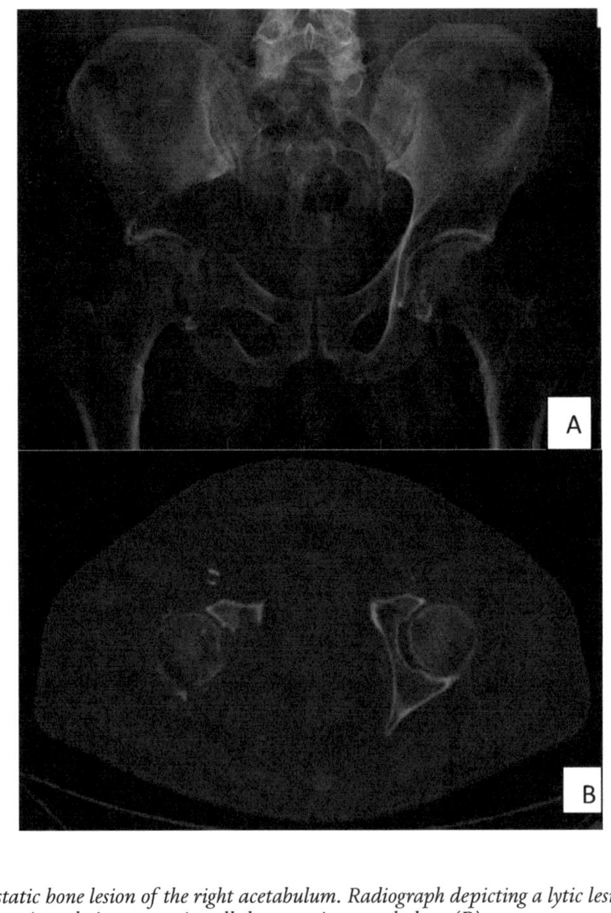

Figure 1.
Lung cancer metastatic bone lesion of the right acetabulum. Radiograph depicting a lytic lesion (A) and axial CT image demonstrating a lesion occupying all the posterior acetabulum (B).

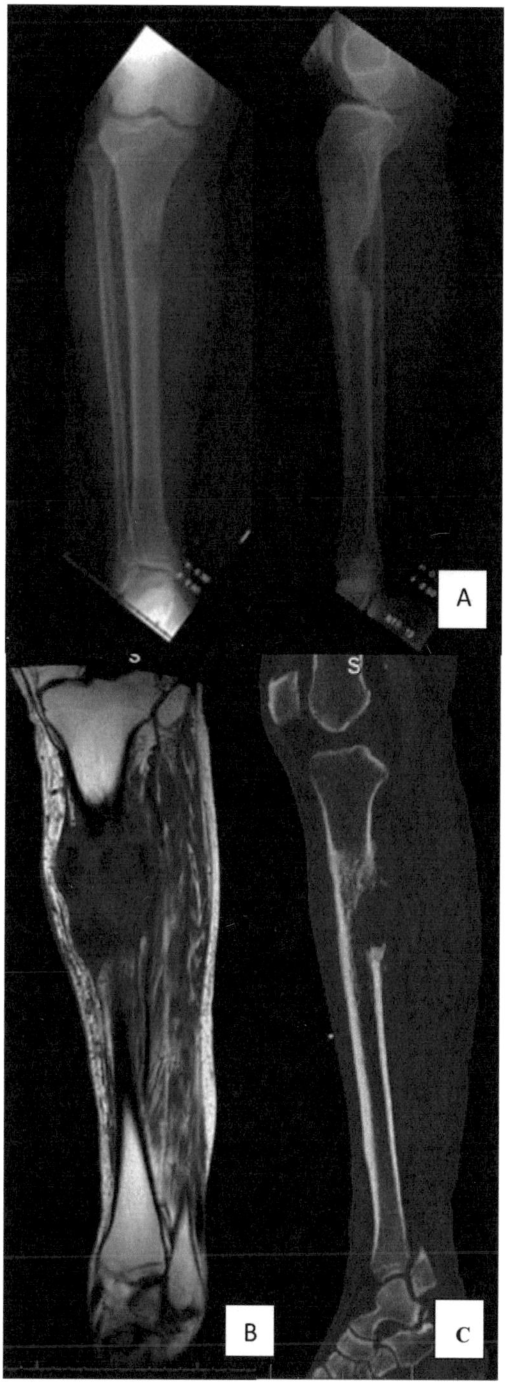

Figure 2.
Distal bone metastasis on a lung cancer patient. Radiograph image demonstrating a lytic lesion in the proximal tibia, anterior–posterior and lateral view (A). MRI image, T1-sequence depicting a low signal lesion with interior necrosis (B). Sagittal view of CT scan image depicting the lytic lesion and soft tissue extension to the posterior compartment of the leg (C).

factors such as PTHrP and interleukin-1 among others that induce bone resorption [19]. Symptoms include nausea and vomiting, anorexia, fatigue, polyuria and polydipsia, and later on seizures, arrhythmia, ileus and even coma. Aggressive hydration and bisphosphonates are the treatment of choice [20].

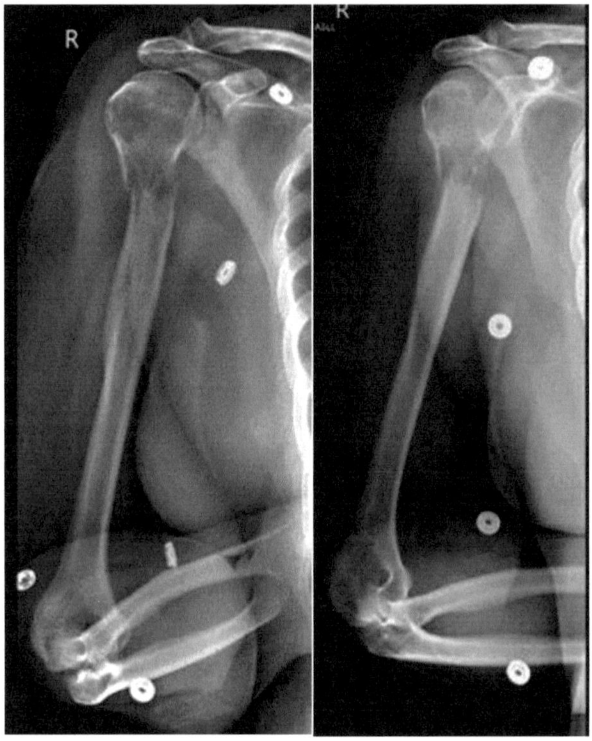

Figure 3.
Radiographic images, anterior–posterior and lateral of proximal right humerus lytic lesion and pathological fracture in a lung cancer patient.

3. Imaging studies

Obtaining dedicated imaging studies is indicated at initial staging or when a patient presents with symptoms such as bone pain. Radiographs are usually obtained as initial exam in the case of symptomatic patients to assess for bone lesions or a pathological fracture. Radiographs are considered of low sensitivity to detect bone lesions since more than 50% of the bone needs to be compromised to be clearly seen on plain films [21]. Lung cancer presents predominately with lytic lesions, although sclerotic and mixed have been described [21, 22]. Additionally, plain films are of low sensitivity to monitor response since it takes 3–6 months for a good response, new bone formation and sclerosis, to be visible [23]. CT scans are more sensitive and depict better resolution of bone trabeculae and cortical bone as well as better definition of sclerotic lesions and bone marrow lesions when present [24]. Usually not obtained as single bone study but rather as part of whole-body staging exams. MRI images in lung cancer patients are usually reserved for the study of the spine vertebral bodies and the potential involvement of the surrounding structures such as spinal cord and nerve roots due to tumor extension [25]. An alternative to assess bone lesions in the entire skeleton is bone scintigraphy, which is usually easily available (**Figure 4**). Bone scintigraphy has high sensitivity and can detect lesions earlier than observed in plan radiographs, however it is unspecific and has a high rate of false positives [26].

PET CT scans are widely used to stage patients and assess treatment response. This study produces high resolution images and detects increased metabolic activity for example in oncologic lesions (**Figure 5**). It has good sensitivity and specificity for metastatic spread diagnosis, allows for the assessment of visceral lesions at the same time and is able to detect bone lesions early [22, 27].

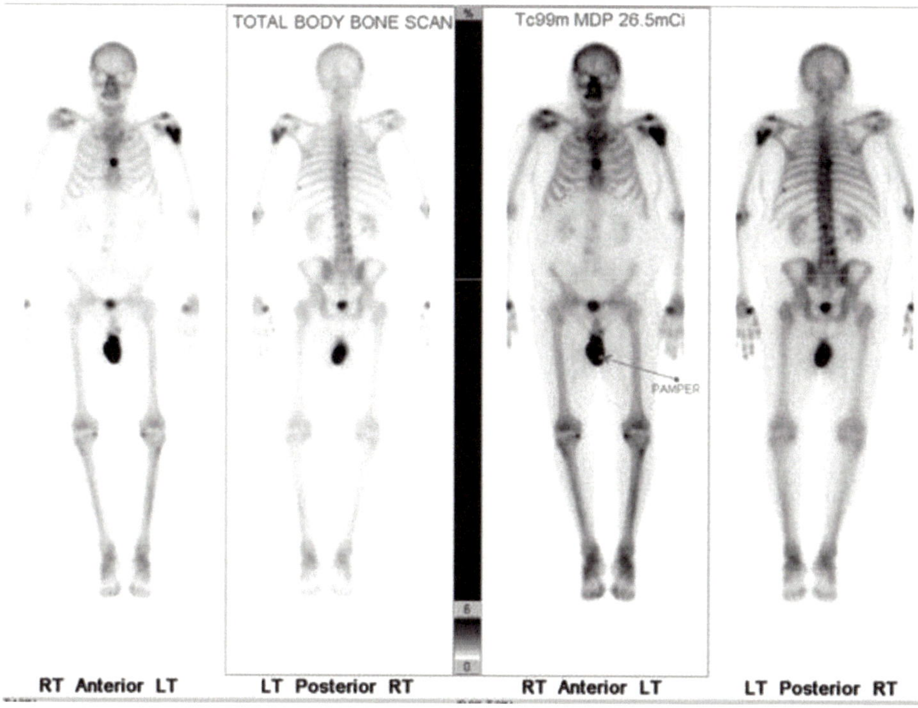

Figure 4.
Bone scintigraphy study with Tecnecium-99 depicting a lesion in the proximal left humerus and sternum.

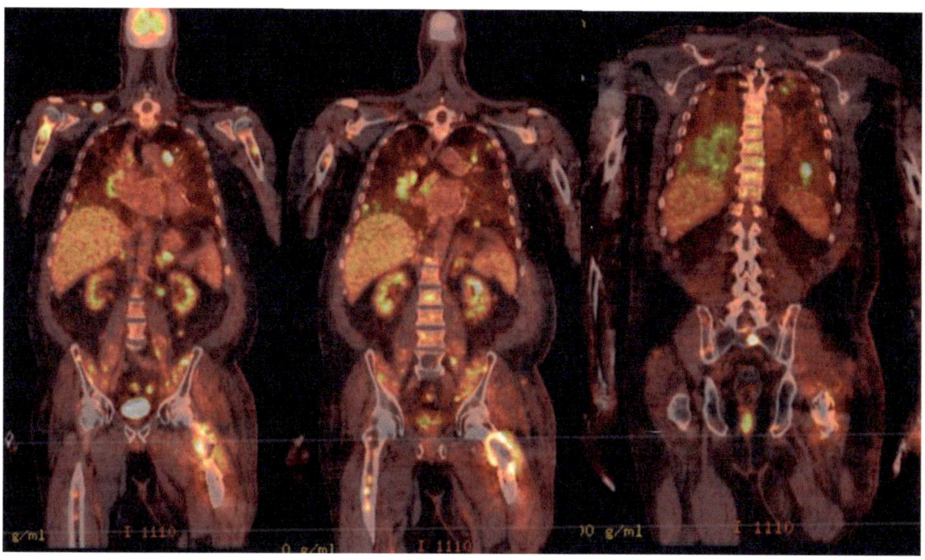

Figure 5.
PET CT images of a lung cancer patient demonstrating several metastatic lesions including the proximal left femur, right femur, proximal right humerus and spine among others.

4. Treatment

Treatment for bone lesions secondary to lung cancer can be divided in systemic and local therapies. The first line of treatment used to be Platinum-based chemotherapy, applied in 4 to 6 cycles followed by a period of observation [28]. Research progress has led to the unveiling of potential new molecular abnormalities passible of targeting treatment, it is estimated that almost 70% of patients with advanced disease may present some of these targetable aberrations [29]. Systemic cancer-directed therapy is discussed in depth in other chapters of this book. In terms of systemic anti bone-resorption-treatments the current recommendations are for the administration of either bisphosphonates or Denosumab [30]. These drugs interfere with the vicious cycle where osteoclasts are stimulated due to an imbalance in local factors produced by the invading tumor cells, leading to a disbalance in the normal bone remodeling process, continuous bone resorption, lytic lesions, bone weakening and eventually a pathological fracture [31]. Inhibitors of bone resorption are known to relief pain, prevent and delay SREs, decrease the number of pathological fractures, have anti-tumor activity by inhibiting tumor cell growth and stimulation programmed cell death; and are the treatment for hypercalcemia as well [32, 33]. Common side effects associated to these drugs are nephrotoxicity, gastrointestinal discomfort and osteonecrosis of the jaw, physician and renal function monitoring are recommended [34].

Local treatments include radiation to the lesion and surgery. Radiotherapy it is used in the setting of bone metastatic spread as a palliative measure to control pain, prevent the progression of lesions into a pathological fracture of limbs, to control lesions locally, prophylactically and therapeutically for spinal cord compression [35]. Dose recommendations and delivery schedules vary and may range from a single fraction with a dose of 8 Gy to higher doses like 30 Gy in 8 to 10 fractions. Most patients achieve pain relief if not a complete response generally occurring in the first 2 weeks of treatment [36]. Bone response when present can be observed 3 to 6 weeks from the end of treatment and the maximum effect is detected after 6 months [37].

Surgery has a narrower indication spectrum in patients with metastatic lung cancer, usually being indicated for pathological or impending fractures, to maintain function and good quality of life and to prevent neurological damage. A bone lesion requiring surgery is an indication of a poorer prognosis on itself, thus the decision of proceeding with surgery and the type of surgery must be contrasted with the complications and the recovery time each procedure will entail. Prior studies have shown that 10% of the patients die within a month of the procedure and almost 80% do so within a year [13]. However, a more recent study has shown that if the patient has a good response to new biologic drug therapies, the one-year survival improves to over 60% making relevant the consideration for more durable orthopedic implants [38].

Surgical treatment of bone lesions of the limbs in general involve fixating the bone with either plates and screws or an intramedullary device. Additionally, in cases where the lesion is more advanced and near a joint, treatment involves resecting the bone and replacing it with an endoprosthetic implant. Each procedure has its own rates of complications and its own rates of hardware failure. Implants may fail for different reasons the most common being disease progression and mechanical fatigue, both are time and disease dependent factors that the surgeon must consider when choosing the most appropriate procedure. Ideally these patients are identified prior to fracture occurrence and a prophylactic fixation can be performed. A simple mechanism to identify impending fractures is through the Mirel's score which considers the characteristics of the patient's pain and the characteristics of the lesion on radiographic images (location, type of lesion, degree of extension) assigning each item a value and the ultimate sum will dictate the treatment between observation and an indication for prophylactic fixation [39]. Likewise, an alternative is the Harrington criteria that considers the size of the lesion, the percentage of cortical destruction, the presence of pain after radiation and the pathologic avulsion of the lesser trochanter to suggest prophylactic fixation of the lesion [40]. Surgical intervention prior to the actual fracture, when indicated, has shown shorter hospital stay, decreased requirements for blood transfusion as well as improved functional outcomes [41, 42]. For femur diaphyseal lesions causing symptoms for an impending pathological fracture, the treatment of choice is a load-sharing intramedullary nail (**Figure 6**). For more extensive lesions where there is soft tissue extension of the bone lesion fixating the bone with plate and screws or a nail can be associated with curettage of the lesion and cement augmentation (**Figure 7**). Additionally, in case where the patient is identified late and there is extensive bone destruction located near a joint, bone resection and replacement may be indicated (**Figure 8**).

A very important aspect of the treatment of these patients, oftentimes forgotten or not given its rightful importance, is pain control. Most patients with metastatic bone cancer will experience moderate to severe pain at some point of their disease [4]. Moreover, pain originating in bones is the most common type of pain these patients experience at may at times seem exaggerated to the actual lesion

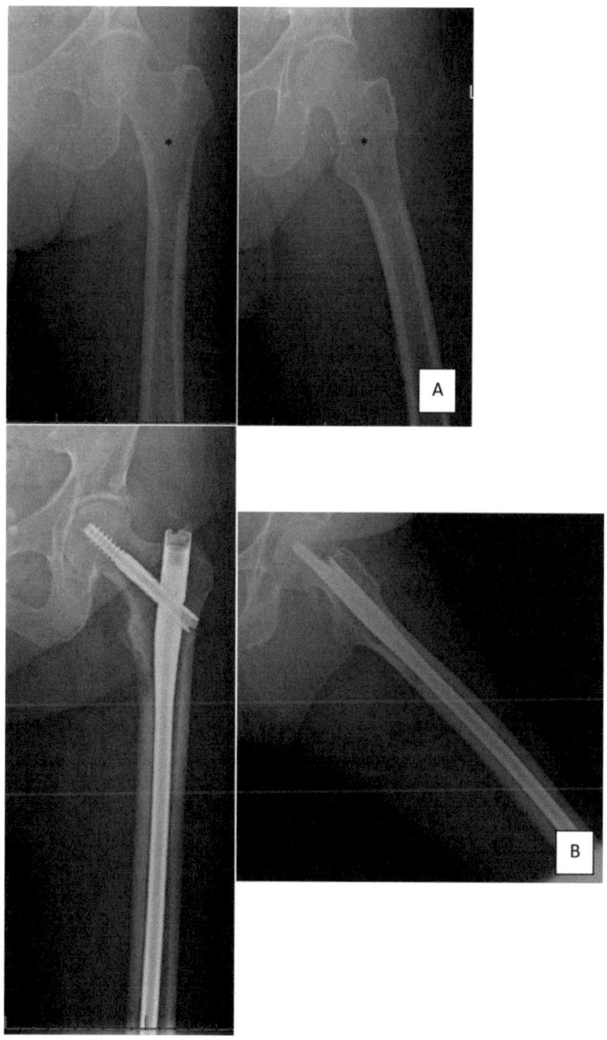

Figure 6.
Lung cancer patient with a lesion in the proximal femur (*) causing symptoms concerning for an impending fracture (A). The patient was treated with prophylactic fixation with an intramedullary long nail (B).

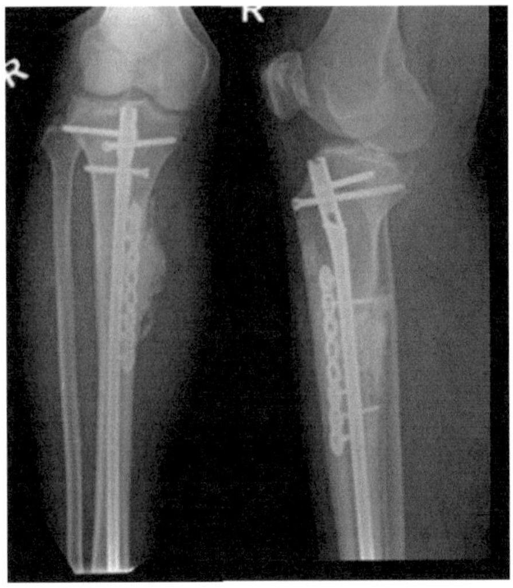

Figure 7.
Lung cancer patient had an extensive lesion in proximal tibia with soft tissue extension. The bone was fixated with a nail and plate and screws with curettage of lesion and cement augmentation. The patient had postoperative radiation of the leison as well.

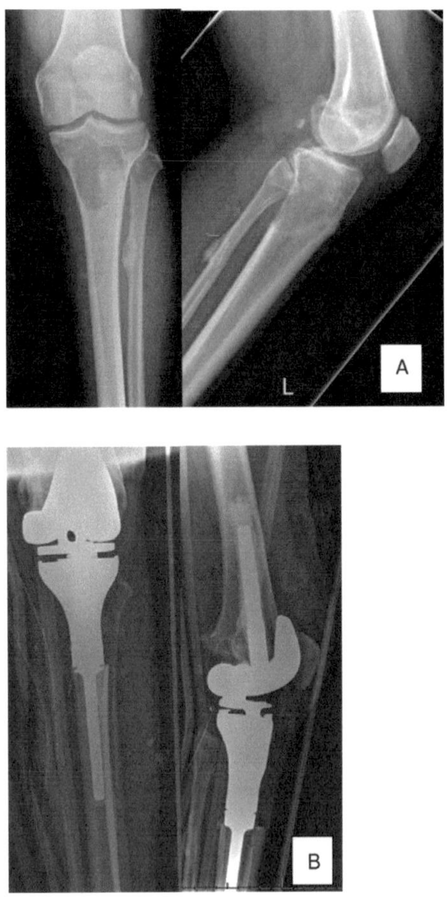

Figure 8.
Patient presented with an extensive proximal tibia lesion close to the knee joint (A). Bone resection and a proximal tibia replacement was performed (B).

proportion [43]. Pain derived from bone metastases is felt as dull, constant and increasing in intensity [43]. This more chronic type of pain is replaced by a more intense and severe pain, breakthrough pain, which is also more difficult to control. Breakthrough pain can occur spontaneously or associated with weight bearing of an affected extremity [44]. It is extremely high in intensity, last for only a few minutes but can repeat itself several times a day, thus can severely affect the function and life quality of the patient [45]. Since the pain mechanisms in bone metastases originated pain are multiple, so are the treatment modalities. Systemic and local therapy such as radiation to a specific lesion may help alleviate the pain by decreasing disease activity and lesion progression [46]. Analgesic treatment is according to the World Health Organization ladder and it can be use in conjunction with bone modifying agents like bisphosphonates or Denosumab, corticoids and anticonvulsant drugs [46].

5. Conclusion

Even though bone metastatic spread in lung cancer used to mean a poor prognosis for those patients, current multimodality therapies continue to improve survival. Awareness and effective treatment of these lesions is paramount to maintain a good quality of life and function. Skeletal events related to bone metastases can severely affect the patient, produce increased costs to the healthcare system and affect survival. Ideally, an oncology orthopedic specialist ought to be included in the multidisciplinary treating team from the moment of diagnosis of bone metastatic spread.

Conflict of interest

The authors state no conflict of interest related to the writing of this chapter.

Author details

Ana C. Belzarena
Oncology Orthopedic Service, Miami Cancer Institute, Baptist Health South Florida, Miami, Florida, United States

*Address all correspondence to: ceciliabel@baptisthealth.net

References

[1] Lung Cancer Statistics: How Common is Lung Cancer. (n.d.). Retrieved January 17, 2021, from https://www.cancer.org/cancer/lung-cancer/about/key-statistics.html

[2] D'Addario G, Fruh M, Reck M, et al. Metastatic non-small-cell lung cancer: ESMO Clinical Practice Guidelines for diagnosis, treatment and follow-up. Ann Oncol 2010; 21Suppl 5v116–v119.

[3] Stinchcombe TE, Lee CB, Socinski MA. Current approaches to advanced-stage non-small-cell lung cancer: first-line therapy in patients with a good functional status. Clin Lung Cancer 2006; 7Suppl 4S111–S117.

[4] Coleman RE. Clinical features of metastatic bone disease and risk of skeletal morbidity. Clin Cancer Res, 2006; 12: 6243s–49s.

[5] Wang CY, Zhang XY. [(99m)Tc-MDP whole body bone imaging in evaluation of the characteristics of bone metastasis of primary lung cancer]. Zhonghua Zhong Liu Za Zhi, 2010; 32: 382-86.

[6] Quint LE, Tummala S, Brisson LJ, et al. Distribution of distant metastases from newly diagnosed non-small cell lung cancer. Ann Thorac Surg 1996; 62: 246-250.

[7] Zhang L, Gong Z. Clinical Characteristics and Prognostic Factors in Bone Metastases from Lung Cancer. Med Sci Monit. 2017; 23: 4087-4094. Published 2017 Aug 24. doi:10.12659/msm.902971.

[8] Nottebaert M, Exner GU, von Hochstetter AR, Schreiber A (1989) Metastatic bone disease from occult carcinoma: a profile. Int Orthop 13(2):119-123.

[9] Le Chevalier T, Cvitkovic E, Caille P, Harvey J, Contesso G, Spielmann M, Rouesse J (1988) Early metastatic cancer of unknown primary origin at presentation. A clinical study of 302 consecutive autopsied patients. Arch Intern Med 148(9):2035-2039.

[10] de Kock I, Mirhosseini M, Lau F, et al. Conversion of Karnofsky Performance Status (KPS) and Eastern Cooperative Oncology Group Performance Status (ECOG) to Palliative Performance Scale (PPS), and the interchangeability of PPS and KPS in prognostic tools. J Palliat Care, 2013; 29: 163-69.

[11] Healey JH, Turnbull AD, Miedema B, Lane JM. Acrometastases. A study of twenty-nine patients with osseous involvement of the hands and feet. J Bone Joint Surg Am. 1986;68(5):743-746.

[12] Pockett RD, Castellano D, McEwan P, et al. The hospital burden of disease associated with bone metastases and skeletal-related events in patients with breast cancer, lung cancer, or prostate cancer in Spain. Eur J Cancer Care (Engl) 2010; 19: 755-760.

[13] Utzschneider S, Wicherek E, Weber P, Schmidt G, Jansson V, Dürr HR. Surgical treatment of bone metastases in patients with lung cancer. Int Orthop. 2011;35(5):731-736. doi:10.1007/s00264-010-1074-9.

[14] Selvaggi G, Scagliotti G. Management of bone metastases in cancer: a review. Clin Rev Oncol Hematol 2005;56:365-78.

[15] Hirsh V, Tchekmedyian NS, Rosen LS, Zheng M, Hei YJ. Clinical benefit of zoledronic acid in patients with lung cancer and other solid tumors: analysis based on history of skeletal complications. Clin Lung Cancer 2004;6:170-174.

[16] Tsuya A, Kurata T, Tamura K, Fukuoka M. Skeletal metastases in non-small cell lung cancer: a retrospective study. Lung Cancer 2007; 57:229-232.

[17] Delea TE, McKiernan J, Brandman J, et al. Impact of skeletal complications on total medical care costs among patients with bone metastases of lung cancer. J Thorac Oncol 2006;1:571-576.

[18] Bender RA, Hansen H. Hypercalcemia in bronchogenic carcinoma. A prospective study of 200 patients. Ann Intern Med 1974;80:205-208.

[19] Rankin W, Grill V, Martin TJ. Parathyroid hormone-related protein and hypercalcemia. Cancer 1997;80:1564-1571.

[20] Major P, Lortholary A, Hon J, et al. Zoledronic acid is superior to pamidronate in the treatment of hypercalcemia of malignancy: a pooled analysis of two randomized, controlled clinical trials. J Clin Oncol 2001;19:558-567.

[21] Choi J, Raghavan M. Diagnostic imaging and image-guided therapy of skeletal metastases. Cancer Control. 2012;19:102-112.

[22] Vassiliou V, Andreopoulos D, Frangos S, Tselis N, Giannopoulou E, Lutz S. Bone metastases: assessment of therapeutic response through radiological and nuclear medicine imaging modalities. Clin Oncol (R Coll Radiol) 2011;23:632-645.

[23] Bäuerle T, Semmler W. Imaging response to systemic therapy for bone metastases. Eur Radiol. 2009;19:2495-2507.

[24] Rosenthal D. Radiologic diagnosis of bone metastases. Cancer 1997;80:1595-607.

[25] Evans A, Robertson J. Magnetic resonance imaging versus radionuclide scintigraphy for screening in bone metastases. Clin Radiol 2000;55:653.

[26] Zhang Y, Zhao C, Liu H, Hou H, Zhang H. Multiple metastasis-like bone lesions in scintigraphic imaging. J Biomed Biotechnol. 2012;2012:957364.

[27] Shreve P, Grossman H, Gross M, Wahl R. Metastatic prostate cancer: initial findings of PET with 2-deoxy-2 (F-18) fluoro-d-glucose. Radiology 1996;199:751-5.

[28] Masters GA Temin S Azzoli CG, et al. Systemic therapy for stage iv non-small-cell lung cancer: American Society of Clinical Oncology Clinical Practice Guideline Update. J Clin Oncol. 2015; 33: 3488-3515.

[29] Tsao AS Scagliotti GV Bunn Jr, PA et al. Scientific advances in lung cancer 2015. J Thorac Oncol. 2016; 11: 613-638.

[30] National Comprehensive Cancer Network. Clinical Practice Guidelines in Oncology (NCCN Guidelines™): Non-small cell lung cancer (version 3.2011). http://www.nccn.org/professionals/physician_gls/f_guidelines.asp

[31] Al Husaini H, Wheatley-Price P, Clemons M, Shepherd FA. Prevention and management of bone metastases in lung cancer: a review. J Thorac Oncol. 2009;4(2):251-259. doi:10.1097/JTO.0b013e31819518fc.

[32] Boissier S, Ferreras M, Peyruchaud O, et al. Bisphosphonates inhibit breast and prostate carcinoma cell invasion, an early event in the formation of bone metastases. Cancer Res 2000;60:2949-2954.

[33] Rosen LS, Gordon D, Tchekmedyian NS, et al. ng-term efficacy and safety of zoledronic acid in the treatment of skeletal metastases in patients with non-small cell lung carcinoma and other solid tumors: a randomized, Phase III, double blind, placebo-controlled trial. Cancer 2004; 100: 2613-2621.

[34] Diel IJ, Bergner R, Grotz KA. Adverse effects of bisphosphonates: current issues. J Support Oncol 2007; 5: 475-482.

[35] Bezjak A. Palliative therapy for lung cancer. Semin Surg Oncol 2003; 21:138-147.

[36] D'Oronzo S, Coleman R, Brown J, Silvestris F. Metastatic bone disease: Pathogenesis and therapeutic options: Up-date on bone metastasis management. J Bone Oncol. 2018;15:004-4. Published 2018 Nov 6. doi:10.1016/j.jbo.2018.10.004.

[37] De Felice F, Piccioli A, Musio D, Tombolini V. The role of radiation therapy in bone metastases management. Oncotarget. 2017;8(15):25691-25699.

[38] Gutowski CJ, Zmistowski B, Fabbri N, Boland PJ, Healey JH. Should the Use of Biologic Agents in Patients With Renal and Lung Cancer Affect Our Surgical Management of Femoral Metastases?. Clin Orthop Relat Res. 2019;477(4):707-714. doi:10.1097/CORR.0000000000000434

[39] Mirels H. Metastatic disease in long bones: a proposed scoring system for diagnosing impending pathologic fractures. Clin Orthop Relat Res. 1989;249:256-264.

[40] Harrington K. Impending pathologic fractures from metastatic malignancy: evaluation and management. Instr Course Lect. 1986;35:357-381.

[41] Morishige M, Muramatsu K, Tominaga Y, Hashimoto T, Taguchi T. Surgical treatment of metastatic femoral fractures: achieving an improved quality of life for cancer patients. Anticancer Res. 2015;35:427-432.

[42] McLynn RP, Ondeck NT, Grauer JN, Lindskog DM. What Is the Adverse Event Profile After Prophylactic Treatment of Femoral Shaft or Distal Femur Metastases?. Clin Orthop Relat Res. 2018;476(12):2381-2388. doi:10.1097/CORR.0000000000000489.

[43] Mercadante S. Malignant bone pain: pathophysiology and treatment. Pain 1997; 69: 1-18.

[44] Zeppetella G. Impact and management of breakthrough pain in cancer. Curr. Opin. Support Palliat. Care. 2009; 3:1-6.

[45] Delaney, A.; Fleetwood–Walker, S.M.; Colvin, L.A.; Fallon, M. Translational medicine: Cancer pain mechanisms and management. Br. J. Anaesth. 2008, 101, 87-94.

[46] Zajączkowska R, Kocot-Kępska M, Leppert W, Wordliczek J. Bone Pain in Cancer Patients: Mechanisms and Current Treatment. Int J Mol Sci. 2019;20(23):6047. Published 2019 Nov 30. doi:10.3390/ijms20236047.

Section 5

Potential Future Directions

Chapter 10

Liquid Biopsy Analysis of Circulating Tumor Biomarkers in Lung Cancer

Peter Ping Lin

Abstract

Risk stratification, prognostication and longitudinal monitoring of therapeutic efficacy in lung cancer patients remains highly challenging. It is imperative to establish robust surrogate biomarkers for identifying eligible patients, predicting and effectively monitoring clinical response as well as timely detecting emerging resistance to therapeutic regimens. Circulating tumor biomarkers, analyzed by liquid biopsy, are primarily composed of nucleic acid-based circulating tumor DNA (ctDNA) and an aneuploid cell-based category of circulating tumor cells (CTCs) and circulating tumor-derived endothelial cells (CTECs). Unlike ctDNA, cancer cells are the origin of all categories of various tumor biomarkers. Involvement of aneuploid CTCs and CTECs in tumorigenesis, neoangiogenesis, tumor progression, cancer metastasis and post-therapeutic recurrence has been substantially investigated. Both CTCs and CTECs possessing an active interplay and crosstalk constitute a unique category of cellular circulating tumor biomarkers. These cells concurrently harbor the intact cancer-related genetic signatures and full tumor marker expression profiles in sync with disease progression and therapeutic process. Recent progress in clinical implementation of non-invasive liquid biopsy has made it feasible to frequently carry out ctDNA analysis and unbiased detection of a full spectrum of non-hematologic circulating rare cells including CTCs and CTECs in lung cancer patients, regardless of variation in heterogeneous cell size and cancer cell surface anchor protein expression. *In situ* phenotypic and karyotypic comprehensive characterization of aneuploid CTCs and CTECs, in combination with single cell-based genotyping and improved ctDNA analyses, will facilitate and benefit multidisciplinary management of lung cancer.

Keywords: CTC, CTEC, ctDNA, therapeutic resistance, aneuploidy, iFISH

1. Introduction

Recent progress in multidisciplinary management of advanced lung cancer has triggered enthusiasm in investigating both prognostic roles of tumor microenvironment (TME) and clinical utilities of liquid biopsy in lung cancer patients [1, 2]. How the tumor-reprogrammed lung TME promotes primary tumor progression and cancer metastasis remains to be further elucidated [1].

Aberrant stromal and infiltrated immune cells, sustained neovascularization, as well as dysfunctional neoangiogenic vasculatures in solid tumors all contribute towards constituting an immunosuppressive TME suitable for cancer cell growth and metastasis [3]. Tumor-derived endothelial cells (TECs) participate in making up the lining of neoangiogenic vasculatures in the TME and accelerating tumor progression [4, 5]. Following their shedding into peripheral blood, $CD31^-$ cancer cells and $CD31^+$ TECs turn into circulating tumor cells (CTCs) [6] and circulating tumor-derived endothelial cells (CTECs) [7, 8], respectively. Beyond peripheral blood, tumor cells and TECs may also disseminate into body fluid including bone marrow (BM), malignant pleural effusion (MPE), ascites and cerebrospinal fluid (CSF), etc. These cells are respectively termed as disseminated tumor cells (DTCs) [9] and disseminated tumor-derived endothelial cells (DTECs). The non-hematologic circulating rare cells, consisting of CTCs, CTECs, DTCs and DTECs, possess the malignancy hallmark of aneuploidy [10–14] and play a fundamental role in tumorigenesis, neoangiogenesis, tumor progression, cancer metastasis and relapse [7, 13].

Liquid biopsy provides applicable and convenient choices for analyzing tumor-derived cells and molecules in cancer patients' circulation system [15], which is particularly adequate for lung cancer as it does not require an invasive and harmful procedure to perform a conventional pathological biopsy on the malignant lesion in lung. Liquid biopsy utilizes non-invasive approaches to reveal the molecular landscape of neoplasm in real time and facilitate management of lung cancer throughout treatment process, from identifying eligible patients, dynamically monitoring therapeutic efficacy to detecting minimal residual disease and emerging resistance [16] with respect to guiding personalized precision therapy [2].

Being as a category of liquid biopsy technologies, analysis of tumor cell genome-derived circulating tumor DNA (ctDNA) has been applied to assist management of advanced stage lung cancer [2, 17]. The cell-free biomarker ctDNA measurements show rapid response to administration of therapeutic agents. Recent advance in molecular genotyping in terms of identifying genetic mutations in ctDNA has successfully guided therapies targeting mutant *EGFR* or the *EML4-ALK* rearrangement in lung cancer patients [18, 19]. However, the specificity and sensitivity of ctDNA assay remain challenging [20, 21]. Compared to ctDNA, CTC has presented its unique advantage in terms of being as an effective response measure of prolonged survival for metastatic cancer patients in multiple clinical studies [22]. It has been realized that aneuploid circulating rare cells constitute a unique category of viable cell-based cellular circulating tumor biomarkers. Those cellular circulating tumor biomarkers contain intact genetic signatures and full protein expression profiles along with tumor progression and throughout clinical treatment process [7, 13]. The clinical relevance of aneuploid circulating rare cells in the context of tumor angiogenesis [23], cancer metastases and prognosis [6, 9] was described elsewhere [9, 24]. Detection of CTCs and CTECs has been clinically applied to prognosticate lung cancer patients [22], evaluate or monitor therapeutic efficacy in both cancer patients [25–27] and patient- or CTC-derived xenograft tumor mouse model (PDX, CDX) [28–31]. Moreover, examination of CTCs and CTECs has been successfully utilized to timely detect emerging therapeutic resistance [32–36] as well as postsurgical cancer relapse [37, 38]. Overall, availability of analysis of circulating rare cells has brought extraordinary depth by allowing feasible frequent examination of the whole intact target cells and their molecular contents including cancer-related DNA, RNA and tumor marker proteins [21]. Other liquid biopsy-relevant genotyping strategies conducted on circulating exosomes, microRNA, mRNA, metabolites and tumor-educated platelets are immature and remain to be further optimized and clinically validated [2, 17].

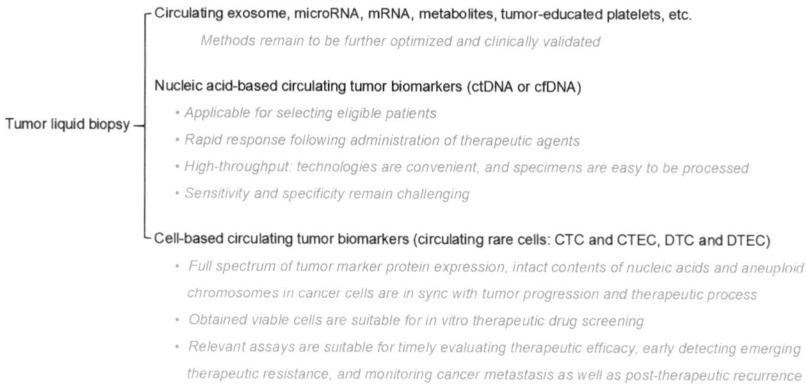

Figure 1.
Categorization of tumor liquid biopsy. Various cellular and molecular approaches are applied in the non-invasive tumor liquid biopsy to detect nucleic acid-based and cell-based circulating tumor biomarkers.

Categorization and clinical utilities of tumor liquid biopsy, primarily composed of nucleic acid-based and cell-based circulating tumor biomarker analyses, are depicted in **Figure 1**.

2. Hypoxic tumor microenvironment in lung cancer

The lung TME is a complex, dynamic system comprised of tangled interactions among carcinoma cells and their surrounding cells in a hypoxic environment [39, 40]. Aside from non-cellular compositions of cytokine and extracellular matrix, the cellular components of the lung cancer TME consist of undifferentiated cancer stem cells (CSCs) [41] and their differentiated progeny tumor cells possessing either intrinsic or induced plasticity [42]. In addition, a variety of cells other than neoplastic cells also localize in the TME, which, able to foster both tumor growth and dissemination, are composed of stromal cells and non-stromal immune cells. Tumor-associated stromal cells consist of cancer-associated fibroblasts (CAFs), pericytes, adipocytes and endothelial cells (ECs) that make up the lining of tumor vasculature. The innate immune cells in the TME encompass dendritic cells, monocytes, macrophages and lymphocytes. The major components of lymphocytes in the TME are tumor-infiltrating T cells which are recognized as a hallmark of cancer [43]. Among different subtypes of T cells in the lung TME, $CD3^+/CD8^+$ cytotoxic T cells and $CD3^+/CD4^+/CD25^+$ regulatory T cells (Tregs) are the most representative subpopulations. Cytotoxic T cells exhibit anti-tumor activity which is negatively regulated by the $FOXP3^+$ immune-suppressive Tregs [44]. Alike prognostic factors of immune cells in the lung TME, the $FOXP3^+$ Tregs correlate with poor prognosis [44] and early recurrence, particularly in node-negative NSCLC patients [45].

Hypoxia, a common phenomenon in malignant neoplasm, leads to acquisition of epithelial-to-mesenchymal transition (EMT) and endothelial-to-mesenchymal transition (EndoMT) phenotypic plasticity by epithelial cancer cells and endothelial cells, respectively. Hypoxia-inducible factor (HIF) pathway is the most distinctive intracellular signaling event that triggers and regulates EMT and EndoMT [7]. HIF pathway is activated in the hypoxic lung TME, resulting in nuclear translocation of HIF-1α and subsequent heterodimerization with HIF-1β in the nucleus [46]. HIF-1α/β heterodimers subsequently interact with NFκB to promote a series of downstream signaling cascades. Hypoxia is, therefore, the vital inducer of EMT and

EndoMT [47, 48] which fundamentally constitute the intracellular central hub of tumor neovascularization and cancer metastasis [7].

In the hypoxic TME, active crosstalk among carcinoma cells and their associated stromal cells accelerates lung cancer development by promoting tumor expansion, invasion and disease progression [49, 50]. The lung hypoxic TME thereby significantly impacts both malignant tumor progression and treatment response. Impaired vascularity and hypoxia will lead to an increased metastasis potential and treatment resistance in lung cancer [39].

3. ctDNA

ctDNA is released from apoptotic or necrotic cancer cells either in the TME of primary/metastatic lesions or in peripheral circulation. ctDNA levels correlate with tumor burden and response to therapy in NSCLC patients [51, 52]. In contrast to normal cells, neoplastic cells possess tumor-specific somatic alternations in the genome. Mutations harbored by ctDNA, including both point mutations and structural alternations (such as genome-wide copy number variations and rearrangements), correspond to that in primary tumors [21].

3.1 Clinical application of ctDNA

Following rapid evolvement of PCR and next generation sequencing (NGS)-based ctDNA analysis, its clinical application as a high-throughput diagnostic test has been facilitated in several areas. **(i)** Early detection of lung cancer: localized lung cancer at early stage sheds DNA into peripheral circulation and detection of methylated ctDNA may help diagnose early stage lung cancer [53]. **(ii)** Tumor genotyping to identify lung cancer patients eligible for mutation-targeted therapies: the most representative example is to examine sensitizing exon 19 deletions and the L858R mutation as well as the resistance mutation T790M in plasma ctDNA. All will guide administration of EGFR-Tyrosine kinase inhibitors (TKIs), such as gefitinib, erlotinib and afatinib to lung cancer patients [18]. **(iii)** Surrogates of therapeutic efficacy: ctDNA dynamics is able to predict benefit of immunotherapy [54] and may also correlate with chemoradiation efficacy in lung cancer patients [55]. **(iv)** Identification of localized lung cancer at high risk of disease relapse: compared to conventional histopathological criteria in identifying post-therapeutic localized lung cancer patients suitable for personalized adjuvant therapeutic setting, cancer personalized profiling by deep sequencing (CAPP-seq) ctDNA analysis is able to detect post-surgical minimal or molecular residual disease (MRD), thereby identifying patients bearing the lowest disease burden eligible for adjuvant therapy [21, 56]. **(v)** Early detection of lung cancer relapse: whole genome analysis of ctDNA may directly identify tumor-derived structural alternations comprised of chromosomal copy number changes and rearrangements, including specific amplification of cancer driver genes (*ERBB2*, *CDK6*, etc.) that correlate with cancer recurrence [57]. In addition, phylogenetic ctDNA profiling was also reported to enable detection of recurrent NSCLC at early stage [58].

3.2 Limitations and improvement of ctDNA analysis

Advances in next generation DNA sequencing technologies have promoted clinical application of ctDNA as a tool to facilitate management of lung cancer, such as earlier detection and improvement of therapeutic outcomes by enabling early intervention, etc. However, limitations of ctDNA have recently attracted increasing attention. Cancer-related genetic contents carried by fractured ctDNA is limited due to its 90–150 base pairs of small fragments [2]. Moreover, in carcinoma patients, little amount of cancer-related ctDNA co-exist with much larger amount of cancer-irrelevant cell free DNA (cfDNA) shed from normal cells in peripheral blood [2, 17]. This raises notable concerns regarding the specificity and sensitivity of ctDNA analysis [20, 21], particularly for low-frequency mutation detection in early stage NSCLC patients [59]. Such concern has been recently further reenforced by copious data analyses co-performed by the American Society of Clinical Oncology (ASCO) and the College of American Pathologists (CAP), indicating that clinical utility and validity of ctDNA in early-stage cancer detection, treatment monitoring, or residual disease detection in a variety of cancer patient are still vague and inconclusive [60]. Extensive clinical studies, performed by the improved technologies with higher sensitivity and specificity, will further validate and reveal clinical utilities of ctDNA.

4. Aneuploid CTCs and CTECs

Almost all different types of tumor biomarkers originate from neoplastic cells. CTCs and CTECs dynamically comprise integral molecular landscape of both cancer-related genetic variations and tumor marker expression along with tumor progression and clinical treatment process.

4.1 Aneuploidy in malignant cancer cells

Aneuploidy refers to either a gain or loss of chromosomes in a cell. Unlike constitutional aneuploidy, somatic aneuploidy is the most common feature of human carcinomas [11, 12]. In particular, aneuploid chromosome 8 (Chr 8) was observed in neoplastic cells of almost all solid tumors, including lung cancer [61].

Aneuploidy is a cellular transformation-related dynamic chromosome mutation event regulated by cell fusion and a number of mitotic genes [7, 62]. Mutations of those mitotic genes were identified in cancer cells, implicating such mutation in induction of mis-chromosome segregated aneuploidy in neoplastic cells [63]. Aberrant ploidy of extra chromosomes in cancer cells was found to relevant to genomic instability [64]. In addition, gain or deletion of hundreds of genes brought by aneuploidy in carcinoma cells results in profound varieties of phenotypes, which further drives cancer development, evolution, heterogeneity, lethal progression, drug resistance and therapy failure [14, 65]. Of extreme importance was the discovery that the degree of aneuploidy is proportional to the grade of malignancy and genetic instability of neoplasm [66, 67], showing that the higher the degree of aneuploidy, the higher the frequency of *KRAS* and *TP53* mutations, and the higher the malignancy grade of cancer cells [62, 67, 68].

4.2 Cytogenetic abnormalities in CTCs and CTECs

In the lung cancer TME, alike aneuploid neoplastic cells, a majority of ECs in tumor vasculature are aneuploid TECs [69] that could be derived from either endothelialization of malignant lung cancer cells or cancerization of stromal ECs [7, 70]. Abnormal neovasculature composed of TECs possesses loosened junctions between ECs, resulting in an increased vascular permeability and transendothelial intravasation as well as extravasation during tumor metastasis. Aneuploid TECs, harboring dual-properties of endothelial vascularization ability and cancerous malignancy [71], were reported to contribute to tumor progression [5]. Following shedding into blood, both CTCs and CTECs adopt molecular properties from their parental cells in the TME of primary lesion, including cytogenetic abnormalities of aneuploidy. Each subcategory of those aneuploid circulating rare cells correlate with distinct clinical endpoints, such as targeted distant cancer metastasis [72, 73] and resistance to chemo- [33, 34] or immunotherapy [36].

5. Co-detection, comprehensive characterization and clinical value of diverse subtypes of lung cancer CTCs and CTECs

5.1 Conventional strategies to detect lung cancer CTCs

Several strategies were applied to attempt to detect CTCs in lung cancer patients [74]. CTC surface anchor protein (such as CD326 EpCAM)-dependent isolation (e.g. CellSearch) and cell size-exclusion filtration to enrich large cell size CTCs (>WBC size) are the most representative conventional approaches. However, it has been realized that clinically relevant small cell size CTCs (≤WBC size), such as mesenchymal CTCs [75], are lost throughout the filtered depletion of WBCs, raising non-negligible concerns with respect to specificity and sensitivity for cell filtration strategy [76, 77], particularly for lung cancer CTC detection [78]. CellSearch technology relies on positive expression of EpCAM and cytokeratin (CK) for isolation and identification, respectively. This method, restricted to both EpCAM and CK double-positive cells, is able to effectively detect CTCs shed from some particular types of solid tumors expressing abundant epithelial marker EpCAM, such as colon, breast and prostate cancers [79]. However, a majority of CTCs in various carcinoma patients exhibit a highly dynamic distribution of EpCAM during cancer progression and metastasis [80, 81]. Additionally, expression of EpCAM and CK is down-regulated during EMT in the process of CTC formation [81, 82]. Furthermore, most lung cancer CTCs exhibit either low or non-expression of EpCAM [83, 84]. Those inherited cell biological "hurdles" inevitably lead to a false negative detection of the "uncapturable" and/or "invisible" lung CTCs by the conventional approach [85]. It is therefore necessary to develop an alternative strategy, beyond restriction to EpCAM and CK double positive expression, to effectively isolate, identify, comprehensively characterize and classify a variety of highly heterogeneous aneuploid circulating rare cells in lung cancer patients.

5.2 *In situ* phenotypic and karyotypic characterization of aneuploid CTCs and CTECs by iFISH

Aside from respectively addressing nucleic acid, tumor marker proteins, or cell morphology alone, a comprehensive strategy integrating subtraction enrichment (SE) and immunostaining-fluorescence *in situ* hybridization (SE-iFISH) has been developed to effectively enrich and identify heterogeneously sized circulating rare cells [8, 61]. Following non-hypotonic removal of RBCs, subtraction enrichment is able to effectively enrich circulating rare cells in varieties of cancer patients including NSCLC and small cell lung cancer (SCLC) [86], regardless of cell size variation and the target cell surface anchor protein expression. Following efficient enrichment, iFISH co-detects tumor marker expression and chromosome aneuploidy in enriched non-hematologic circulating rare cells (CRCs) [61]. Besides, iFISH is also able to detect aneuploid hematologic rare cells derived from lymphoma and myeloma ($CD45^+$, aneuploid in Chr 12). As depicted in **Figure 2**, the most representative populations of the primary entity of non-hematologic aneuploid circulating rare cells, identified by iFISH, are CTCs/CTECs in peripheral blood and DTCs/DTECs in

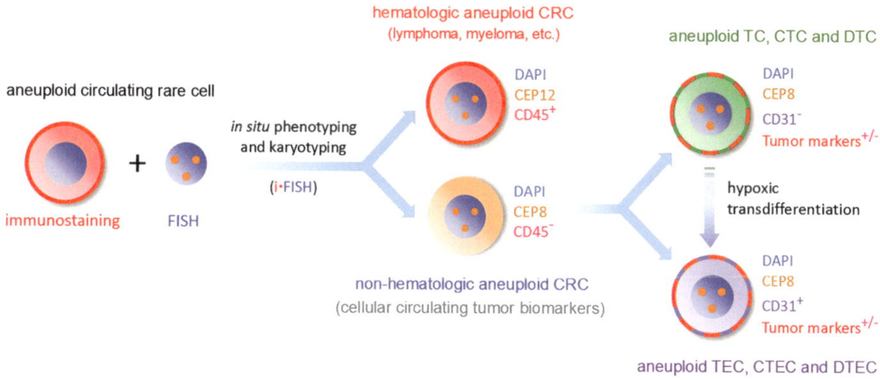

Figure 2.
Categorization of aneuploid circulating rare cells comprehensively identified and characterized by iFISH. Aneuploid circulating rare cells (CRCs) are classified into hematologic and non-hematologic categories. The former class is composed of lymphoma, myeloma, etc. which are aneuploid in chromosome 12. The non-hematologic category consists of CD31⁻ CTCs and CD31⁺ CTECs in blood, DTCs as well as disseminated TECs (DTECs) in body fluid (bone marrow, malignant pleural effusion, ascites, cerebrospinal fluid, etc.). The aneuploid non-hematologic CRCs, either expressing tumor markers or not, constitute a unique category of cell-based cellular circulating tumor biomarkers. In the hypoxic environment, some CD31⁻ tumor cells (TCs) may transdifferentiate into CD31⁺ TECs either in vivo *or* in vitro.

body fluid. Under hypoxic conditions, some $CD31^-$ tumor cells (TCs) could transdifferentiate into $CD31^+$ TECs, both *in vivo* and *in vitro* [7, 87, 88].

Based upon the degree of aneuploidy, tumor marker protein expression and cell morphology (large, small, cluster or microemboli), each category of circulating rare cells can be classified into diverse subtypes. Each subtype of cells respectively possesses distinct clinical values.

5.3 Clinical significance of CTCs and CTECs in lung cancer

5.3.1 Quantification

Clinical utilities of detecting CTCs and CTECs in management of NSCLC and SCLC have been investigated along the axis of "early diagnosis–treatment–relapse" [89]. Though low-dose CT (LDCT) screening was reported to reduce lung cancer mortality in low-risk populations [90, 91], its extensive application is limited due to relatively low sensitivity in high-risk populations [17, 90], unavailability of frequent re-examinations within a short period as well as socio-economic affordability. As a diagnostic marker of lung cancer, non-invasive and periodic detection of CTCs and CTECs may provide a compensatory choice to allow an effective early diagnosis of lung cancer [17, 92–94]. Multiple studies indicated that lung cancer CTCs could be detected several months prior to radiographic appearance of the primary lesion [74, 95].

With respect to diagnosed lung cancer patients, the quantity of CTCs was found to correlate with patients' pathological staging as well as amount of cytokeratin 19-derived Cyfra 21–1 in plasma [86, 96]. CTC is a risk stratification parameter for NSCLC in terms of distant metastasis [73, 97]. Prognostic values of CTCs in therapeutic lung cancer patients were published elsewhere [86, 98], indicating that baseline lung CTC counts were associated with patients' poor prognosis and response to treatment [99]. Compared to evaluation of therapeutic efficacy performed by CT scanning and RECIST criteria, quantitative change in CTCs occurs ahead of conventional medical imaging examination [86, 100], suggesting that cellular response to therapeutic regimens is more sensitive than observable size variation in imaged tumor mass.

Close attention has been recently focused on whether surgical resection may promote a quantitative increase in lung cancer CTCs. Although a study performed by the EpCAM-dependent strategy indicated that surgical approaches did not impact CTC quantity [101], the conclusion was uncertain due to the reality that the applied technology was biased in restricting to CK and EpCAM double-positive CTCs which account for only a very small proportion of overall lung CTCs. Nonetheless, several studies performed by others using different technical platforms indicated that surgical manipulation indeed increased CTC quantity either in pulmonary venous (PV) blood during surgery [102, 103] or in post-surgical patients' peripheral blood [104]. Increased CTCs in PV were reported to associate with patients' poor prognosis [103, 105]. Similar to association of post-surgical hepatocellular carcinoma (HCC) CTCs with cancer relapse [38], detection of CTCs in PV during operation or in post-surgical peripheral blood also enables early detection of lung cancer recurrence, particularly in the post-resected lung cancer patients [37, 106–108].

5.3.2 Molecular characterization

In addition to enumerating cell number alone, molecular characterization of DNA, RNA, chromosomes and proteins in circulating rare cells has been carried out to investigate the clinical relevance of molecular landscape in diverse subcategories of lung CTCs and CTECs [36, 93, 109].

Tumor-associated DNA copy number aberrations (CNAs) profiling illustrated distinctive genetic features in chemosensitive and chemorefractory SCLC CTCs [110], that will be beneficial to patients' personalized precision therapy. Besides DNA, the quantity of several tumor markers' mRNA, such as CEA mRNA in both pre- and post-surgical NSCLC patients, may serve as an independent prognosticator for poor prognosis [111].

Compared to a significant reduction in risk of mortality in post-surgical NSCLC patients who had near-diploid tumors [68, 112], subjects possessing aneuploidy in lung cancer cells exhibited a significant increase in risk of death [112]. Recent studies demonstrated that aneuploidy plays a critical role in chemoresistance in gastric cancer patients [33, 34] as well as in metastatic "patient-derived xenograft tumor mouse models" (mPDX) exhibiting primary gastric cancer metastasizing to lung [30]. For instance, gastric CTCs with trisomy 8 were found to possess intrinsic chemoresistance, whereas multiploid (≥pentasomy 8) CTCs displayed acquired resistance to cisplatin. It is logical to speculate that aneuploid lung cancer CTCs may share the similar property of aneuploidy-related therapeutic resistance.

Efficient identification of lung cancer patients eligible for targeted therapies remains a challenging topic. Compared to conventional detection of *ALK* rearrangement on biopsy specimen with respect to identifying subjects for crizotinib treatment, detection performed on CTCs to examine *ALK* rearrangement provides a better alternative in terms of rapidity and repeatability [13, 113, 114]. Targeted therapy on epidermal growth factor receptor (EGFR) tyrosine kinase inhibitors (gefitinib and erlotinib TKIs) has been profoundly applied to eligible NSCLC patients. Single cell-based analysis of genetic abnormalities, such as exon 19 deletion/*EGFR* L858R TKI-sensitizing mutation [115] and T790M TKI-resistance mutation in CTCs, could serves as an adequate alternative to identify eligible patients [116] and timely monitor emerging acquired therapeutic resistance to TKIs throughout therapy [117, 118]. Interestingly, compared to the 33% positive detection rate of *EGFR* L858R in ctDNA, 92% of the same cohort showed such mutation in their CTCs [117].

Next-generation sequencing (NGS) successfully guided *in vitro* drug screenings carried out on the cultured primary CTCs [119]. One study demonstrated that NGS performed on the cultured metastatic tumor cells which were enriched from cerebrospinal fluid in breast cancer patients led pinpointing of chemotherapeutic agent palbociclib (the synthetic CDK4/6 inhibitor) upon identifying single nucleotide variant (SNV) in those cells [120]. A similar *in vitro* therapeutic drug screening strategy performed on 3D cultured CTCs was reported to help direct potent lung cancer precision therapy [121]. In addition to analyzing DNA mutations in pooled CTCs, the single-cell based DNA [29] or RNA sequencing [31] performed on chemosensitive and chemoresistant CTC-derived xenografts (CDX) demonstrated that intratumoral heterogeneity (ITH), which was constituted of coexisting subpopulations of cancer cells with heterogeneous gene expression, led to the development of platinum-resistance in SCLC patients [29, 31]. A similar study performed by others on SCLC PDX and CDX confirmed that these models were able to capture the mutational landscape and functional traits from their primary donor tumors [28].

Aside from genetic and karyotypic characterization, phenotypic analysis of tumor marker protein expression in CTCs provides additional prognosticating value. For instance, EpCAM and Vimentin are the epithelial and mesenchymal markers of EMT and EndoMT, respectively [122, 123], both showing particular clinical outcomes in carcinoma patients. $EpCAM^+$ CTCs and DTCs are able to lead oligometastasis to lung in breast carcinoma patients [72]. Moreover, CTCs expressing EpCAM correlate with poor prognosis in lung cancer patients [84]. $Vimentin^+$ CTC is another independent prognosticator for poor prognosis and survival. Positive detection of $Vimentin^+$ CTCs at baseline has been recently reported to associate with lung cancer's hepatic metastasis and patients' poor prognosis [73].

5.3.3 Clinical utilities of co-detection of CTCs and CTECs

Most efforts made on liquid biopsy have, so far, been primarily focusing on CTCs. In comparison with CTCs, the aneuploid $CD31^+$ CTECs, harboring mixed properties of epithelium, endothelium, mesenchyme, aneuploidy, malignancy and mobility, are expected to perform an important role in tumorigenesis, progression, metastasis and neovascularization [7]. Since the existence of CTECs in cancer patients was reported for the first time [8], clinical values of CTECs in a variety of carcinoma patients have been illustrated [7, 36, 93, 124]. Compared to CTCs, lung cancer CTECs appear to be more relevant to therapeutic resistance and disease progression. Particularly, in NSCLC patients subjected to the checkpoint blockade immunotherapy (nivolumab), unlike nivolumab-sensitive $PD\text{-}L1^+$ CTCs which revealed a quantitative decrease following treatment, the number of post-immunotherapeutic aneuploid $PD\text{-}L1^+$ CTECs increased. Patients possessing post-immunotherapeutic aneuploid $PD\text{-}L1^+$ CTECs showed a significantly shorter PFS compared to those without $PD\text{-}L1^+$ CTECs [36]. Innovative attempts to therapeutically target CTEC-relevant EndoMT and aneuploidy will vitally impact aneuploid CTECs and ultimately improve lung cancer patients' treatment efficacy [125, 126]. As a novel and mobile therapeutic target, elimination of CTECs in cancer patients is expected to promote an effective obstruction in cancer metastasis.

Detection and clinical values of advanced molecular characterization of lung cancer CTCs and CTECs are summarized in **Table 1**.

To maximize clinical values of CTCs and CTECs, it is ideal to co-characterize all three elements of nucleic acids, tumor marker protein expression and cellular morphology in target cells. Such three-in-one comprehensive co-detection and molecular characterization of aneuploid circulating rare cells will effectively and

Clinical values of lung cancer CTCs and CTECs	References
Early diagnosis	[17, 74, 92, 93, 95]
Pathological staging	[86, 96]
Identification of eligible patients (TKIs, *ALK* crizotinib)	[13, 114, 116]
In vitro therapeutic drug screening	[120, 121]
Under treatment	
Risk assessment for distant metastasis	[73, 97]
Prognosis	[72, 73, 84, 86, 98–100, 112]
Post-surgery (prognostic value)	[102–105]
Timely monitoring therapeutic resistance	[31, 36, 110, 117, 118]
Early detection of recurrence	[37, 74, 106–108]
Advanced molecular characterization	
Aneuploidy and *ALK* rearrangement	[13, 112–114]
Co-detection of aneuploidy and tumor marker expression in CTCs and CTECs (iFISH)	[8, 36, 61]
CTC-derived xenograft (CDX)	[28, 29, 31]
Single cell-based DNA sequencing	[28, 29, 110, 116, 118]
Single cell-based RNA sequencing	[31]

Table 1.
Clinical utilities of detecting lung cancer CTCs and CTECs.

efficiently assist modern multidisciplinary management of lung cancer with respect to early-stage screening, identification of eligible patients, selection and optimization of therapeutic regimen, risk stratification, minimal residual disease detection, timely evaluation of therapeutic efficacy, monitoring treatment resistance and early detection of post-therapeutic recurrence.

6. Conclusions

Both aneuploid $CD31^+$ CTECs and $CD31^-$ CTCs compose a unique pair of cellular circulating tumor biomarkers that have an active crosstalk and interplay in circulation, thus promoting lymphogenous and hematogenous cancer metastasis as well as disease progression. CTECs, bearing properties of malignancy, vascularization and mobility, serve as a significant, versatile player in tumor neovascularization and cancer metastasis. Clinical implementation of advanced co-detection and comprehensive characterization of all diverse subtypes of aneuploid CTCs and CTECs, in combination with single cell-based genetic signature profiling and improved ctDNA analysis will help improve and profit current and future cancer research and precision management of patients with a variety of carcinomas, including, but not limited to, lung cancer.

Acknowledgements

Author thanks staffs at Cytelligen (San Diego, CA, USA; www.cytelligen.com) and Cytointelligen (China Medical City, Taizhou, Jiangsu, China; www.cytointelligen.com) for providing assistance. Author also thanks Alexander Y. Lin for helping improve the drafted manuscript.

Conflict of interest

i•FISH® is the registered trademark of Cytelligen. Dr. Peter P. Lin is the president at Cytelligen. No additional COI to be disclosed.

Author details

Peter Ping Lin
Cytelligen, San Diego, CA 92121, USA

*Address all correspondence to: plin@cytelligen.com

References

[1] Altorki NK, Markowitz GJ, Gao D, Port JL, Saxena A, Stiles B, McGraw T, Mittal V: The lung microenvironment: an important regulator of tumour growth and metastasis. *Nat Rev Cancer* 2019, 19(1):9-31.

[2] Guibert N, Pradines A, Favre G, Mazieres J: Current and future applications of liquid biopsy in nonsmall cell lung cancer from early to advanced stages. *Eur Respir Rev* 2020, 29:190052.

[3] Quail DF, Joyce JA: Microenvironmental regulation of tumor progression and metastasis. *Nat Med* 2013, 19(11):1423-1437.

[4] Hida K, Hida Y, Amin DN, Flint AF, Panigrahy D, Morton CC, Klagsbrun M: Tumor-associated endothelial cells with cytogenetic abnormalities. *Cancer Res* 2004, 64(22):8249-8255.

[5] Hida K, Maishi N, Annan DA, Hida Y: Contribution of Tumor Endothelial Cells in Cancer Progression. *Int J Mol Sci* 2018, 19(5):1272.

[6] Cristofanilli M, Budd GT, Ellis MJ, Stopeck A, Matera J, Miller MC, Reuben JM, Doyle GV, Allard WJ, Terstappen LW *et al*: Circulating tumor cells, disease progression, and survival in metastatic breast cancer. *N Engl J Med* 2004, 351(8):781-791.

[7] Lin PP: Aneuploid Circulating Tumor-Derived Endothelial Cell (CTEC): A Novel Versatile Player in Tumor Neovascularization and Cancer Metastasis. *Cells* 2020, 9(6):1539.

[8] Lin PP, Gires O, Wang DD, Li L, Wang H: Comprehensive *in situ* co-detection of aneuploid circulating endothelial and tumor cells. *Sci Rep* 2017, 7(1):9789.

[9] Wang H, Stoecklein NH, Lin PP, Gires O: Circulating and disseminated tumor cells: diagnostic tools and therapeutic targets in motion. *Oncotarget* 2017, 8(1):1884-1912.

[10] Ben-David U, Amon A: Context is everything: aneuploidy in cancer. *Nat Rev Genet* 2020, 21(1):44-62.

[11] Gordon DJ, Resio B, Pellman D: Causes and consequences of aneuploidy in cancer. *Nat Rev Genet* 2012, 13(3):189-203.

[12] Kops GJ, Weaver BA, Cleveland DW: On the road to cancer: aneuploidy and the mitotic checkpoint. *Nat Rev Cancer* 2005, 5(10):773-785.

[13] Lin PP: Aneuploid CTC and CEC. *Diagnostics (Basel)* 2018, 8(2):26.

[14] Sansregret L, Swanton C: The Role of Aneuploidy in Cancer Evolution. *Cold Spring Harb Perspect Med* 2017, 7(1):a028373.

[15] Alix-Panabieres C, Pantel K: Circulating Tumor Cells: Liquid Biopsy of Cancer. *Clin Chem* 2013, 59(1):110-118.

[16] Meador CB, Lovly CM: Liquid biopsies reveal the dynamic nature of resistance mechanisms in solid tumors. *Nat Med* 2015, 21(7):663-665.

[17] Rolfo C, Russo A: Liquid biopsy for early stage lung cancer moves ever closer. *Nat Rev Clin Oncol* 2020, 17(9):523-524.

[18] Bernabe R, Hickson N, Wallace A, Blackhall FH: What do we need to make circulating tumour DNA (ctDNA) a routine diagnostic test in lung cancer? *Eur J Cancer* 2017, 81:66-73.

[19] Madsen AT, Winther-Larsen A, McCulloch T, Meldgaard P, Sorensen BS: Genomic Profiling of Circulating Tumor DNA Predicts Outcome and

Demonstrates Tumor Evolution in ALK-Positive Non-Small Cell Lung Cancer Patients. *Cancers (Basel)* 2020, 12(4).

[20] Elazezy M, Joosse SA: Techniques of using circulating tumor DNA as a liquid biopsy component in cancer management. *Comput Struct Biotechnol J* 2018, 16:370-378.

[21] Haber DA, Velculescu VE: Blood-based analyses of cancer: circulating tumor cells and circulating tumor DNA. *Cancer Discov* 2014, 4(6):650-661.

[22] Heller G, McCormack R, Kheoh T, Molina A, Smith MR, Dreicer R, Saad F, de Wit R, Aftab DT, Hirmand M *et al*: Circulating Tumor Cell Number as a Response Measure of Prolonged Survival for Metastatic Castration-Resistant Prostate Cancer: A Comparison With Prostate-Specific Antigen Across Five Randomized Phase III Clinical Trials. *J Clin Oncol* 2018, 36(6):572-580.

[23] Bertolini F, Shaked Y, Mancuso P, Kerbel RS: The multifaceted circulating endothelial cell in cancer: towards marker and target identification. *Nat Rev Cancer* 2006, 6(11):835-845.

[24] Joosse SA, Gorges TM, Pantel K: Biology, detection, and clinical implications of circulating tumor cells. *EMBO Mol Med* 2015, 7(1):1-11.

[25] Alix-Panabieres C, Pantel K: Clinical Applications of Circulating Tumor Cells and Circulating Tumor DNA as Liquid Biopsy. *Cancer Discov* 2016, 6(5):479-491.

[26] Pawlikowska P, Faugeroux V, Oulhen M, Aberlenc A, Tayoun T, Pailler E, Farace F: Circulating tumor cells (CTCs) for the noninvasive monitoring and personalization of non-small cell lung cancer (NSCLC) therapies. *J Thorac Dis* 2019, 11(Suppl 1):S45-S56.

[27] Shishido SN, Carlsson A, Nieva J, Bethel K, Hicks JB, Bazhenova L, Kuhn P: Circulating tumor cells as a response monitor in stage IV non-small cell lung cancer. *J Transl Med* 2019, 17(1):294.

[28] Drapkin BJ, George J, Christensen CL, Mino-Kenudson M, Dries R, Sundaresan T, Phat S, Myers DT, Zhong J, Igo P *et al*: Genomic and Functional Fidelity of Small Cell Lung Cancer Patient-Derived Xenografts. *Cancer Discov* 2018, 8(5):600-615.

[29] Hodgkinson CL, Morrow CJ, Li Y, Metcalf RL, Rothwell DG, Trapani F, Polanski R, Burt DJ, Simpson KL, Morris K *et al*: Tumorigenicity and genetic profiling of circulating tumor cells in small-cell lung cancer. *Nat Med* 2014, 20(8):897-903.

[30] Jiang J, Wang DD, Yang M, Chen D, Pang L, Guo S, Cai J, Wery JP, Li L, Li H *et al*: Comprehensive characterization of chemotherapeutic efficacy on metastases in the established gastric neuroendocrine cancer patient derived xenograft model. *Oncotarget* 2015, 6(17):15639-15651.

[31] Stewart CA, Gay CM, Xi Y, Sivajothi S, Sivakamasundari V, Fujimoto J, Bolisetty M, Hartsfield PM, Balasubramaniyan V, Chalishazar MD *et al*: Single-cell analyses reveal increased intratumoral heterogeneity after the onset of therapy resistance in small-cell lung cancer. *Nat Cancer* 2020, 1:423-436.

[32] Klameth L, Rath B, Hochmaier M, Moser D, Redl M, Mungenast F, Gelles K, Ulsperger E, Zeillinger R, Hamilton G: Small cell lung cancer: model of circulating tumor cell tumorospheres in chemoresistance. *Sci Rep* 2017, 7(1):5337.

[33] Li Y, Zhang X, Liu D, Gong J, Wang DD, Li S, Peng Z, Wang X, Lin PP, Li M *et al*: Evolutionary Expression

of HER2 Conferred by Chromosome Aneuploidy on Circulating Gastric Cancer Cells Contributes to Developing Targeted and Chemotherapeutic Resistance. *Clin Cancer Res* 2018, 24(21):5261-5271.

[34] Li YL, Zhang XT, Ge S, Gao J, Gong JF, Lu M, Zhang QY, Cao YS, Wang DD, Lin PP *et al*: Clinical significance of phenotyping and karyotyping of circulating tumor cells in patients with advanced gastric cancer. *Oncotarget* 2014, 5(16):6594-6602.

[35] Pailler E, Faugeroux V, Oulhen M, Mezquita L, Laporte M, Honore A, Lecluse Y, Queffelec P, NgoCamus M, Nicotra C *et al*: Acquired Resistance Mutations to ALK Inhibitors Identified by Single Circulating Tumor Cell Sequencing in ALK-Rearranged Non-Small-Cell Lung Cancer. *Clin Cancer Res* 2019, 25(22):6671-6682.

[36] Zhang L, Zhang X, Liu Y, Zhang T, Wang Z, Gu M, Li Y, Wang DD, Li W, Lin PP: PD-L1$^+$ aneuploid circulating tumor endothelial cells (CTECs) exhibit resistance to the checkpoint blockade immunotherapy in advanced NSCLC patients. *Cancer Lett* 2020, 469:355-366.

[37] Bayarri-Lara C, Ortega FG, Cueto Ladron de Guevara A, Puche JL, Ruiz Zafra J, de Miguel-Perez D, Ramos AS, Giraldo-Ospina CF, Navajas Gomez JA, Delgado-Rodriguez M *et al*: Circulating Tumor Cells Identify Early Recurrence in Patients with Non-Small Cell Lung Cancer Undergoing Radical Resection. *PloS One* 2016, 11(2):e0148659.

[38] Wang L, Li Y, Xu J, Zhang A, Wang X, Tang R, Zhang X, Yin H, Liu M, Wang DD *et al*: Quantified postsurgical small cell size CTCs and EpCAM$^+$ circulating tumor stem cells with cytogenetic abnormalities in hepatocellular carcinoma patients determine cancer relapse. Quantified postsurgical small cell size CTCs and EpCAM$^+$ circulating tumor stem cells with cytogenetic abnormalities in hepatocellular carcinoma patients determine cancer relapse. *Cancer Lett* 2018, 412:99-107.

[39] Graves EE, Maity A, Le Q-T: The Tumor Microenvironment in Non-Small Cell Lung Cancer. *Semin Radiat Oncol* 2010, 20:156-163.

[40] Whiteside TL: The tumor microenvironment and its role in promoting tumor growth. *Oncogene* 2008, 27(45):5904-5912.

[41] Plaks V, Kong N, Werb Z: The cancer stem cell niche: how essential is the niche in regulating stemness of tumor cells? *Cell Stem Cell* 2015, 16(3):225-238.

[42] Tang DG: Understanding cancer stem cell heterogeneity and plasticity. *Cell Res* 2012, 22(3):457-472.

[43] Balkwill F, Mantovani A: Inflammation and cancer: back to Virchow? *Lancet* 2001, 357(9255):539-545.

[44] Shang B, Liu Y, Jiang S, Liu Y: Prognostic value of tumorinfiltrating FoxP3$^+$ regulatory T cells in cancers: a systematic review and meta-analysis. *Sci Rep* 2015, 5:15179.

[45] Shimizu K, Nakata M, Hirami Y, Yukawa T, Maeda A, Tanemoto K: Tumor-Infiltrating Foxp3+ Regulatory T Cells are Correlated with Cyclooxygenase-2 Expression and are Associated with Recurrence in Resected Non-small Cell Lung Cancer. *J Thorac Oncol* 2010, 5:585-590.

[46] Ziello JE, Jovin IS, Huang Y: Hypoxia-Inducible Factor (HIF)-1 regulatory pathway and its potential for therapeutic intervention in malignancy and ischemia. *Yale J Biol Med* 2007, 80(2):51-60.

[47] Choi KJ, Nam JK, Kim JH, Choi SH, Lee YJ: Endothelial-to-mesenchymal

transition in anticancer therapy and normal tissue damage. *Exp Mol Med* 2020, 52(5):781-792.

[48] Zhang L, Huang G, Li X, Zhang Y, Jiang Y, Shen J, Liu J, Wang Q, Zhu J, Feng X *et al*: Hypoxia induces epithelial-mesenchymal transition via activation of SNAI1 by hypoxia-inducible factor -1alpha in hepatocellular carcinoma. *BMC Cancer* 2013, 13:108.

[49] Liu T, Han C, Wang S, Fang P, Ma Z, Xu L, Yin R: Cancer-associated fibroblasts: an emerging target of anti-cancer immunotherapy. *J Hematol Oncol* 2019, 12(1):86.

[50] Shiga K, Hara M, Nagasaki T, Sato T, Takahashi H, Takeyama H: Cancer-Associated Fibroblasts: Their Characteristics and Their Roles in Tumor Growth. *Cancers (Basel)* 2015, 7(4):2443-2458.

[51] Chae YK, Davis AA, Agte S, Pan A, Simon NI, Iams WT, Cruz MR, Tamragouri K, Rhee K, Mohindra N *et al*: Clinical Implications of Circulating Tumor DNA Tumor Mutational Burden (ctDNA TMB) in Non-Small Cell Lung Cancer. *Oncologist* 2019, 24(6):820-828.

[52] Lee Y, Park S, Kim WS, Lee JC, Jang SJ, Choi J, Choi CM: Correlation between progression-free survival, tumor burden, and circulating tumor DNA in the initial diagnosis of advanced-stage EGFR-mutated non-small cell lung cancer. *Thorac Cancer* 2018, 9(9):1104-1110.

[53] Liang W, Zhao Y, Huang W, Gao Y, Xu W, Tao J, Yang M, Li L, Ping W, Shen H *et al*: Non-invasive diagnosis of early-stage lung cancer using high-throughput targeted DNA methylation sequencing of circulating tumor DNA (ctDNA). *Theranostics* 2019, 9(7):2056-2070.

[54] Moding EJ, Liu Y, Nabet BY, Chabon JJ, Chaudhuri AA, Hui AB, Bonilla RF, Ko RB, Yoo CH, Gojenola L *et al*: Circulating tumor DNA dynamics predict benefit from consolidation immunotherapy in locally advanced non-small-cell lung cancer. *Nat Cancer* 2020, 1:176-183.

[55] Corradetti MN, Torok JA, Hatch AJ, Xanthopoulos EP, Lafata K, Jacobs C, Rushing C, Calaway J, Jones G, Kelsey CR *et al*: Dynamic Changes in Circulating Tumor DNA During Chemoradiation for Locally Advanced Lung Cancer. *Adv Radiat Oncol* 2019, 4(4):748-752.

[56] Chaudhuri AA, Chabon JJ, Lovejoy AF, Newman AM, Stehr H, Azad TD, Khodadoust MS, Esfahani MS, Liu CL, Zhou L *et al*: Early Detection of Molecular Residual Disease in Localized Lung Cancer by Circulating Tumor DNA Profiling. *Cancer Discov* 2017, 7(12):1394-1403.

[57] Leary RJ, Sausen M, Kinde I, Papadopoulos N, Carpten JD, Craig D, O'Shaughnessy J, Kinzler KW, Parmigiani G, Vogelstein B *et al*: Detection of chromosomal alterations in the circulation of cancer patients with whole-genome sequencing. *Sci Transl Med* 2012, 4(162):162ra154.

[58] Abbosh C, Birkbak NJ, Wilson GA, Jamal-Hanjani M, Constantin T, Salari R, Le Quesne J, Moore DA, Veeriah S, Rosenthal R *et al*: Phylogenetic ctDNA analysis depicts early-stage lung cancer evolution. *Nature* 2017, 545(7655):446-451.

[59] Abbosh C, Birkbak NJ, Swanton C: Early stage NSCLC - challenges to implementing ctDNA-based screening and MRD detection. *Nat Rev Clin Oncol* 2018, 15(9):577-586.

[60] Merker JD, Oxnard GR, Compton C, Diehn M, Hurley P, Lazar AJ, Lindeman N, Lockwood CM, Rai AJ, Schilsky RL *et al*: Circulating Tumor DNA Analysis in Patients With Cancer: American Society of Clinical

Oncology and College of American Pathologists Joint Review. *J Clin Oncol* 2018, 36:1631-1641.

[61] Lin PP: Integrated EpCAM-independent subtraction enrichment and iFISH strategies to detect and classify disseminated and circulating tumors cells. *Clin Transl Med* 2015, 4(1):38.

[62] Krajcovic M, Overholtzer M: Mechanisms of ploidy increase in human cancers: a new role for cell cannibalism. *Cancer Res* 2012, 72(7):1596-1601.

[63] Sen S: Aneuploidy and cancer. *Curr Opin Oncol* 2000, 12(1):82-88.

[64] Passerini V, Ozeri-Galai E, de Pagter MS, Donnelly N, Schmalbrock S, Kloosterman WP, Kerem B, Storchova Z: The presence of extra chromosomes leads to genomic instability. *Nat Commun* 2016, 7:10754.

[65] Stopsack KH, Whittaker CA, Gerke TA, Loda M, Kantoff PW, Mucci LA, Amon A: Aneuploidy drives lethal progression in prostate cancer. *Proc Natl Acad Sci USA* 2019, 116:11390-11395.

[66] Duesberg P, Rausch C, Rasnick D, Hehlmann R: Genetic instability of cancer cells is proportional to their degree of aneuploidy. *Proc Natl Acad Sci USA* 1998, 95(23):13692-13697.

[67] Kronenwett U, Huwendiek S, Ostring C, Portwood N, Roblick UJ, Pawitan Y, Alaiya A, Sennerstam R, Zetterberg A, Auer G: Improved grading of breast adenocarcinomas based on genomic instability. *Cancer Res* 2004, 64(3):904-909.

[68] Danielsen HE, Pradhan M, Novelli M: Revisiting tumour aneuploidy - the place of ploidy assessment in the molecular era. *Nat Rev Clin Oncol* 2016, 13(5):291-304.

[69] Hida K, Klagsbrun M: A new perspective on tumor endothelial cells: unexpected chromosome and centrosome abnormalities. *Cancer Res* 2005, 65(7):2507-2510.

[70] Chen HF, Wu KJ: Endothelial Transdifferentiation of Tumor Cells Triggered by the Twist1-Jagged1-KLF4 Axis: Relationship between Cancer Stemness and Angiogenesis. *Stem Cells Int* 2016, 2016:6439864.

[71] Wagner MJ, Ravi V, Menter DG, Sood AK: Endothelial cell malignancies: new insights from the laboratory and clinic. *NPJ Precis Oncol* 2017, 1(1):11.

[72] Liu X, Li J, Cadilha BL, Markota A, Voigt C, Huang Z, Lin PP, Wang DD, Dai J, Kranz G *et al*: Epithelial-type systemic breast carcinoma cells with a restricted mesenchymal transition are a major source of metastasis. *Sci Adv* 2019, 5(6):eaav4275.

[73] Wang Y, Liu Y, Zhang L, Tong L, Gao Y, Hu F, Lin PP, Li B, Zhang T: Vimentin expression in circulating tumor cells (CTCs) associated with liver metastases predicts poor progression-free survival in patients with advanced lung cancer. *J Cancer Res Clin Oncol* 2019, 145(12):2911-2920.

[74] Hofman V, Heeke S, Marquette CH, Ilié M, Hoffman P: Circulating Tumor Cell Detection in Lung Cancer: But to What End? *Cancers (Basel)* 2019, 11:262.

[75] Ito H, Inoue H, Kimura S, Ohmori T, Ishikawa F, Gohda K, Sato J: Prognostic impact of the number of viable circulating cells with high telomerase activity in gastric cancer patients: a prospective study. *Int J Oncol* 2014, 45(1):227-234.

[76] Alunni-Fabbroni M, Sandri MT: Circulating tumour cells in clinical practice: Methods of detection and possible characterization. *Methods* 2010, 50(4):289-297.

[77] Coumans FA, van Dalum G, Beck M, Terstappen LW: Filter characteristics influencing circulating tumor cell enrichment from whole blood. *PloS One* 2013, 8(4):e61770.

[78] Marquette CH, Boutros J, Benzaquen J, Ferreira M, Pastre J, Pison C, Padovani B, Bettayeb F, Fallet V, Guibert N: Circulating tumour cells as a potential biomarker for lung cancer screening: a prospective cohort study. *Lancet Respir Med* 2020, 8:709-716.

[79] Yu M, Stott S, Toner M, Maheswaran S, Haber DA: Circulating tumor cells: approaches to isolation and characterization. *J Cell Biol* 2011, 192(3):373-382.

[80] Driemel C, Kremling H, Schumacher S, Will D, Wolters J, Lindenlauf N, Mack B, Baldus SA, Hoya V, Pietsch JM *et al*: Context-dependent adaption of EpCAM expression in early systemic esophageal cancer. *Oncogene* 2014, 33:4904-4915.

[81] Gires O, Stoecklein NH: Dynamic EpCAM expression on circulating and disseminating tumor cells: causes and consequences. *Cell Mol Life Sci:CMLS* 2014, 71(22):4393-4402.

[82] Yu M, Bardia A, Wittner BS, Stott SL, Smas ME, Ting DT, Isakoff SJ, Ciciliano JC, Wells MN, Shah AM *et al*: Circulating breast tumor cells exhibit dynamic changes in epithelial and mesenchymal composition. *Science* 2013, 339(6119):580-584.

[83] Krebs MG, Hou JM, Sloane R, Lancashire L, Priest L, Nonaka D, Ward TH, Backen A, Clack G, Hughes A *et al*: Analysis of circulating tumor cells in patients with non-small cell lung cancer using epithelial marker-dependent and -independent approaches. *J Thorac Oncol* 2012, 7(2):306-315.

[84] Wit SD, Dalum GV, Lenferink ATM, Tibbe AGJ, Hiltermann TJN, Groen HJM, Rijn CJMV, Terstappen LWMM: The detection of $EpCAM^+$ and $EpCAM^-$ circulating tumor cells. *Sci Rep* 2015, 5:12270.

[85] Grover PK, Cummins AG, Price TJ, Roberts-Thomson IC, Hardingham JE: Circulating tumour cells: the evolving concept and the inadequacy of their enrichment by EpCAM-based methodology for basic and clinical cancer research. *Ann Oncol* 2014, 25(8):1506-1516.

[86] Wu C, Hao H, Li L, Zhou X, Guo Z, Zhang L, Zhang X, Zhong W, Guo H, Bremner RM *et al*: Preliminary investigation of the clinical significance of detecting circulating tumor cells enriched from lung cancer patients. *J Thorac Oncol* 2009, 4(1):30-36.

[87] Liu Z, Qi L, Li Y, Zhao X, Sun B: VEGFR2 regulates endothelial differentiation of colon cancer cells. *BMC Cancer* 2017, 17(1):593.

[88] Wang X, Xu W, Wang S, Yu F, Feng J, Wang X, Zhang L, Lin J: Transdifferentiation of human MNNG/HOS osteosarcoma cells into vascular endothelial cells in vitro and in vivo. *Oncol Rep* 2017, 38(5):3153-3159.

[89] Foy V, Fernandez-Gutierrez F, Faivre-Finn C, Dive C, Blackhall F: The clinical utility of circulating tumour cells in patients with small cell lung cancer. *Transl Lung Cancer Res* 2017, 6(4):409-417.

[90] Okereke IC, Nishi S, Zhou J, Goodwin JS: Trends in lung cancer screening in the United States, 2016-2017. *J Thorac Dis* 2019, 11(3):873-881.

[91] Shieh Y, Bohnenkamp M: Low-Dose CT Scan for Lung Cancer Screening: Clinical and Coding Considerations. *Chest* 2017, 152(1):204-209.

[92] Ilie M, Hofman V, Long-Mira E, Selva E, Vignaud J-M, Padovani B, Mouroux J, Marquette C-H, Hofman P: "Sentinel" Circulating Tumor Cells Allow Early Diagnosis of Lung Cancer in Patients with Chronic Obstructive Pulmonary Disease. *PloS One* 2014, 9:e111597.

[93] Lei Y, Sun N, Zhang G, Liu C, Lu Z, Huang J, Zhang C, Zang R, Che Y, Mao S *et al*: Combined detection of aneuploid circulating tumor-derived endothelial cells and circulating tumor cells may improve diagnosis of early stage non-small-cell lung cancer. *Clin Transl Med* 2020:e128.

[94] Tanaka F, Yoneda K, Kondo N, Hashimoto M, Takuwa T, Matsumoto S, Okumura Y, Rahmani S, Tsubota N, Tsujimura T *et al*: Circulating Tumor Cell as a Diagnostic Marker in Primary Lung Cancer. *Clin Cancer Res* 2009, 15:6980-6986.

[95] Seijo LM, Peled N, Ajona D, Boeri M, Field JK, Sozzi G, Pio R, Zulueta JJ, Spira A, Massion PP *et al*: Biomarkers in Lung Cancer Screening: Achievements, Promises, and Challenges. *J Thorac Oncol* 2019, 14(3):343-357.

[96] Chen Q, Ge F, Cui W, Wang F, Yang Z, Guo Y, Li L, Bremner RM, Lin PP: Lung cancer circulating tumor cells isolated by the EpCAM-independent enrichment strategy correlate with Cytokeratin 19-derived CYFRA21-1and pathological staging. *Clinica Chimica Acta* 2013, 419:57-61.

[97] Hanssen A, Riebensahm C, Mohme M, Joosse SA, Velthaus JL, Berger LA, Bernreuther C, Glatzel M, Loges S, Lamszus K *et al*: Frequency of Circulating Tumor Cells (CTC) in Patients with Brain Metastases: Implications as a Risk Assessment Marker in Oligo-Metastatic Disease. *Cancers (Basel)* 2018, 10(12).

[98] Naito T, Tanaka F, Ono A, Yoneda K, Takahashi T, Murakami H, Nakamura Y, Tsuya A, Kenmotsu H, Shukuya T *et al*: Prognostic Impact of Circulating Tumor Cells in Patients with Small Cell Lung Cancer. *J Thorac Oncol* 2012, 7:512-519.

[99] Punnoose EA, Atwal S, Liu W, Raja R, Fine BM, Hughes BGM, Hicks RJ, Hampton GM, Amler LC, Pirzkall A *et al*: Evaluation of Circulating Tumor Cells and Circulating Tumor DNAinNon–Small Cell Lung Cancer: Association with Clinical Endpoints in a Phase II Clinical Trial of Pertuzumab and Erlotinib. *Clin Cancer Res* 2012, 18:2391-2401.

[100] Krebs MG, Hou JM, Ward TH, Blackhall FH, Dive C: Circulating tumour cells: their utility in cancer management and predicting outcomes. *Ther Adv Med Oncol* 2010, 2(6):351-365.

[101] Tamminga M, de Wit S, van de Wauwer C, van den Bos H, Swennenhuis JF, Klinkenberg TJ, Hiltermann TJN, Andree KC, Spierings DCJ, Lansdorp PM *et al*: Analysis of Released Circulating Tumor Cells During Surgery for Non-Small Cell Lung Cancer. *Clin Cancer Res* 2020, 26(7):1656-1666.

[102] Hashimoto M, Tanaka F, Yoneda K, Takuwa T, Matsumoto S, Okumura Y, Kondo N, Tsubota N, Tsujimura T, Tabata C *et al*: Significant increase in circulating tumour cells in pulmonary venous blood during surgical manipulation in patients with primary lung cancer. *Interact Cardiovasc Thorac Surg* 2014, 18(6):775-783.

[103] Li Y, Cheng X, Chen Z, Liu Y, Liu Z, Xu S: Circulating tumor cells in peripheral and pulmonary venous blood predict poor long-term survival in resected non-small cell lung cancer patients. *Sci Rep* 2017, 7(1):4971.

[104] Sawabata N, Funaki S, Hyakutake T, Shintani Y, Fujiwara A, Okumura M: Perioperative circulating tumor cells in surgical patients with non-small cell lung cancer: does surgical manipulation dislodge cancer cells thus allowing them to pass into the peripheral blood? *Surg Today* 2016, 46(12):1402-1409.

[105] Murlidhar V, Reddy RM, Fouladdel S, Zhao L, Ishikawa MK, Grabauskiene S, Zhang Z, Lin J, Chang AC, Carrott P *et al*: Poor Prognosis Indicated by Venous Circulating Tumor Cell Clusters in Early-Stage Lung Cancers. *Cancer Res* 2017, 77(18):5194-5206.

[106] Chemi F, Rothwell DG, McGranahan N, Gulati S, Abbosh C, Pearce SP, Zhou C, Wilson G, Jamal-Hanjani M, Birkbak N *et al*: Pulmonary venous circulating tumour cell dissemination before tumour resection and disease relapse. *Nat Med* 2019, 25:1534-1539.

[107] Chinniah C, Aguarin L, Cheng P, Decesaris C, Cutillo A, Berman AT, Frick M, Doucette A, Cengel KA, Levin W *et al*: Early Detection of Recurrence in Patients with Locally Advanced Non-small Cell Lung Cancer via Circulating Tumor Cell Analysis. *Clin Lung Cancer* 2019, 20:384-390.

[108] Wu C-Y, Lee C-L, Wu C-F, Fu J-Y, Yang C-T, Wen C-T, Liu Y-H, Liu H-P, Hsieh JC-H: Circulating Tumor Cells as a Tool of Minimal Residual Disease Can Predict Lung Cancer Recurrence: A longitudinal, Prospective Trial. *Diagnostics (Basel)* 2020, 10:144.

[109] Hanssen A, Wagner J, Gorges TM, Taenzer A, Uzunoglu FG, Driemel C, Stoecklein NH, Knoefel WT, Angenendt S, Hauch S *et al*: Characterization of different CTC subpopulations in non-small cell lung cancer. *Sci Rep* 2016, 6:28010.

[110] Carter L, Rothwell DG, Mesquita B, Smowton C, Leong HS, Fernandez-Gutierrez F, Li Y, Burt DJ, Antonello J, Morrow CJ *et al*: Molecular analysis of circulating tumor cells identifies distinct copy-number profiles in patients with chemosensitive and chemorefractory small-cell lung cancer. *Nat Med* 2017, 23:114-119.

[111] Yamashita J, Matsuo A, Kurusu Y, Saishoji T, Hayashi N, Ogawa M: Preoperative evidence of circulating tumor cells by means of reverse transcriptase-polymerase chain reaction for carcinoembryonic antigen messenger RNA is an independent predictor of survival in non-small cell lung cancer: a prospective study. *J Thorac Cardiovasc Surg* 2002, 124(2):299-305.

[112] Choma D, Daures JP, Quantin X, Pujol JL: Aneuploidy and prognosis of non-small-cell lung cancer: a meta-analysis of published data. *Br J Cancer* 2001, 85(1):14-22.

[113] Faugeroux V, Pailler E, Auger N, Taylor M, Farace F: Clinical Utility of Circulating Tumor Cells in ALK-Positive Non-Small-Cell Lung Cancer. *Front Oncol* 2014, 4:281.

[114] Pailler E, Adam J, Barthelemy A, Oulhen M, Auger N, Valent A, Borget I, Planchard D, Taylor M, Andre F *et al*: Detection of circulating tumor cells harboring a unique ALK rearrangement in ALK-positive non-small-cell lung cancer. *J Clin Oncol* 2013, 31(18):2273-2281.

[115] Lee VH, Tin VP, Choy TS, Lam KO, Choi CW, Chung LP, Tsang JW, Ho PP, Leung DK, Ma ES *et al*: Association of exon 19 and 21 EGFR mutation patterns with treatment outcome after first-line tyrosine kinase inhibitor in metastatic non-small-cell lung cancer. *J Thorac Oncol* 2013, 8(9):1148-1155.

[116] Park SM, Wong DJ, Ooi CC, Kurtz DM, Vermesh O, Aalipour A,

Suh S, Pian KL, Chabon JJ, Lee SH *et al*: Molecular profiling of single circulating tumor cells from lung cancer patients. *Proc Natl Acad Sci USA* 2016, 113(52):E8379-E8386.

[117] Maheswaran S, Sequist LV, Nagrath S, Ulkus L, Brannigan B, Collura CV, Inserra E, Diederichs S, Iafrate AJ, Bell DW *et al*: Detection of mutations in EGFR in circulating lung-cancer cells. *N Engl J Med* 2008, 359(4):366-377.

[118] Ran R, Li L, Wang M, Wang S, Zheng Z, Lin PP: Determination of EGFR mutations in single cells microdissected from enriched lung tumor cells in peripheral blood. *Anal Bioanal Chem* 2013, 405(23):7377-7382.

[119] Yu M, Bardia A, Aceto N, Bersani F, Madden MW, Donaldson MC, Desai R, Zhu H, Comaills V, Zheng Z *et al*: Cancer therapy. Ex vivo culture of circulating breast tumor cells for individualized testing of drug susceptibility. *Science* 2014, 345(6193):216-220.

[120] Li X, Zhang Y, Ding J, Wang M, Li N, Yang H, Wang K, Wang D, Lin PP, Li M *et al*: Clinical significance of detecting CSF-derived tumor cells in breast cancer patients with leptomeningeal metastasis. *Oncotarget* 2018, 9(2):2705-2714.

[121] Xu Z, Gao Y, Hao Y, Li E, Wang Y, Zhang J, Wang W, Gao Z, Wang Q: Application of a microfluidic chip-based 3D co-culture to test drug sensitivity for individualized treatment of lung cancer. *Biomaterials* 2013, 34(16):4109-4117.

[122] Lamouille S, Xu J, Derynck R: Molecular mechanisms of epithelial-mesenchymal transition. *Nat Rev Mol Cell Biol* 2014, 15(3):178-196.

[123] Munz M, Baeuerle PA, Gires O: The emerging role of EpCAM in cancer and stem cell signaling. *Cancer Res* 2009, 69(14):5627-5629.

[124] Ma G, Jiang Y, Liang M, Li J, Mao X, Veeramootoo JS, Xia T, Liu X, Wang S: Dynamic monitoring of $CD45^-$/$CD31^+$/$DAPI^+$ circulating endothelial cells aneuploid for chromosome 8 during neoadjuvant chemotherapy in locally advanced breast cancer. *Ther Adv Med Oncol* 2020, 12:1-14.

[125] Man S, Sanchez Duffhues G, Ten Dijke P, Baker D: The therapeutic potential of targeting the endothelial-to-mesenchymal transition. *Angiogenesis* 2019, 22(1):3-13.

[126] Manchado E, Malumbres M: Targeting aneuploidy for cancer therapy. *Cell* 2011, 144(4):465-466.

Chapter 11

Lung Cancer Oncotherapy through Novel Modalities: Gas Plasma and Nanoparticle Technologies

Milad Rasouli, Nadia Fallah and Kostya (Ken) Ostrikov

Abstract

Cold atmospheric pressure plasma (CAP) is emerging as new healthcare technology and it has a high potential through physical and chemical effects for cancer treatment. Recently, CAP, plasma activated liquid (PAL), and nanomaterial have been significant advances in oncotherapy. Reactive oxygen-nitrogen species (RONS), electrical field, and other agents generated by CAP interact with cells and induce selective responses between the malignant and normal cells. Nanomedicine enhances therapeutic effectiveness and decreases the side effects of traditional treatments due to their target delivery and dispersion in tumor tissue. There are various nanocarriers (NCs) which based on their properties can be used for the delivery of different agents. The combination of gas plasma and nanomaterials technologies is a new multimodal treatment in cancer treatment, therefore, is expected that the conjunction of these technologies addresses many of the oncology challenges. This chapter provides a framework for current research of NC and gas plasma therapies for lung cancer. Herein, we focus on the application of gas plasmas and nanotechnology to drug and gene delivery and highlight several outcomes of its. The types and features of the mentioned therapeutics strategy as novel classes for treating lung cancer individually and synergistic were examined.

Keywords: gas plasma, nanocarrier, reactive oxygen and nitrogen species (RONS), selectivity, lung cancer

1. Introduction

Lung cancer is the most commonly diagnosed cancer and the leading cause of cancer death worldwide, with a survival of only 15% of cancer patients 5 years after diagnosis. Eighty-five percent of lung cancers are classified as non-small lung cells, including adenocarcinoma (ADC), squamous cell carcinoma (SCC), and large cell cancer, with 75% being diagnosed in advanced stages [1].

Due to the failure of common chemotherapeutic agents, resistance to them in lung cancer patients, and given the high mortality rate of this type of cancer, urgent need for new therapies that overcome drug resistance [2]. Alternative treatments must have fewer side effects and are more effective.

Gas plasma is a cocktail of chemical and physical factors including short and long-lived RONS, ions, electrons, UV photons, and electric fields. One of the important practical applications of plasmas lies in the future, in the field of medicine. Plasma medicine is an emerging strategy for widespread applications such as oncotherapy, wound healing, virology, biofilm, implant surfaces, and dentistry [3]. Plasma oncology that uses gas plasma technology for cancer treatment, is one of the newest and most promising multimodal therapies in cancer treatment [4]. Cancer treatment by plasma in two methods direct exposure and plasma-activated liquid (PAL) in the form of in vitro and in vivo have developed and had an impressive effect [5]. Responses of cancer cells to CAP respectively from 2004 to 2019, are apoptosis, growth inhibition, cytoskeletal damage, selective cancer cell death, cell cycle arrest, DNA, mitochondrial damage, growth inhibition in vivo, increased intracellular ROS, a selective increase of ROS, immunogenic cancer cell death, cell-based H_2O_2 generation, and currently, selectivity mechanism based on primary and secondary singlet oxygen [6].

Multimodal or combination cancer therapies can provide better treatment outcomes for patients. CAP can be used as a novel method because it combines electromagnetic, chemical, and thermal compounds in mild doses. It also combines well with other methods to produce beneficial synergistic effects [7].

Advances in nanotechnology have led to the rapid development of the synthesis, characterization, and application of nanocarriers (NCs) in cancer treatment [8]. Nanomaterials, due to their unique properties, can provide benefits such as clinical diagnosis, heat treatment, and body imaging, so they are a good candidate for pharmaceutical systems. One of the most important advantages associated with NC systems is their ability to withstand physiological stress or improve biological stability and their oral consumption, which makes them more attractive than other delivery strategies [9]. To be several innovative drug delivery methods are used in cancer treatment. A wide range of nanocomposites based on synthetic polymers, proteins, lipids, and organic and inorganic particles have been used to treat cancer specifically to deliver drugs specifically to solid tumors. A carrier offers many benefits such as protection against damage to the bloodstream, better drug solubility, increased drug stability, targeted drug delivery, reduction of toxic effects, and drug improvement. Permeability and preservation of the enhanced effect have long been considered as the main mechanism to facilitate the preferential accumulation of nanoparticles in tumor tissues compared to normal tissues [8–10].

CAP and nanoparticles have been known that alone or simultaneous with conventional therapies to covers wide ranges of oncotherapies challenges. There are interesting similarities and contrasts in their interaction with living cells and tissues, and these are directly related to the characteristics and scope of their therapeutic modality, especially chemical reactivity, selective action against pathogens and cancer cells, immunity to healthy cells and tissues, and transmission. It is time to consider synergies and the simultaneous combination of plasma-nanoparticles and their associated benefits for the development of effective therapies that improved selective efficacy and high safety for modern medicine. Here, a detailed overview of the advantages and limitations of nanomedicine and plasma medicine as novel technologies are presented and then we enumerate some of the main possibilities of synergy between nanotechnology and plasma technology for lung cancer treatment [11–14].

2. Gas plasma as an oncotherapeutics agent

2.1 Definition and application of gas plasma

Gas (also known as physical) plasma is the fourth state of matter and represents a quasi-neutral gas of charged and neutral particles that exhibits collective behavior. The plasma is categorized into three types of hot, warm, and non-thermal (cold) plasmas [15]. CAP has recently become a promising solution to a range of challenges due to its diverse applications in healthcare, environmental remediation and pollution control, materials processing, electrochemistry, nanomaterial synthesis, and more have been considered [16]. Cold (non-thermal) plasma is a cocktail of chemical and physical agents such as short-lived reactive species, long-lived reactive species, electromagnetic field, and ultraviolet radiation [17]. Plasma treatment is transferring of these reactive agents to targets or samples. Generation, interaction and transferring of reactive agents from plasma to the target as shown in **Figure 1**, contains multidisciplinary areas including plasma physics, plasma chemistry, solution chemistry, and biochemistry [18].

These reactive agents cause the plasma to have promising biological effects. Gas plasma as an emerging therapeutic implication has attracted attention recently in various fields of medicine. Cancer treatment, wound healing, dental hygiene, bacteria eradication, and blood coagulation are some of the promising fields for plasma treatment [17]. When CAP devices for cancer application are developed and optimized plasma sources, biologically relevant plasma components, physical and chemical characterization, and application adapted designed are the most important aspects before in vivo and clinical application that should be considered [19].

On the other hand, a mixture of specific factors including device parameters (treatment area, flow rate, working gas, gas composition, shielding for tuning), process parameters (treatment time, incubation time, direct vs. indirect, distance to effluent, throughput), cell type (normal vs. cancer), morphology and physiology, surface receptor expression, volume and content of liquids, chemical composition of liquids, physiological state and disease, and penetration depth influencing the impact and efficiency of gas plasma performance [20].

Redox flux increase to cells, multimodality nature, mild effect, flexibility in use, and dose-dependent effect as primary features of CAP cause to unique clinical properties of plasma including selectivity for cancer cells, enhancing cancer chemosensitivity, stimulation of the immune system, elimination of cancer stem cells, and halting cancer metastasis [3].

2.2 Selectivity mechanism of CAP and PAM

The inefficacy of utilized approaches in oncotherapy has turned cancer into a chronic disease. Conventional anti-cancer agents lack the selectivity towards normal and cancer cells and target over than malignant tumors. Targeting normal cells and pathways that are necessary for the survival of its limited application of common modalities. As a result, new oncotherapeutics strategies must have high selectivity performance [8, 14].

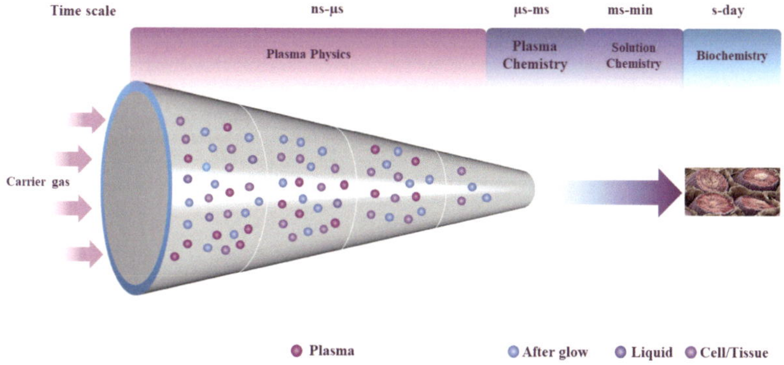

Figure 1.
Generation, interaction and transferring of reactive agents from plasma to the biological target.

Possible mechanisms that have been proposed for selective effects are based on the fundamental difference between normal and cancer cells. In contrast to normal cells that do not metabolize glucose for lactation in the presence of oxygen, cancer cells have different and abnormal metabolism and even metabolize glucose for lactation in the presence of oxygen (aerobic glycolysis). This effect, known as the Warburg effect, is one of the most important metabolic differences in normal and cancerous cells. Therefore, cancer cells are more sensitive to the accumulation of ROS than normal cells [21]. The ROS play a key role in conventional cancer treatments such as chemotherapy and radiation therapy. Among them, hydrogen peroxide can be considered as the most basic and important species [22]. Cold plasma is also being integrated with the production of RONS in the context of therapeutic methods based on redox reactions. Nevertheless, despite the similarities at least in the level of reactive oxygen species between the mechanism of CAP and other anticancer drugs, CAP by generating RNS distinguishes itself from other treatments [23].

The selectivity mechanism of CAP and PAM between the normal and cancerous cells has been discussed in previous studies. Several factors influence the selective effect of CAP and PAM, such as the expression of aquaporins or cholesterol or the ability to protect against oxidative stress by the anti-oxidative system to determine how many RONS can enter the cell and interfere with intracellular signaling pathways. Bauer and Graves in recent years suggested that activation of intercellular Hypochlorous acid (HOCl) signaling which after catalase inactivation through subsequent generate primary and secondary $^1O_2$ by the interaction of long-lived species in PAM have a key role in the selectivity of CAP and PAM [24, 25]. Keidar and colleagues proposed that the key role in selectivity for expression of aquaporin levels and suggested that the high level of aquaporin that makes the more hydrogen peroxide (H_2O_2) derived plasma as a key anticancer RONS, penetrates the cell and initiate apoptosis. In other words, cancer cells are more vulnerable than normal cells due to the high expression of aquaporin on cytoplasmic membranes [26, 27]. Van der Paal et al. suggested that RONS enter into normal and cancer cells according to the corresponding cholesterol fraction of their cell membrane. Since cancer cells have lower cholesterol fraction compared to normal cells, they are most affected [28, 29]. Despite all the studies that have been done, the selectivity of CAP and PAM is still a matter of scientific debate and there is no consensus in the community.

Bauer et al. have recently presented a mechanism for selectivity of CAP and PAM that includes three steps. The generation of primary and secondary singlet oxygen which is inactivated membrane-associated catalase (step1), penetration of H_2O_2 through aquaporins (step2), and at the final step causes cell death through the mitochondrial pathway of apoptosis by the reactivated HOCl or $^\bullet NO/ONOO^-$ – mediated apoptosis-inducing signaling. $^1O_2$, which can be considered an important role in the selectivity of CAP and PAM, is produced primarily from hydrogen peroxide and nitrite that are two long-lived species in PAM, and in the second stage, $^1O_2$ is generated from H_2O_2 and $ONOO^-$ due to NOX1 (membrane) and NOS (intracellular) respectively (**Figure 2**) [24, 25, 30, 31].

2.3 Gas plasma for lung cancer oncotherapy

Even though a concise time has been passed since the initial discovery of plasma oncotherapy, we are seeing tremendous progress in this field, and day to day the hope of becoming a treatment option for clinical practice is increasing. The effect of gas plasma on all types of cancer including oral cancer, hepatic cancer, skin cancer, glioblastoma, breast cancer, pancreatic cancer, ovarian cancer, neuroblastoma,

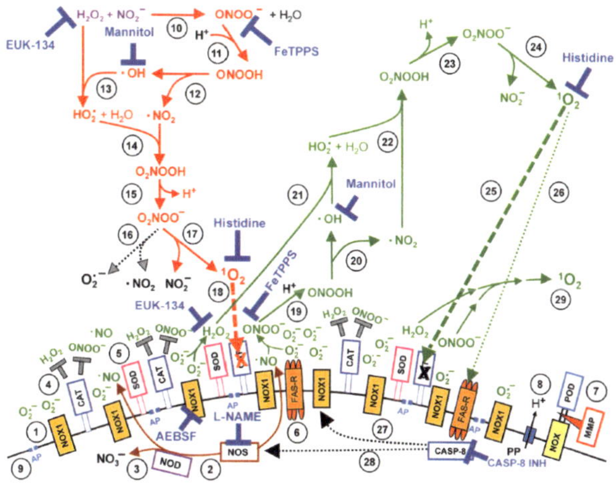

Figure 2.
Apoptosis induction by CAP/PAM is mediated by the generation of primary and secondary singlet oxygen ($^1O_2$). NADPH oxidase 1 (NOX1) is expressed in the membrane of tumor cells and generates extracellular superoxide anions ($O_2^{\bullet-}$) (#1). NO synthase (NOS) (#2) generates $^\bullet$NO which can be either oxidated by $^\bullet$NO dioxygenase (NOD) (#3) or pass through the cell membrane. Membrane-associated catalase (#4) protects tumor cells towards intercellular RONS-mediated signaling. Comodulatory SOD (#5) is required to prevent $O_2^{\bullet-}$- mediated inhibition of catalase. Further important elements in the membrane are the FAS receptor (#6), dual oxidase (DUOX) (#7), from which a peroxidase domain (POD) is split through matrix metalloprotease, proton pumps (#8) and aquaporins (#9). H_2O_2 and NO_2^- derived from CAP treatment and stable in PAM interact and generate peroxynitrite ($ONOO^-$) (#10). In the vicinity to membrane-associated proton pumps $ONOO^-$ is protonated to peroxynitrous acid (ONOOH) (#11) and decomposes into $^\bullet NO_2$ and $^\bullet$OH radicals (#12). $^\bullet$OH radicals react with H_2O_2, resulting in the formation of hydroyperoxyl radicals ($HO_2^\bullet$) (#13). The subsequent generation of peroxynitric acid (O_2NOOH) (#14) and peroxynitrate (O_2NOO^-) (#15) allows for the generation of "primary singlet oxygen" ($^1O_2$) (#17). Primary $^1O_2$ causes local inactivation of membrane-associated catalase (#18). Surviving H_2O_2 and $ONOO^-$ at the site of inactivated catalase are the source for sustained generation of "secondary $^1O_2$" through reactions #19- #24. Secondary $^1O_2$ may either inactivate further catalase molecules (#25) and thus trigger autoamplification of $^1O_2$ generation (#29), or activate the FAS receptor (#26) and in this way enhance the activities of NOX1 and NOS. This enhances the efficiency of secondary $^1O_2$ generation. The site of action of specific inhibitors and scavengers are indicated. Please find details on the elements on the surface of tumor cells in ref.s, on singlet oxygen generation in ref.s, and on intercellular apoptosis-inducing signaling after catalase inactivation in ref.s. this figure was obtained with permission from [25] under the terms of creative commons CC BY license.

prostate cancer, head and neck cancer, lung cancer, osteosarcoma, leukemia, and colorectal cancer have been studied at least in in-vitro levels. The volume of work has expanded greatly in recent years and has even expanded to the evaluation stage of plausible action mechanism of plasma, which was described in detail in the previous section. Another factor that has led to great hope in this field is the apparent success of plasma for a wide range of cancers. In particular, enhancing chemosensitivity and selectivity respecting to cancer cells of plasma in comparison to routinely treatments were remarkable achievements for plasma.

Lung cancer treatment studies approximately include 10% of plasma oncology research. Although most studies still are limited to laboratory and animal work, the initial outcomes show high plasma potential for the treatment of lung cancer. In this section, in addition to reviewing the studies, we enumerate the limitations and try to enumerate some of the possibilities of future work. Here, we review all of the current research on lung cancer treatment by CAP.

2.3.1 The impact of plasma device and process parameters on lung cancer cells

The nature of plasma is such that the cocktail of plasma device parameters affects the oxidation potential and its performance when interacting with the target [32]. **Figure 3** is documented depicts a set of all the factors that are important for plasma therapy. If it is still unknown to us how chemical and physical factors affect target or sample, but in general it can be said that all the factors mentioned in the figure, affect plasma-target interaction. However, it is impossible to explain explicitly these issues, especially the plasma dose is a debate for plasma medicine society.

Lung cancer also has been evaluated by a variety of plasma oncology factors. Preliminary works only examining the effects of plasma device and process parameters including working gas, flow rate, applied voltage, frequency, and treatment time. Therefore, the authors try to investigate the effects of the physical factors of different plasma devices on cancer cells and only evaluated the cell death and did not study to determine the molecular mechanism of CAP.

Huang et al. attempt to evaluate the efficiency of gas plasma on lung cancer cell lines. Device and process parameters such as increasing applied power and prolonging exposure time, respectively, influence the efficiency of gas plasma on A549 cancer cells. In addition, introduced OH, O, N_2, N^+, Ar, Ar^+, and Ar^{2+} radicals that generated with plasma as responsible for cell deactivation [33].

Akhlaghi et al. more focused on device parameters and examine the effects of the gas mixture, gas flow rate, applied voltage, and distance from the nozzle on the two lung cancer cell lines. 3 T3 cell line related to the fibroblast was also evaluated. The authors argue that except for the gas flow rate other mentioned parameters can affect the efficacy of plasma. In particular, treatment time plays a decisive role in the viability of cancer and normal cells [34].

A549 lung cancer cells evaluated with mDBD plasma. Karki et al. believe that mDBD plasma can localized target lung cancer. Also, the cell culture medium temperature did not exceed 26°C. The production of reactive oxygen and nitrogen species inhibits cell migration and is thought to be the main factor in the plasma process and induces apoptosis in lung cancer cells [35].

Various plasma devices have been used to treat lung cancer. Most of these devices are made by the research teams themselves and rarely meet the required standards for medical devices. Details of the multiple plasma devices used for lung cancer are summarized in **Table 1**.

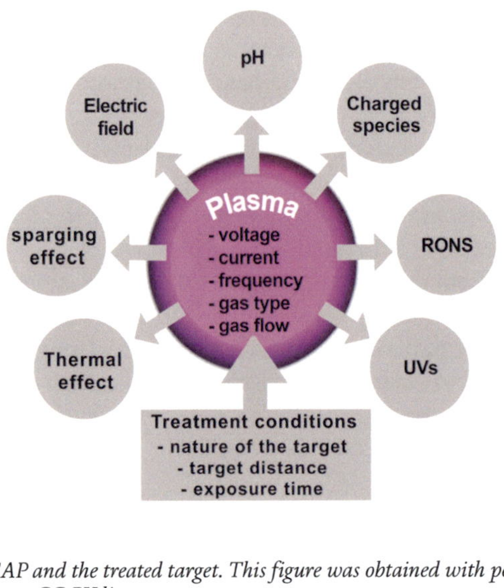

Figure 3.
The interaction between CAP and the treated target. This figure was obtained with permission from [32] under the terms of creative commons CC BY license.

Device	Type	Gas	Voltage (kV)	Frequency (kHz)	Treatment time (min)	Distance (cm)	Slm	Ref
Microplasma	Jet	He	6–9	32	0.03–0.33	1	0.01–0.1	[36]
Plasma jet	Jet	He	2–5	n.a	0.5	1	11	[37]
NTP device	DBD	He	12	24	1–3	0.5	1.33	[38]
Plasma needle	Jet	Ar	30	11.55	0–6	n.a	0.9	[33]
Plasma jet	Jet	He/O_2	1.8	50	0.16	0.5	0.5	[39]
mDBD plasma	Jet	Air	12	1	0–2	0.1	n.a	[40]
APPJ	Jet	He	7	39.5	0–0.5	n.a	1	[41]
CAP device	Jet	He	8	25	n.a	2	4	[42]
NTAPPJ	Jet	Ar	4	19.5	0–2	1.1	3	[43]
NEAPP	DBD	Ar	10	0.06	3	0.3	2	[44]
Plasma device	DBD	Air	0.08	0.06	0–5	0.4	n.a	[45]
APPJ	Jet	He	0.7–1.1	35	0.16	1	0.1	[46]

Table 1.
Overview detail of plasma devices for lung cancer oncotherapy.

2.3.2 The selective effects of gas plasma oncotherapy towards lungs normal and cancer cells

Followed by the initial studies, plasma oncology research continued with the addition of healthy cells. With the addition of normal cells, the selective effect of gas plasma oncotherapy was added to the set of plasma oncology studies. Lung cancer, as one of the most challenging cancers, was one of these cancers on which the selective effect of plasma was investigated. Here is a review of several works that were placed in this category.

In a highly interesting work, Keidar et al. examined the selective effects of cold plasma in vitro and in vivo on different types of cancer. That study demonstrated the selective effect of cold plasma on the normal human bronchial epithelial (NHBE) and lung cancer (SW900) cell lines. Beyond negligible thermal effects of plasma therapy, their study suggests cell adhesion, cell proliferation, growth regulation, and cell death in cancer processes, are selectively deregulated by non-thermal plasma modality. Besides, the possibility of improved survival, reductions in tumor volumes, and paradigm shift in cancer therapy through cold plasma treatment were reported for the first time in this study [37].

Kim et al. to investigate the influence of cold plasma on TC-1 mouse lung carcinoma cells (ATCC No. JHU-1) and mouse fibroblast CL.7 cells (ATCC TIB-80), developed a highly flexible microplasma jet device comprising hollow-core optical fibers of three different sizes. Under different experimental conditions, plasma induce dose-dependent apoptosis and did not affect a necrotic response in the cultured cells. Also, plasma plume size is a dominant factor in the efficacy of plasma. On the other hand, TC-1 tumor cells were more sensitive to plasma exposure than CL.7 fibroblast cells under these experimental conditions. Therefore, under these plasma dose conditions, plasma oncology can be used as a selective treatment for TC-1 tumor cells with no harm to CL.7 fibroblast cells [36].

A previous study also has reported selectivity of gas plasma towards normal (BEAS-2B, HEK293T) and cancer (A549) cells. The generation of intracellular reactive oxygen species (ROS) in cancer cells is higher than in normal cells and this difference is the main cause for the selectivity of gas plasma oncotherapy [46].

2.3.3 Plasma activated liquid for lung cancer treatment

On the other hand, in recent years, due to some limitations of direct plasma treatment such as the inability to penetrate the tissue, maintenance problems, etc. A new type of plasma therapy in the form of the plasma-activated liquid has developed. Exposure of liquids (medium, water, PBS, and ...) to plasma plume and add these activating liquids to the biological samples or living tissue recently received attention as a plasma treatment modality [47]. As adjuvant oncotherapy, Cheng et al. used plasma activated medium (PAM) for investigating the impact of gas plasma on benign mesothelial cells, CL1–5 and A549, normal fibroblasts, and cancer-associated fibroblasts (CAFs) cells. To evaluate PAM as a treatment method that can be used in clinical applications, its effectiveness was compared with hyperthermochemotherapy. This study revealed PAM selectively inhibits the proliferation of lung cancer cells and these effects are related to the produced H_2O_2 and NO_2^- in the culture medium [43].

Another study in this regard has dealt in detail with the various interactions and factors affecting the process of plasma therapy. An important role of the composition of culture medium and maintainability of activated medium for at least one week in −80 C are some of the interesting results of this study. PAM accompanied by ER stress induces caspase-independent apoptosis in A549 lung cancer cells through down-regulated anti-apoptosis proteins, activating PARP-1, and AIF release. H_2O_2 as a long live reactive oxygen species plays an important role in the whole process of plasma therapy [44].

The last literature regarding the application of PAM for lung cancer was done by Kumar et al. The temperature and pH culture medium not changed significantly after activating via discharge. The concentration of H_2O_2 as a key indicator at the different numbers of pulsed plasma discharge was measured. It was observed that lung cancer cells were more susceptible to PAM and PAM selectivity induces apoptosis in lung cancer cells [48].

2.3.4 The underlying molecular mechanism induced by gas plasma in lung cancer

Recently, studies in this field have entered a new arena and in some cases, mechanism of action also study. In recent years, with the expansion of the understanding of plasma redox research, has entered a new phase and the mechanism of plasma function with a focus on RONS, as determining factors in the treatment process are evaluated. Herein, we discuss the role of generated RONS by CAP. It can be seen that plasma has appeared successful in more studies and has been able to selectively induce apoptosis in cancer cells.

A noteworthy study by Yang et al. has investigated the molecular mechanism of gas plasma effects on A549 and H1299 cells. The most striking result to emerge from the data is that miR-203a/BIRC5 axis was affected by gas plasma. The miR-203a targets BIRC5 which plays a critical role in angiogenesis, proliferation, and regulating the cell cycle in cancer cells. Therefore, Gas plasma with upregulation miR-203a suppressed proliferation and promoted apoptosis in A549 and H1299 cells [41].

Ma et al. evaluated the effects of gas plasma and the contribution of reactive oxygen and nitrogen and plausible molecular mechanism on human lung adenocarcinoma epithelial (A549). Due to cell types and different plasma doses, they conclude that various cell types indicated different sensitivity under plasma irradiation. Although H_2O_2 has a vital role but other ROS or RNS such as NO_3^-, $HO^\bullet$, etc. generated by plasma also be involved in the mechanism of it. Plasma induces cell death, apoptosis, DNA damage, and mitochondrial dysfunction and these are related to generated reactive species in the culture medium. Although CAP and PAM exhibit similar performance at low doses, at high doses PAM exhibits less toxicity compared to CAP [38].

Along with the physical characterization, the molecular mechanism of plasma on human lung adenocarcinoma cell lines (A549) was examined by Joh et al. Besides, the flow rate and working gas mixture in detail evaluated. This study provides new insights into the physical characterization of gas plasma. The overproduction of ROS induces DNA damage accompanied with high expression of p53 [39].

Karki et al. utilized 3D collagen matrices to assess apoptotic cell death of A549 lung cancer cells by applying gas plasma. They found generated reactive oxygen and nitrogen species reduces the viability of A549 lung cancer cells. Gas plasma has a greater impact on the superficial surface of 3D matrices but by penetrating deep into the 3D matrix, its effect is reduced [40].

The last work of this group explored the selective effect of gas plasma oncotherapy on both A549 as lung adenocarcinoma and MRC-5 as lung fibroblast cells. Besides, the extracellular concentration of reactive oxygen and nitrogen, cell cycle analysis, and the expression of genes related to apoptosis were investigated. Although gas plasma significantly targets cancer cells, the viability of normal cells is also reduced. Cancer cells in comparison to normal cells had higher expression of apoptosis-related genes (H2AX, BAX, 53, Caspase-8, and ATM) and greater penetrated intracellular RONS [49].

The most interesting finding of another study is related to the potential mechanism of gas plasma on A549 cells. The authors utilize the microarray approach in detail to examine the cellular response to stress, cell cycle, apoptotic process, and other cellular functions response to plasma irradiation for the first time. The author concluded changes in MEKK, GADD, FOS, and JUN gene expression that causes p53 and mitogen-activated protein kinase (MAPK) signaling pathways activation. From the results related to the expression of related genes cellular differentiation and proliferation also was observed [50].

The basic contention of Panngom et al. which was obtained from a study on H460 and HCC1588 (human lung cancer cell lines) and two human lung normal cell lines (MRC5 and L132) is that Gas plasma can preferentially kill cancerous lung cancer cells. Data from apoptosis-related assays consistent with cell death revealed H460 cancer cells more affected in comparison to MRC5 normal cells by plasma treatment. In the shorter treatment time, plasma selectively targets cancer cells and normal cells are not affected but at the longer plasma exposure time, the viability of two cancer and normal cells approximately equally reduces. The core finding of this work introduces a new strategy for lung cancer treatment through mitochondria targeting. On the other hand, although, they point to the possibility of intrinsic and extrinsic apoptosis pathways, they emphasize mitochondria-mediated apoptosis [45]. Finally, according to Ma et al. Heme oxygenase-1 (HO-1) as a target could be considered for the future oncotherapeutics modalities. This exciting result comes from that gas plasma via generation of ROS inhibits Nrf2/HO-1 pathway in A549 cells [51].

3. Nanoparticle based delivery system for lung cancer treatment

The term nanotechnology describes a wide range of nanometer-scale technologies with widespread applications in various medical and industrial areas.

Nanotechnology involves the production and application of physical, chemical, and biological systems at scales ranging from individual atoms or molecules to about 100 nanometers, as well as the integration of resulting nanostructures into larger systems [9]. Now, the convergence of disciplines (chemistry, biology, electronics, physics, engineering, etc.) has led to multiple applications in the treatment of diseases including cancer, the production of materials, computer chips, medical diagnostics, and healthcare, energy, biotechnology, space exploration, and security issues. Therefore, nanotechnology is expected to have a significant impact on our economy and society over the next 10 to 15 years, and to become more important in the long run as more scientific and technological advances are made. It is the convergence of science on the one hand and the growing diversity of applications on the other that is advancing the potential of nanotechnologies. In fact, their greatest impact may come from an unexpected combination of previously separate aspects [10].

Drug delivery in nanoscale with advances in nanotechnology has had an impressive effect on clinical therapeutics in comparison with conventional chemotherapy in the last two decades. NCs have made from different materials such as organic nanocarriers, inorganic nanocarriers, and a combination of both as shown in the composition section of **Figure 4**. Lipid-based nanocarriers and polymeric frameworks are known as organic nanocarriers, while quantum dots and silica nanoparticles are inorganic nanocarriers [52, 53].

Nanotechnology is a science for the production of carriers at a nanometer scale, and Nanomedicine is an important field of academic research causing clinical and commercial development. NCs must have certain properties to be efficiently transmitted; 1) because they are used in this method for delivery of drugs to specific targets and cells, for decreasing side effects and damaging impact on normal cells should have a specific antibody on their surface that binds to a specific marker on cancer cells as shown in targeting section of **Figure 4** [54], 2) NCs should not arouse the immune system, to prevent of their degradable before receiving by tumor cells [55], 3) and the entrance of NCs into solid tumors and release of agents based on the characteristic of NCs and cancer cell.

Drug release is controlled by many external and internal stimuli, e.g. temperature, pH, ionic strength, sound, redox, and electric or magnetic fields that improve the targeted therapy [56]. Good biocompatibility, low toxicity, high stability, size, shape and surface charge of NCs have a crucial role in their biological performance. There are various methods for preparing NCs, agents can encapsulate in the matrix or the core of NCs and also in some cases can chemically bind to the surface of NCs [57].

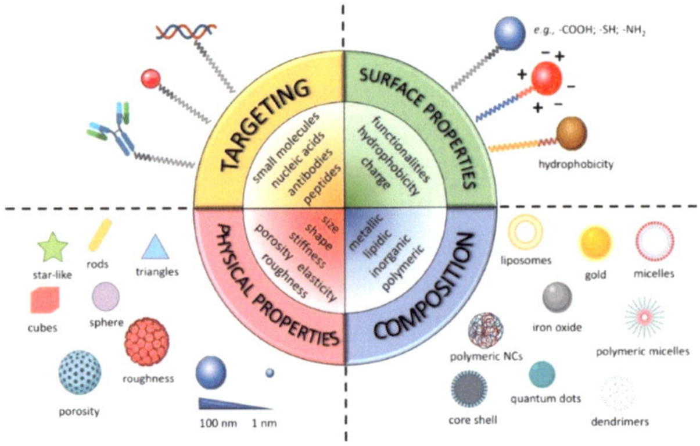

Figure 4.
Physical and chemical properties of nanocarriers. This figure was obtained with permission from [52] under the terms of creative commons CC BY license.

Gene delivery along with drug delivery is used for cancer treatment. Increase the production of some proteins or downregulation (or silencing) of some genes with the use of antisense or siRNA are the basis of this treatment. Low toxicity is the dedicated property of this type of therapy [58].

In this section, we have classified a few numbers of performed research for lung cancer treatment based on their type of NC. Most of these studies have been implemented in the level of in vitro and in vivo and evaluating cellular uptake, cytotoxicity, apoptosis, volume and growth of tumors. From my point of view, some of them have the potential to enter the clinical trial phase. For some of them is necessary to study more about the drugs and nanocarriers action mechanism in tumor tissue, which should be further studied.

3.1 Organic nanocarriers

3.1.1 Lipid-based nanocarriers

Recently lipids are very popular systems for the delivery of drugs to target tissues. There are different types of lipids, that use in this drug delivery system such as oils, waxes, cholesterol, sterols, triglycerides, phospholipids and fat soluble vitamins. Lipid-based NCs due to the electrostatic interaction between the polar phospholipid head and the solvent have spherical shape. The flexible nature of lipid-based NCs like liposomes helps them to squeeze large particles into small intercellular pores. Neutral surface charge of nanoparticles causing their Instability. The inside surface of blood vessels and cells contains many negatively charged components such as glycocalyx, so Lipid-based NCs surface charge is designed positive for better absorption to target cells [59, 60].

Some of the studies that use lipid-based NCs gathered below, for comparison the level of the studies and effectiveness of different types of lipid-based NCs in recent years. A549 cells are the most usable cells for in vitro and in vitro (A549 tumor-bearing mice) experiments that are treated with different kinds of drugs and agents conjugated with lipid-based NCs. An increase in cellular uptake, cytotoxicity and apoptosis and a decrease in tumor growth and volume were the most common results obtained from in vitro and in vivo experiments respectively.

In 2018 Kabary et al. produced layer-by-layer (LbL) lipid nanoparticles (NPs) by lactoferrin (LF) and hyaluronic acid (HA) to deliver berberine (BER) and rapamycin (RAP) for the treatment of lung cancer. NPs with capsulated agents increase cytotoxicity against A549 lung cancer cells by rising up the entrance of drugs to the cells. Drug release was controlled by binding BER to sodium lauryl sulfate (SLS) and production of BER-hydrophobic ion pair (BER-HIP). LF and HA on the surface of lipid NPs caused the stability of them. These NPs protected RAP against hydrolysis and augment its stability in phosphate buffered saline (PBS). In vivo experiments also indicate the growth of tumor was inhibited, and RAP can decrease the angiogenesis by inhibiting vascular endothelial growth factor (VEGF) and BER has an inhibition effect on angiogenesis and tumor progression via blocking of various pro-inflammatory and angiogenic factors. To mice fed HA/LF-LbL-RAP-BER/SLS-NPs, the level of Ki-67 as a proliferation marker was reduced in tumors in comparison with control [61].

Overexpression of nuclear factor E2–related factor 2 (Nrf2) caused drug resistance in lung cancer. Therefore, in other research, hyaluronic acid-based nanostructured lipid carriers (NLCs) for specific targeting via CD44 receptor in cancer cells was used to increase the effect of apigenin (APG) as an Nrf2 inhibitor. After treatment of A549 cells with this NC, cells became sensitive to docetaxel (DTX) and cell toxicity increased. HA-APG-NLCs also induced apoptosis in treated A549 cells (**Figure 5**) [62].

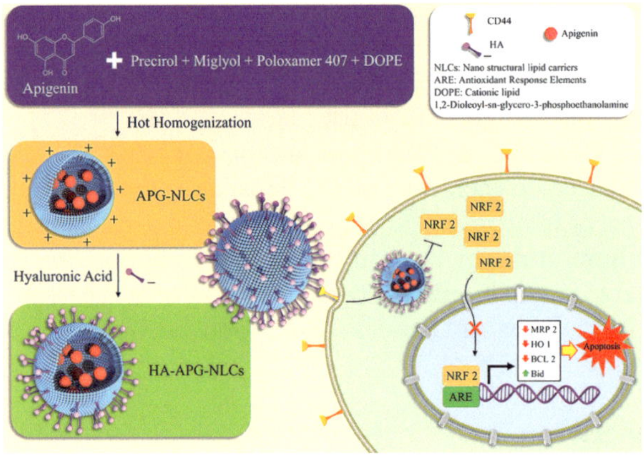

Figure 5.
Schematic of targeted hyaluronic acid-based lipid nanoparticle for delivery of apigenin in lung cancer cells. This figure was obtained with permission from [62] under the terms of creative commons CC BY license.

Also in 2019, Cetuximab (CET), paclitaxel (PTX) and 5-Demethylnobiletin (DMN) conjugated to nano lipid carriers (NLCs) (CET-PTX/DMN-NLCs). A549 cell viability after treatment by CET-PTX/DMN-NLCs decreased, and the anti-tumor effect was evaluated by in vivo experiment on Lung tumor xenografts mice [63].

Moreover, EGFR-targeted lipid polymeric nanoparticles (LPNs) conjugated to EGF-PEG-DSPE ligand in the outer layer and encapsulated cisplatin (CDDP) and doxorubicin (DOX) in the core and phospholipid layer respectively. While this nanocarrier reaches to target tissue DOX released faster than CDDP. Cytotoxicity showed a dose-dependent manner in this study. Accumulation in the heart and kidney are very lower than tumor tissue, and tumor volume and growth decreased significantly after treatment [64].

Wang and colleagues used Tf modified redox-sensitive lipid-polymer hybrid nanoparticles enclosed Afatinib (Afa) (Tf-SS-Afa-LPNs). There is a positive relation between GSH concentration and drug release. Cell proliferation was inhibited after treatment by Tf-SS-Afa-LPNs, and in vivo experiments showed afatinib accumulate more in the lung and lead to antitumor activity in it [65].

According to a recent report in 2020, for treatment of small-cell lung cancer (SCLC) polyphenol curcumin (Cc) as a natural drug bind to polysaccharide-cloaked lipidic nanocarriers (Cc@CLNs). This nanocarrier has some properties that stand out it from others: potential of penetration to the cell membrane, resistance to degradation of pepsin and trypsin, increase cellular uptake and bioavailability. Absorption of Cc@CLNs was analyzed by in situ experiments in rats and results showed uptake increased through Cc@CLNs compared with free Cc. For in vitro experiment H446 cells were cultured, the viability of cells showed time- and dose-dependent behavior. Cc@CLNs induced cell apoptosis and also augment the value of the intracellular ROS. Also, Cc@CLNs causing a decrease of the levels of the SCLC stem cell markers CD133 and ABCG2. SCLC H446 tumor-bearing mice after treatment via Cc@CLNs showed a lower tumor size and weight [66].

Besides, the properties of lipid NCs also make them suitable for gene delivery, so in 2019 a study was performed on MiR-660 upregulating. MiR-660 has known as a tumor suppressor miRNA in lung cancer cells and also can block the migration and invasion of tumor cells. P53 as a tumor suppressor gene regulate by mouse double minute 2 (MDM2) and inhibition of MDM2 play an important role in suppression of tumor growth both in vitro and in vivo (patient-derived xenograft (PDX) models of lung cancer). In this study Coated Cationic Lipid-nanoparticles (CCL) were used to deliver miRNA-660 (CCL660). Results demonstrated by overexpression of miRNA-660 tumor growth decreased, and by a reduction in MDM2, anti-cancer activity of P53 was confirmed and expression of miR-660 blocked H460 metastatic lung cancer cells [67].

3.1.2 Polymeric nanocarriers (PNCs)

Biodegradable polymers such as poly(lactic acid) (PLA), poly(lactic-co-glycolic) acid (PLGA), gelatin, albumin, chitosan, polycaprolactone, and poly-alkyl-cyano-acrylates are the most popular inexpensive polymers that are used in synthesizes of NCs. [68]. These solid structures released drugs in response to pH, light and redox potential [69].

Production of PNCs in detail brought in previous references that those who are interested to know more can refer to them. There are various PNCs that we mentioned some of them in the following, they have covalent and non-covalent interaction with specific proteins to improve and compensate for PNCs problems such as poor solubility and poor bioavailability [70]. Investigation of studies in the last 2 years demonstrates that these NCs play a significant role in the treatment of lung cancer. In vitro and in vivo studies demonstrated PNCs are without any problem (e.g., toxicity) to cells and host. Results of gathered studies indicated PNCs are more common and effective in comparison with lipid-based NCs. Due to their high diversity, different ranges of drugs and agents are connected to them to deliver to lung cells of tumors. In vitro experiments in PNCs showed high internalization and cytotoxicity and disrupt some crucial cancer signaling. Moreover, as mentioned in the Lipid-based NCs section in vivo experiments in PNCs indicated a reduction in tumor growth and volume and more drug dispersion in lung tumors.

In 2019, Quercetin (QR) loaded on T7 surface-functionalized PEGylated liposomes that contained soy-phosphatidylcholine (SPC) was used for an experiment on A549, MRC-5 cells and A549-Luc orthotopic lung tumor-bearing BALB/c nude mice. Increasing cytotoxicity, cellular uptake and rate of penetration in 3D lung tumor spheroids and induction of apoptotic effect and inhibition of tumor growth were the results of this study [71].

In another research, polypyrrole (Ppy)–polyethylenimine (PEI) nanocomplex (NC) was evaluated for the delivery system. One of the problems of Ppy for synthesizing of NC was its poor insolubility in water. For solving this problem some agents such as heparin, polyvinyl acetate, and chitosan were used for coating this polymer and increased their stability. Negatively charged lung cancer cells absorbed cationic Ppy–PEI NC and leading to less damage to surrounding cationic inflammatory tissue. Mitochondria dysfunction and ROS (Ppy–PEI NC could produce few ROS and hydrogen peroxide) are two important factors that causing cell apoptotic process [72].

Gong et al. used a pH-responsive methoxyl poly(ethylene glycol)-poly (aspartyl(dibutylethylenediamine)-co-phenylalanine) (mPEG-P(Asp(DBA)-co-Phe)) for delivery of afatinib as inhibition of epidermal growth factor (EGFR) and doxorubicin as a DNA-damaging chemotherapeutic to A549 lung cancer cells. Results showed by pH reduction, the release of both of them increased also they could cytotoxicity and apoptotic in cancer cells, and in vivo experiments indicated tumor growth and volume decreased in treatment mice [73].

Biodegradable PLGA NCs are another PNC that encapsulates the erlotinib cyclodextrin (Erlo-CD) complex. Enhanced cellular uptake caused higher cytotoxicity.

This NC leads to erlotinib resistant A549 cells became sensitive to erlotinib and tumor growth and metastasis decreased. Evaluating caspase-3 and caspase-7 activity showed inducing apoptosis in A549 cells, and 3D-spheroid cell culture was utilized for better mimics the physiological solid tumor [74].

On the other hand, various PNCs recently were evaluated. Alectinib as a clinical drug with adverse side effects used for target therapy in ALK-positive NSCL with dual-targeted (magnetic/TAT) NCs that made by poly (ethylene glycol) (PEG) and poly (hexyl ethylene phosphate) (PHEP). Magnetic targeting causing the exit of alectinib from vessels into tumor tissue and TAT targeting enhances tumor cellular uptake [75].

Moreover, in a recent study PNCs (PLGA) encapsulate sorafenib (SF) used for the treatment of NSCLC. Sorafenib is an inhibitor of Ras/Raf/MEK/ERK and has an anti-tumor activity via downregulation of the VEGFR-2/platelet-derived growth factor receptor (PDGFR)-β. Tumor accumulation, cytotoxicity and local release are other properties of SF NP [76].

S-HAp nanospheres with PEG and folic acid (FA) is another pH-responsive NC that delivers DOX to tumor tissues [77].

pH and redox-sensitive NPs is another PNC made from PEG-SS-PBAE-PLGA (PSPP) to encapsulate the platinum complexes of curcumin (Pt-Cc@PSPPN). Pt-Cc@PSPPN showed excellent stability. In A549 cells, cytotoxicity and apoptotic effect increased due to higher cellular uptake, and in vivo experiments, on A549 xenograft tumor-bearing nude mice indicated local bio distribution and antitumor activity of Pt-Cc@PSPPN. For anti-metastasis effect, CD31, VEGF, and MMP2 antibodies were evaluated and indicated metastasis inhibition [78].

Also in 2020, PEG-PLGA NPs enclosed febuxostat (FBX) (FBX–PLGA–PEG). The viability of A549 cells decreased. Evaluating of caspase 3 activity showed treatment by FBX–PLGA–PEG induced cellular apoptotic and cell cycle arrest [79].

In other investigations, Vaidya and colleagues indicated a kind of NPs made from PEI as a cationic stabilizer and coating bovine serum albumin (BSA) for a reduction in toxicity, controlled quinacrine (QA) release and accumulation of particles in the target region. Higher cellular uptake, cellular cytotoxicity, apoptosis and cell cycle arrest achieved in A549 cells. These results were obtained by evaluating p53, p21, LC3B, p62 and cleaved caspase-3. To better predict the physiological interaction in cytotoxicity and cell viability, the 3D-spheroid cell culture study was performed [80].

Another property of polymers, PEG–PLA and Pluronic P105 could encapsulate PTX (PEG–PLA/P105/PTX micelles). PEG–PLA/P105/PTX micelles combined with ambroxol (Ax) causing toxicity in A549 cells. PEG–PLA/P105/PTX micelles in combination with Ax lead to anticancer effect and excellent biodistribution [81].

Interestingly, PNCs have also been reported to be able to gen delivery, for example in 2019 siVEGF and chemotherapeutics etoposide (ETO) encapsulated by PEGylated histidine-grafted chitosan-lipoic acid (PHCL). Internalization in A549 cells treated by PHCL-Lip/ETO-siVEGF augmented, and by downregulation of VEGF via siVEGF cellular uptake enhanced and proliferation and metastasis decreased. For assessment of the ability of NPs in penetrating, A549 tumor spheroids were constructed (**Figure 6**) [82].

In another experiment, Cyanine 3 (Cy3)-labeled siRNA conjugated to HA-modified chitosan NPs (sCS NPs-HA) was prepared to use for experiment on A549 cells and xenograft tumor model female BALB/c mice. Cy3-labeled siRNA specifically delivered to A549 cells due to the CD44 receptor by sCS NPs-HA, and caused inhibition in cell proliferation by downregulation in BCL2. In vivo experiments showed tumor size and growth reduction [83].

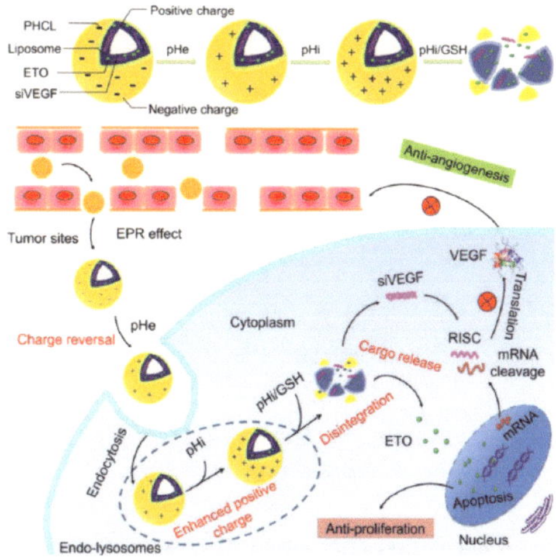

Figure 6.
VEGF siRNA and etoposide delivery via multi-functional nanoparticles for non-small cell lung cancer treatment. This figure was obtained with permission from [82] under the terms of creative commons CC BY license.

3.2 Inorganic nanocarriers

3.2.1 Quantum dots

Quantum Dots (QDs) by nanocrystal structure are semiconductors that gave them the ability to emit fluorescence from visible to infrared wavelengths. Surface modification of QDs gave them the potential in cancer imaging which is essential for choosing the appropriate cancer therapy [84]. Among the features of QDs are the following: do not react with drugs, have a high capacity for drugs encapsulated, low toxicity, good biocompatibility, strength and stability. In addition to the properties mentioned, their very small size (2–10 nm in diameter) makes them very efficient in drug delivery for lung cancer therapy [85].

One of the cases of QD-NCs as a system delivery is a ZnO QDs-based pH-responsive which coated by dicarboxyl-terminated PEG to increase the stability was prepared. CD44 as a marker in A549 cancer cells bind to HA that exist in ZnO QDs, and DOX by covalent interaction was loaded on ZnO QDs. In acidic endosome/lysosome, Zn^{2+} in ZnO QDs controlled the release of DOX that both of them used for lung cancer therapy via antitumor effect [86].

DOX and Cyclosporin (CsA) loaded on photoluminescent Graphene QDs encapsulated mesoporous NPs (GND@MSNs). Cell cytotoxicity was evaluated in A549 and HEL-299 Cells. GND@MSNs+DOX + CsA by inducing DNA damage causing apoptosis and cell cycle arrest [87].

3.2.2 Mesoporous silica nanocarriers (MSNCs)

MSNCs can be loading a variety of drugs and agents. The size of these carriers is crucial for effective drug delivery. The pore size in MSNs can be different, and internalization and biodistribution are related to the shape of them [88]. For instance, DOX deliver by an NC system made from d-a-tocopheryl polyethylene glycol 1000 succinate (TPGS)-functionalized polydopamine-coated MSNCs (MSNs-DOX@PDA-TPGS). This system released drugs in response to a decrease in pH. Both the A549 cells and drug-resistant A549 cells were tested for evaluating cytotoxicity and cellular uptake. Charge of the tumor cell membrane is negative

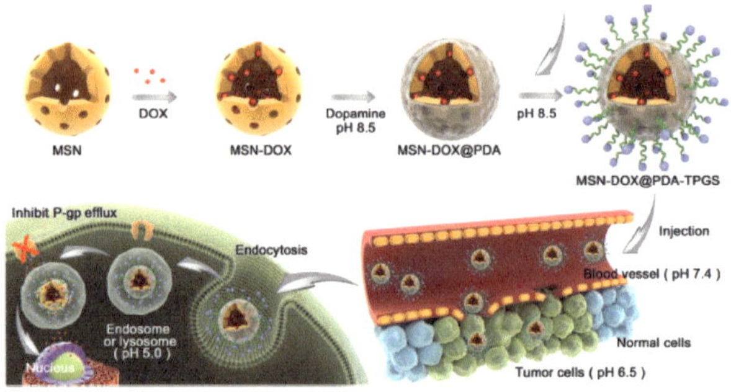

Figure 7.
TPGS-functionalized mesoporous silica nanocarrier for DOX delivery against lung cancer cells. This figure was obtained with permission from [89] under the terms of creative commons CC BY license.

and these NPs because free amines and ammonium groups of TPGSNH2 are slightly positive that enhance cellular uptake. The existence of TPGS is a factor for reducing drug resistance. Histological analysis showed the antitumor activity of MSNs-DOX@PDA-TPGS (**Figure 7**) [89].

4. Gas plasma in conjunction with nanoparticle for lung cancer treatment

Advances in digital technologies have created new opportunities for diagnosing, managing and treating disease. Several examples of advanced nanotechnology and digital technology have already been approved for the diagnosis and treatment of diseases. Plasma therapy, which has emerged as new healthcare technology, shows great potential for treating many diseases, including cancers with few or even no side effects [90].

In addition to the need to develop new healthcare methods, it is crucial to improve the efficacy of existing clinical used strategies such as chemotherapy drugs. The reality is that we need a solution to sustainable development in oncotherapies. This can only be achieved by combining existing and future methods. Plasma technology alone or in conjunction with nanomaterials shows high potential benefits along with chemotherapeutic strategies, minimizes side effects and increases the selectivity performance. On the other hand, the combination of plasma and nanotechnology leads to a multidisciplinary healthcare package that significantly improves the treatment outcomes of the disease and reduces the economic burden for healthcare in the community, as well as many solves problems related to the health care system (**Figure 8**) [10, 14, 17, 91].

Gas plasma and nanotechnology are the basis for the launch of future oncotherapetics agents. Synergistic effects of CAP, PAM and NCs with conventional therapy like chemotherapy, radiation therapy, pulsed electric fields, and plant origin have been discussed in recent years to improve the effectiveness of these methods. CAP and NPs and are fabricated independently and often along different ways to meet a range of biomedical challenges.

There are interesting similarities in their interaction with living cells and tissues, and these are directly related to the characteristics and scope of their therapeutic solutions, especially chemical reactivity, selective action against pathogens and cancer cells, immunity to healthy cells and tissues, and transmission. Targeted drugs are reflected by them into diseased tissues. It is time to consider synergies and the simultaneous combination of plasma-nanoparticles and their associated benefits for the development of effective therapies improved selective effects and high safety for modern oncology. In this section of the chapter, we focus on the created opportunities for linking plasma technologies and nanocarriers in lung cancer treatment [8–12].

There is only two work about the application of gas plasma and nanoparticle combination in lung cancer oncotherapy. Yu et al. first explored the targeted delivery of a PTX loaded PLGA-based delivery system by magnetic iron oxide nanoparticles (MNPs) in conjunction with plasma treatment. After encapsulating PTX within nanoparticle release of PTX to tumor significantly was modified.

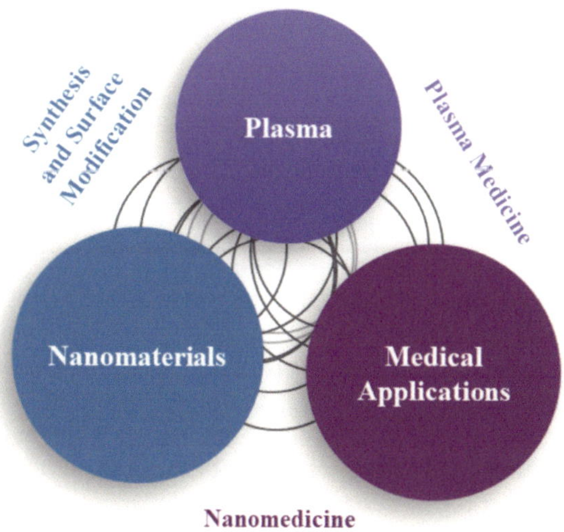

Figure 8.
Gas plasma, nanomaterials and their interaction alongside the medical applications of these two technologies.

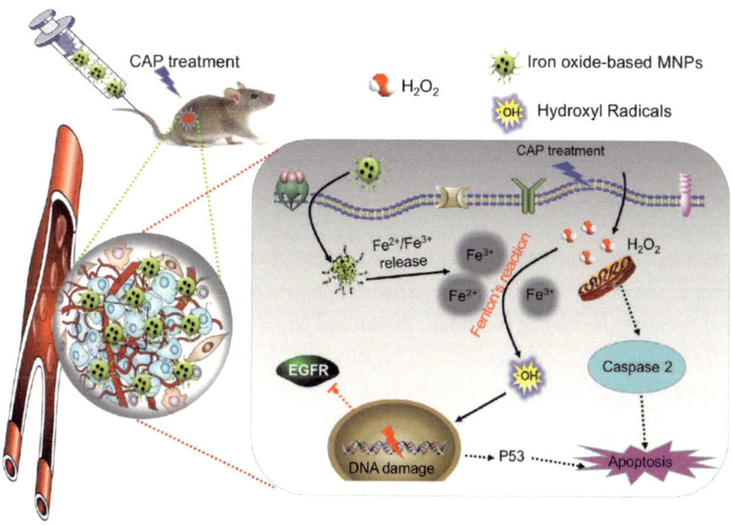

Figure 9.
Molecular mechanisms of MNPs enhancing tumor-selective killing effect of CAP. CAP-originated reactive species will cause a noticeable rise of intracellular H_2O_2, Fe^{2+}/Fe^{3+} released from the lysosome containing MNPs could catalyze H_2O_2 into OH., which cause the injury of cancer cells, such as inducing mitochondria-mediated apoptosis and double strand DNA breaks. This figure was obtained with permission from [92] under the terms of creative commons CC BY license.

Cytotoxic effects of various combinations of the gas plasma, PTX, PTX-loaded electrosprayed nanoparticles, and nanoparticle/plasma evaluated in the multimodal treatment of lung cancer cells. The data verify that plasma increased production of ROS enhanced the efficacy of nanoparticle, and induce apoptosis in A549 cancer cells [42].

Recently this group shines new light on these debates through an examination of lung cancer treatment's underlying mechanism. This study set out to compare and gain further understanding of the mechanism of the gas plasma alone and in combination with iron oxide-based MNPs treatment modalities. The simultaneous combination of gas plasma and MNPs is more promising in inhibiting the proliferation and induction of apoptosis. Plasma via depressing pERK and pAKT inhibited lung cancer cells but synergizing of two modalities induced EGFR downregulation. These results were also confirmed by inhibition of tumor xenograft growth. Finally, plasma and MNPs are highly promising combination treatments for aggressive forms of lung cancer (**Figure 9**) [92].

5. Conclusion and perspective

Cancer is increasingly becoming a chronic disease and has the lower success of a clinical trial among other diseases. As the current trend continues, lung cancer will remain a major challenge to healthcare systems. Therefore, investing in new technologies is essential to overcome this challenge. Many of the previous works about plasma oncotherapy for lung cancer have been performed at the in-vitro level. Therefore, there is still a long way to go before studies close to clinical applications, but in the short term, due to the achieved promising results, multimodal nature of plasma, the ability to synergistically with conventional drugs, it has given us great hope.

Nanocarriers for drug delivery system seems to be a reliable strategy for the biopharmaceutical industry. They have many advantages over conventional therapies and they have a bright future due to their inherent properties. The recent advances achieve in experimental researches such as in vitro (2D/3D cell culture), in vivo and ex vivo of tumor-target nanocarriers make it possible for use of this strategy for clinical trials for use as monotherapies or in combination with chemotherapeutics and it is necessary to standardize this new therapy, till could be approved and suitable for use in humans. This requires that research move from formulation-based approach and laboratory work towards patient-centered experiments.

Advances in nanotechnology and gas plasma have given us hope for cancer treatment. These technologies target the tumor selectively and the combination of gas plasma and nanotechnology have the potential to revolutionize cancer therapy. The integration of plasma science, chemistry, engineering, and oncology proved to be a powerful approach to cancer research, leading to technological and medical breakthroughs. To fully realize the promise of plasma and nanotechnologies in oncology, funding from government agencies and International Research Centers should be specifically targeted towards research at the intersection of these disciplines. Indeed, Investments have been made in this area in recent years, but it not enough due to the high potential of these two technologies.

Given current problems with various non-standard devices and nanoparticles, current investments should be targeted at the first step in developing standardization of plasma devices and nanoparticles. The second phase is the commercialization of nano and plasma technology.

Conflict of interest

The authors have no conflict of interest to declare.

Acronyms and Abbreviations

CAP	Cold Atmospheric pressure Plasma
PAL	Plasma Activated Liquid
RONS	Reactive Oxygen-Nitrogen Species
NSCLC	Non-Small Lung Cells
ADC	Adenocarcinoma
SCC	Squamous Cell Carcinoma
PAM	Plasma-Activated Medium
NCs	Nanocarriers
HOCl	Hypochlorous acid
H_2O_2	Hydrogen peroxide
NHBE	normal human bronchial epithelial
MAPK	mitogen-activated protein kinase
CAFs	Cancer-Associated Fibroblasts
LbL	Layer-By-Layer
NPs	Nanoparticles
LF	Lactoferrin
HA	Hyaluronic Acid
BER	Berberine
RAP	Rapamycin
SLS	Sodium Lauryl Sulfate
HIP	hydrophobic ion pair
PBS	Phosphate Buffered Saline
VEGF	Vascular Endothelial Growth Factor
Nrf2	Nuclear Factor E2–Related Factor 2
NLCs	Nanostructured Lipid Carriers
APG	Apigenin
DTX	Docetaxel
CET	Cetuximab
PTX	Paclitaxel
DMN	5-Demethylnobiletin
LPNs	Lipid Polymeric Nanoparticles
CDDP	Cisplatin
Afa	Afatinib
SCLC	Small-Cell Lung Cancer
Cc	Curcumin
MDM2	Mouse Double Minute 2
CCL	Coated Cationic Lipid-nanoparticles
PLA	Poly Lactic Acid
PLGA	Poly Lactic-co-Glycolic Acid
SPC	Soy-Phosphatidylcholine
Ppy	Polypyrrole
(mPEG-P(Asp(DBA)-co-Phe))	Methoxyl Poly Ethylene Glycol-Poly Aspartyl Dibutylethylenediamine-Co-Phenylalanine
EGFR	Epidermal Growth Factor
Erlo-CD	Erlotinib Cyclodextrin

APT	Aptamer
PEG	Poly Ethylene Glycol
PHEP	Poly Hexyl Ethylene Phosphate
SF	Sorafenib
PDGFR	Platelet-Derived Growth Factor Receptor
FA	Folic Acid
FBX	Febuxostat
PEI	Polyethyleneimine
BSA	Bovine Serum Albumin
QA	Quinacrine
ETO	Etoposide
PHCL	PEGylated Histidine-grafted Chitosan-Lipoic acid
QDs	Quantum Dots
CsA	Cyclosporin
MSNCs	Mesoporous Silica Nanocarriers
TPGS	Tocopheryl Polyethylene Glycol 1000 Succinate
MNPs	Magnetic Iron Oxide Nanoparticles

Author details

Milad Rasouli[1*], Nadia Fallah[2] and Kostya (Ken) Ostrikov[3]

1 Institute for Plasma Research and Department of Physics, Kharazmi University, Tehran, Iran

2 Department of Cellular and Molecular Biology, Faculty of Biological Science, Kharazmi University, Tehran, Iran

3 School of Chemistry and Physics and Institute for Health and Biomedical Innovation, Queensland University of Technology, Brisbane QLD, Australia

*Address all correspondence to: miladrasouli@outlook.com

References

[1] Oudkerk, M., Liu, S., Heuvelmans, M.A. et al. Lung cancer LDCT screening and mortality reduction — evidence, pitfalls and future perspectives. Nat Rev Clin Oncol (2020). doi:10.1038/s41571-020-00432-6

[2] Dhawan, A., Nichol, D., Kinose, F. et al. Collateral sensitivity networks reveal evolutionary instability and novel treatment strategies in ALK mutated non-small cell lung cancer. Sci Rep 7, 1232 (2017). doi:10.1038/s41598-017-00791-8

[3] Xiaofeng Dai, Kateryna Bazaka, Derek J. Richard, Erik (Rik) W. Thompson, Kostya (Ken) Ostrikov, The Emerging Role of Gas Plasma in Oncotherapy, Trends in Biotechnology, Volume 36, Issue 11, 2018, Pages 1183-1198, ISSN 0167-7799, https://doi.org/10.1016/j.tibtech.2018.06.010

[4] Yan D, Wang Q, Adhikari M, Malyavko A, Lin L, Zolotukhin DB, Yao X, Kirschner M, Sherman JH, Keidar M. A physically triggered cell death via transbarrier cold atmospheric plasma cancer treatment. ACS Applied Materials & Interfaces. 2020 Jul 10;12(31):34548-63. DOI: 10.1021/acsami.0c06500

[5] Dai, X, Zhang, Z, Zhang, J, Ostrikov, K. Dosing: The key to precision plasma oncology. Plasma Process Polym. 2020; 17:e1900178. doi:10.1002/ppap.201900178

[6] Michael Keidar, Dayun Yan, Isak I. Beilis, Barry Trink, Jonathan H. Sherman, Plasmas for Treating Cancer: Opportunities for Adaptive and Self-Adaptive Approaches, Trends in Biotechnology, Volume 36, Issue 6, 2018, Pages 586-593, ISSN 0167-7799, doi:10.1016/j.tibtech.2017.06.013.

[7] Dai X, Bazaka K, Thompson E, Ostrikov K. Cold Atmospheric Plasma: A Promising Controller of Cancer Cell States, Cancers. MDPI AG; 2020 Nov 13;12(11):3360. Available from: http://dx.doi.org/10.3390/cancers12113360

[8] Peer, D., Karp, J., Hong, S. et al. Nanocarriers as an emerging platform for cancer therapy. Nature Nanotech 2, 751-760 (2007). doi:10.1038/nnano.2007.387

[9] Shi J, Kantoff PW, Wooster R, Farokhzad OC. Cancer nanomedicine: progress, challenges and opportunities. Nature Reviews Cancer. 2017 Jan;17(1):20. doi:10.1038/nrc.2016.108

[10] Jinjun Shi, Alexander R. Votruba, Omid C. Farokhzad, and Robert Langer, Nanotechnology in drug delivery and tissue engineering: from discovery to applications. Nano Letters 2010 10 (9), 3223-3230, DOI: 10.1021/nl102184c

[11] Liu, D, Szili, EJ, Ostrikov, K(K). Plasma medicine: Opportunities for nanotechnology in a digital age. Plasma Process Polym. 2020; 17:e2000097. doi:10.1002/ppap.202000097

[12] Dai X, Yu L, Zhao X, Ostrikov KK. Nanomaterials for oncotherapies targeting the hallmarks of cancer. Nanotechnology. 2020 Sep;31(39):392001. https://doi.org/10.1088/1361-6528/ab99f1

[13] Kaushik N, Kaushik N, Linh N, GhimireB,PengkitA,SornsakdanuphapJ, et al. Plasma and Nanomaterials: Fabrication and Biomedical Applications. Nanomaterials [Internet]. MDPI AG; 2019 Jan 14;9(1):98. DOI: 10.3390/nano9010098

[14] Kong MG, Keidar M, Ostrikov K. Plasmas meet nanoparticles—where synergies can advance the frontier of medicine. Journal of Physics D: Applied Physics. 2011 Apr

14;44(17):174018. https://doi.org/10.1088/0022-3727/44/17/174018

[15] Chen, F. F. & Chen, F. F. Erratum to: Introduction to Plasma Physics and Controlled Fusion. Introduction to Plasma Physics and Controlled Fusion (2018). doi:10.1007/978-3-319-22309-4_11

[16] Weltmann, K-D, Kolb, JF, Holub, M, et al. The future for plasma science and technology. Plasma Process Polym. 2019;16:e1800118, doi:10.1002/ppap.201800118

[17] Bekeschus, S, Favia, P, Robert, E, von Woedtke, T. White paper on plasma for medicine and hygiene: Future in plasma health sciences. Plasma Process Polym. 2019;16:e1800033, doi:10.1002/ppap.201800033

[18] Lu X, Naidis GV, Laroussi M, Reuter S, Graves DB, Ostrikov K. Reactive species in non-equilibrium atmospheric-pressure plasmas: Generation, transport, and biological effects. Physics Reports. 2016 May 4;630:1-84. https://doi.org/10.1016/j.physrep.2016.03.003

[19] von Woedtke T, Emmert S, Metelmann HR, Rupf S, Weltmann KD. Perspectives on cold atmospheric plasma (CAP) applications in medicine. Physics of Plasmas. 2020 Jul 13;27(7):070601. http://doi.org/10.1063/5.0008093

[20] Schmidt A, Bekeschus S. Redox for repair: cold physical plasmas and Nrf2 signaling promoting wound healing. Antioxidants. 2018 Oct;7(10):146. doi:10.3390/antiox7100146

[21] Kalyanaraman B. Teaching the basics of cancer metabolism: Developing antitumor strategies by exploiting the differences between normal and cancer cell metabolism. Redox biology. 2017 Aug 1;12:833-42. http://doi.org/10.1016/j.redox.2017.04.018

[22] Lopez-Lázaro M. Dual role of hydrogen peroxide in cancer: possible relevance to cancer chemoprevention and therapy. Cancer letters. 2007 Jul 8;252(1):1-8. http://doi.org/10.1016/j.canlet.2006.10.029

[23] Khlyustova, A., Labay, C., Machala, Z. et al. Important parameters in plasma jets for the production of RONS in liquids for plasma medicine: A brief review. Front. Chem. Sci. Eng. 13, 238-252 (2019). doi:10.1007/s11705-019-1801-8

[24] Bauer, G., Sersenová, D., Graves, D.B. et al. Cold Atmospheric Plasma and Plasma-Activated Medium Trigger RONS-Based Tumor Cell Apoptosis. Sci Rep 9, 14210 (2019). doi:10.1038/s41598-019-50291-0

[25] Bauer, G., Sersenová, D., Graves, D.B. et al. Dynamics of Singlet Oxygen-Triggered, RONS-Based Apoptosis Induction after Treatment of Tumor Cells with Cold Atmospheric Plasma or Plasma-Activated Medium. Sci Rep 9, 13931 (2019). doi:10.1038/s41598-019-50329-3

[26] Yan D, Sherman JH, Keidar M. Cold atmospheric plasma, a novel promising anti-cancer treatment modality. Oncotarget. 2017 Feb 28;8(9):15977. doi: 10.18632/oncotarget.13304

[27] Yan D, Talbot A, Nourmohammadi N, Sherman JH, Cheng X, Keidar M. Toward understanding the selective anticancer capacity of cold atmospheric plasma—A model based on aquaporins. Biointerphases. 2015 Dec 22;10(4):040801. DOI: https://doi.org/10.1116/1.4938020

[28] Van der Paal J, Neyts EC, Verlackt CC, Bogaerts A. Effect of lipid peroxidation on membrane permeability of cancer and normal cells subjected to oxidative stress. Chemical science. 2016;7(1):489-98. DOI: 10.1039/C5SC02311D

[29] Van der Paal, J., Verheyen, C., Neyts, E. et al. Hampering Effect of Cholesterol on the Permeation of Reactive Oxygen Species through Phospholipids Bilayer: Possible Explanation for Plasma Cancer Selectivity. Sci Rep 7, 39526 (2017). https://doi.org/10.1038/srep39526

[30] Bauer G. The synergistic effect between hydrogen peroxide and nitrite, two long-lived molecular species from cold atmospheric plasma, triggers tumor cells to induce their own cell death. Redox biology. 2019 Sep 1;26:101291. DOI: https://doi.org/10.1016/j.redox.2019.101291

[31] Bauer G. Intercellular singlet oxygen-mediated bystander signaling triggered by long-lived species of cold atmospheric plasma and plasma-activated medium. Redox biology. 2019 Sep 1;26:101301. DOI: https://doi.org/10.1016/j.redox.2019.101301

[32] Busco G, Robert E, Chettouh-Hammas N, Pouvesle JM, Grillon C. The emerging potential of cold atmospheric plasma in skin biology. Free Radical Biology and Medicine. 2020 Oct 8. https://doi.org/10.1016/j.freeradbiomed.2020.10.004

[33] Huang J, Chen W, Li H, Wang XQ, Lv GH, Khohsa ML, Guo M, Feng KC, Wang PY, Yang SZ. Deactivation of A549 cancer cells in vitro by a dielectric barrier discharge plasma needle. Journal of Applied Physics. 2011 Mar 1;109(5):053305. DOI: https://doi.org/10.1063/1.3553873

[34] Akhlaghi M, Rajaei H, Mashayekh AS, Shafiae M, Mahdikia H, Khani M, Hassan ZM, Shokri B. Determination of the optimum conditions for lung cancer cells treatment using cold atmospheric plasma. Physics of Plasmas. 2016 Oct 20;23(10):103512. DOI: https://doi.org/10.1063/1.4964899

[35] Karki SB, Yildirim-Ayan E, Eisenmann KM, Ayan H. Miniature dielectric barrier discharge nonthermal plasma induces apoptosis in lung cancer cells and inhibits cell migration. BioMed research international. 2017 Jan 24;2017. DOI: https://doi.org/10.1155/2017/8058307

[36] Kim JY, Ballato J, Foy P, Hawkins T, Wei Y, Li J, Kim SO. Apoptosis of lung carcinoma cells induced by a flexible optical fiber-based cold microplasma. Biosensors and Bioelectronics. 2011 Oct 15;28(1):333-8. https://doi.org/10.1016/j.bios.2011.07.039

[37] Keidar, M., Walk, R., Shashurin, A. et al. Cold plasma selectivity and the possibility of a paradigm shift in cancer therapy. Br J Cancer 105, 1295-1301 (2011). https://doi.org/10.1038/bjc.2011.386

[38] Ma, J, Zhang, H, Cheng, C, Shen, J, Bao, L, Han, W. Contribution of hydrogen peroxide to non-thermal atmospheric pressure plasma induced A549 lung cancer cell damage, Plasma Process Polym, 2017; 14:e1600162. https://doi.org/10.1002/ppap.201600162

[39] Joh, H., Choi, J., Kim, S. et al. Effect of additive oxygen gas on cellular response of lung cancer cells induced by atmospheric pressure helium plasma jet. Sci Rep 4, 6638 (2014). https://doi.org/10.1038/srep06638

[40] Karki SB, Gupta TT, Yildirim-Ayan E, Eisenmann KM, Ayan H. Investigation of non-thermal plasma effects on lung cancer cells within 3D collagen matrices. Journal of Physics D: Applied Physics. 2017 Jul 14;50(31):315401. https://doi.org/10.1088/1361-6463/aa7b10

[41] Yang Y, Li D, Li Y, Jiang Q, Sun R, Liu J, Wu F, Miao J, Ni L, Shi X, Huang C. Low-Temperature Plasma Suppresses Proliferation and Induces Apoptosis in Lung Cancer Cells by Regulating the miR-203a/BIRC5 Axis.

Onco Targets Ther. 2020;13:5145-5153, https://doi.org/10.2147/OTT.S244853

[42] Hongli Yu, Yonghong Wang, Saisai Wang, Xujing Li, Wentong Li, Dejun Ding, Xiaoming Gong, Michael Keidar, and Weifen Zhang, ACS Applied Materials & Interfaces 2018 10 (50), 43462-43471. DOI: 10.1021/acsami.8b16487

[43] Cheng, YJ., Lin, CK., Chen, CY. et al. Plasma-activated medium as adjuvant therapy for lung cancer with malignant pleural effusion. Sci Rep 10, 18154 (2020). https://doi.org/10.1038/s41598-020-75214-2

[44] Adachi T, Tanaka H, Nonomura S, Hara H, Kondo SI, Hori M. Plasma-activated medium induces A549 cell injury via a spiral apoptotic cascade involving the mitochondrial–nuclear network. Free Radical Biology and Medicine. 2015 Feb 1;79:28-44. https://doi.org/10.1016/j.freeradbiomed.2014.11.014

[45] Panngom, K., Baik, K., Nam, M. et al. Preferential killing of human lung cancer cell lines with mitochondrial dysfunction by nonthermal dielectric barrier discharge plasma. Cell Death Dis 4, e642 (2013). https://doi.org/10.1038/cddis.2013.168

[46] Ja Kim S, Min Joh H, Chung TH. Production of intracellular reactive oxygen species and change of cell viability induced by atmospheric pressure plasma in normal and cancer cells. Applied Physics Letters. 2013 Oct 7;103(15):153705. https://doi.org/10.1063/1.4824986

[47] Zhou R, Zhou R, Wang P, Xian Y, Mai-Prochnow A, Lu X, Cullen PJ, Ostrikov KK, Bazaka K. Plasma-activated water: generation, origin of reactive species and biological applications. Journal of Physics D: Applied Physics. 2020 May 19;53(30):303001. https://doi.org/10.1088/1361-6463/ab81cf

[48] Kumar N, Park JH, Jeon SN, Park BS, Choi EH, Attri P. The action of microsecond-pulsed plasma-activated media on the inactivation of human lung cancer cells. Journal of Physics D: Applied Physics. 2016 Feb 17;49(11):115401. https://doi.org/10.1088/0022-3727/49/11/115401

[49] Karki, S.B., Gupta, T.T., Yildirim-Ayan, E. et al. Miniature Non-thermal Plasma Induced Cell Cycle Arrest and Apoptosis in Lung Carcinoma Cells. Plasma Chem Plasma Process 40, 99-117 (2020). https://doi.org/10.1007/s11090-019-10037-2

[50] Hou, J., Ma, J., Yu, K.N. et al. Non-thermal plasma treatment altered gene expression profiling in non-small-cell lung cancer A549 cells. BMC Genomics 16, 435 (2015). https://doi.org/10.1186/s12864-015-1644-8

[51] Ma J, Yu KN, Cheng C, Ni G, Shen J, Han W. Targeting Nrf2-mediated heme oxygenase-1 enhances non-thermal plasma-induced cell death in non-small-cell lung cancer A549 cells. Archives of biochemistry and biophysics. 2018 Nov 15; 658:54-65. https://doi.org/10.1016/j.abb.2018.09.015

[52] Salvioni L, Rizzuto MA, Bertolini JA, Pandolfi L, Colombo M, Prosperi D. Thirty years of cancer nanomedicine: Success, frustration, and hope. Cancers. 2019 Dec;11(12):1855. https://doi.org/10.3390/cancers11121855

[53] Senapati, S., Mahanta, A.K., Kumar, S. et al. Controlled drug delivery vehicles for cancer treatment and their performance. Sig Transduct Target Ther. 2018; 3(7). https://doi.org/10.1038/s41392-017-0004-3

[54] Hans ML, Lowman AM. Biodegradable nanoparticles for drug delivery and targeting. Current Opinion in Solid State and Materials Science. 2002 Aug 1;6(4):319-27. https://doi.org/10.1016/S1359-0286(02)00117-1

[55] La-Beck NM, Gabizon AA. Nanoparticle interactions with the immune system: clinical implications for liposome-based cancer chemotherapy. Frontiers in immunology. 2017 Apr 6; 8:416. https://doi.org/10.3389/fimmu.2017.00416

[56] Lee JH, Yeo Y. Controlled drug release from pharmaceutical nanocarriers. Chemical engineering science. 2015 Mar 24; 125:75-84. https://doi.org/10.1016/j.ces.2014.08.046

[57] Kumari A, Yadav SK, Yadav SC. Biodegradable polymeric nanoparticles based drug delivery systems. Colloids and surfaces B: biointerfaces. 2010 Jan 1;75(1):1-8. https://doi.org/10.1016/j.colsurfb.2009.09.001

[58] Mohammadinejad R, Dehshahri A, Madamsetty VS, Zahmatkeshan M, Tavakol S, Makvandi P, Khorsandi D, Pardakhty A, Ashrafizadeh M, Afshar EG, Zarrabi A. In vivo gene delivery mediated by non-viral vectors for cancer therapy. Journal of Controlled Release. 2020 Sep 10; 325:249-75. https://doi.org/10.1016/j.jconrel.2020.06.038

[59] Mishra DK, Shandilya R, Mishra PK. Lipid based nanocarriers: a translational perspective. Nanomedicine: Nanotechnology, Biology and Medicine. 2018 Oct 1;14(7):2023-50. https://doi.org/10.1016/j.nano.2018.05.021

[60] Yingchoncharoen P, Kalinowski DS, Richardson DR. Lipid-based drug delivery systems in cancer therapy: what is available and what is yet to come. Pharmacological reviews. 2016 Jul 1;68(3):701-87. https://doi.org/10.1124/pr.115.012070

[61] Kabary DM, Helmy MW, Elkhodairy KA, Fang JY, Elzoghby AO. Hyaluronate/lactoferrin layer-by-layer-coated lipid nanocarriers for targeted co-delivery of rapamycin and berberine to lung carcinoma. Colloids and Surfaces B: Biointerfaces. 2018 Sep 1;169:183-94. https://doi.org/10.1016/j.colsurfb.2018.05.008

[62] Mahmoudi S, Ghorbani M, Sabzichi M, Ramezani F, Hamishehkar H, Samadi N. Targeted hyaluronic acid-based lipid nanoparticle for apigenin delivery to induce Nrf2-dependent apoptosis in lung cancer cells. Journal of Drug Delivery Science and Technology. 2019 Feb 1;49:268-76. https://doi.org/10.1016/j.jddst.2018.11.013

[63] Guo S, Zhang Y, Wu Z, Zhang L, He D, Li X, Wang Z. Synergistic combination therapy of lung cancer: Cetuximab functionalized nanostructured lipid carriers for the co-delivery of paclitaxel and 5-Demethylnobiletin. Biomedicine & Pharmacotherapy. 2019 Oct 1;118:109225. https://doi.org/10.1016/j.biopha.2019.109225

[64] Nan Y. Lung carcinoma therapy using epidermal growth factor receptor-targeted lipid polymeric nanoparticles co-loaded with cisplatin and doxorubicin. Oncology reports. 2019 Nov 1;42(5):2087-96. https://doi.org/10.3892/or.2019.7323

[65] Wang J, Su G, Yin X, Luo J, Gu R, Wang S, Feng J, Chen B. Non-small cell lung cancer-targeted, redox-sensitive lipid-polymer hybrid nanoparticles for the delivery of a second-generation irreversible epidermal growth factor inhibitor—Afatinib: In vitro and in vivo evaluation. Biomedicine & Pharmacotherapy. 2019 Dec 1;120:109493. https://doi.org/10.1016/j.biopha.2019.109493

[66] Xie X, Li Y, Zhao D, Fang C, He D, Yang Q, Yang L, Chen R, Tan Q, Zhang J. Oral administration of natural polyphenol-loaded natural polysaccharide-cloaked lipidic nanocarriers to improve efficacy against small-cell lung cancer. Nanomedicine:

Nanotechnology, Biology and Medicine. 2020 Oct 1;29:102261. https://doi.org/10.1016/j.nano.2020.102261

[67] Moro M, Di Paolo D, Milione M, Centonze G, Bornaghi V, Borzi C, Gandellini P, Perri P, Pastorino U, Ponzoni M, Sozzi G. Coated cationic lipid-nanoparticles entrapping miR-660 inhibit tumor growth in patient-derived xenografts lung cancer models. Journal of Controlled Release. 2019 Aug 28;308:44-56. https://doi.org/10.1016/j.jconrel.2019.07.006

[68] Ahuja R, Panwar N, Meena J, Singh M, Sarkar DP, Panda AK. Natural products and polymeric nanocarriers for cancer treatment: a review. Environmental Chemistry Letters. 2020 Jul 25:2021-2030. https://doi.org/10.1007/s10311-020-01056-z

[69] Venditti I. Morphologies and functionalities of polymeric nanocarriers as chemical tools for drug delivery: A review. Journal of King Saud University-Science. 2019 Jul 1;31(3):398-411. https://doi.org/10.1016/j.jksus.2017.10.004

[70] Abasian P, Ghanavati S, Rahebi S, Nouri Khorasani S, Khalili S. Polymeric nanocarriers in targeted drug delivery systems: A review. Polymers for Advanced Technologies. 2020 Dec;31(12):2939-54. https://doi.org/10.1002/pat.5031

[71] Riaz MK, Zhang X, Wong KH, Chen H, Liu Q, Chen X, Zhang G, Lu A, Yang Z. Pulmonary delivery of transferrin receptors targeting peptide surface-functionalized liposomes augments the chemotherapeutic effect of quercetin in lung cancer therapy. International journal of nanomedicine. 2019;14:2879. https://dx.doi.org/10.2147%2FIJN.S192219

[72] Chiang CW, Chuang EY. Biofunctional core-shell polypyrrole–polyethylenimine nanocomplex for a locally sustained photothermal with reactive oxygen species enhanced therapeutic effect against lung cancer. International journal of nanomedicine. 2019;14:1575. https://dx.doi.org/10.2147%2FIJN.S163299

[73] Gong, HY., Chen, YG., Yu, XS. et al. Co-delivery of Doxorubicin and Afatinib with pH-responsive Polymeric Nanovesicle for Enhanced Lung Cancer Therapy. Chin J Polym Sci. 2019;37:1224-1233. https://doi.org/10.1007/s10118-019-2272-6

[74] Vaidya B, Parvathaneni V, Kulkarni NS, Shukla SK, Damon JK, Sarode A, Kanabar D, Garcia JV, Mitragotri S, Muth A, upta V. Cyclodextrin modified erlotinib loaded PLGA nanoparticles for improved therapeutic efficacy against non-small cell lung cancer. International journal of biological macromolecules. 2019 Feb 1;122:338-47. https://doi.org/10.1016/j.ijbiomac.2018.10.181

[75] Zeng F, Xu B, Zhu H, Wu S, Liao G, Xie D, Huang L, Qiao G, Yang X, Zhou H. A cascade dual-targeted nanocarrier for enhanced alectinib delivery to ALK-positive lung cancer. Biomaterials science. 2020;8(22):6404-13. https://doi.org/10.1039/D0BM00970A

[76] hukla, S.K., Kulkarni, N.S., Farrales, P. et al. Sorafenib Loaded Inhalable Polymeric Nanocarriers against Non-Small Cell Lung Cancer. Pharm Res. 2020;37(67). https://doi.org/10.1007/s11095-020-02790-3

[77] Li W, Han F, Liu H, Niu X, Shi L. The synthesis of sulfate doped hydroxyapatite for enhanced drug loading and chemotherapeutic drug delivery towards lung cancer treatment. Ceramics International. 2020 Dec 15;46(18):28578-84. https://doi.org/10.1016/j.ceramint.2020.08.015

[78] Chen Y, Chen C, Zhang X, He C, Zhao P, Li M, Fan T, Yan R, Lu Y, Lee RJ, Khan MW. Platinum complexes of curcumin delivered by dual-responsive polymeric nanoparticles improve chemotherapeutic efficacy based on the enhanced anti-metastasis activity and reduce side effects. Acta Pharmaceutica Sinica B. 2020 Jun 1;10(6):1106-21. https://doi.org/10.1016/j.apsb.2019.10.011

[79] Alfaifi, M.Y., Shati, A.A., Elbehairi, S.E.I. et al. Anti-tumor effect of PEG-coated PLGA nanoparticles of febuxostat on A549 non-small cell lung cancer cells. 3 Biotech. 2020;10(133). https://doi.org/10.1007/s13205-020-2077-x

[80] Vaidya B, Kulkarni NS, Shukla SK, Parvathaneni V, Chauhan G, Damon JK, Sarode A, Garcia JV, Kunda N, Mitragotri S, Gupta V. Development of inhalable quinacrine loaded bovine serum albumin modified cationic nanoparticles: Repurposing quinacrine for lung cancer therapeutics. International Journal of Pharmaceutics. 2020 Mar 15;577:118995. https://doi.org/10.1016/j.ijpharm.2019.118995

[81] He W, Xiao W, Zhang X, Sun Y, Chen Y, Chen Q, Fang X, Du S, Sha X. Pulmonary-Affinity Paclitaxel Polymer Micelles in Response to Biological Functions of Ambroxol Enhance Therapeutic Effect on Lung Cancer. International Journal of Nanomedicine. 2020;15:779. https://dx.doi.org/10.2147%2FIJN.S229576

[82] Li F, Wang Y, Chen WL, Wang DD, Zhou YJ, You BG, Liu Y, Qu CX, Yang SD, Chen MT, Zhang XN. Co-delivery of VEGF siRNA and etoposide for enhanced anti-angiogenesis and anti-proliferation effect via multi-functional nanoparticles for orthotopic non-small cell lung cancer treatment. Theranostics. 2019;9(20):5886. https://dx.doi.org/10.7150%2Fthno.32416

[83] Zhang W, Xu W, Lan Y, He X, Liu K, Liang Y. Antitumor effect of hyaluronic-acid-modified chitosan nanoparticles loaded with siRNA for targeted therapy for non-small cell lung cancer. International Journal of Nanomedicine. 2019;14:5287. https://dx.doi.org/10.2147%2FIJN.S203113

[84] Zhang H, Yee D, Wang C. Quantum dots for cancer diagnosis and therapy: biological and clinical perspectives. 2008;3(1):83-91. https://doi.org/10.2217/17435889.3.1.83

[85] Zhao, MX., Zhu, BJ. The Research and Applications of Quantum Dots as Nano-Carriers for Targeted Drug Delivery and Cancer Therapy. Nanoscale Res Lett. 2016;11(207). https://doi.org/10.1186/s11671-016-1394-9

[86] Cai X, Luo Y, Zhang W, Du D, Lin Y. pH-Sensitive ZnO quantum dots–doxorubicin nanoparticles for lung cancer targeted drug delivery. ACS applied materials & interfaces. 2016 Aug 31;8(34):22442-50. https://doi.org/10.1021/acsami.6b04933

[87] Chen F, Zhang H, Jiang L, Wei W, Liu C, Cang S. Enhancing the cytotoxic efficacy of combined effect of doxorubicin and Cyclosporin encapsulated photoluminescent graphene dotted mesoporous nanoparticles against lung cancer cell-specific drug targeting for the nursing care of cancer patients. Journal of Photochemistry and Photobiology B: Biology. 2019 Sep 1;198:111578. https://doi.org/10.1016/j.jphotobiol.2019.111578

[88] Narayan R, Nayak UY, Raichur AM, Garg S. Mesoporous silica nanoparticles: A comprehensive review on synthesis and recent advances. Pharmaceutics. 2018 Sep;10(3):118. https://doi.org/10.3390/pharmaceutics10030118

[89] Cheng W, Liang C, Xu L, Liu G, Gao N, Tao W, Luo L, Zuo Y, Wang X, Zhang X, Zeng X. TPGS-functionalized

polydopamine-modified mesoporous silica as drug nanocarriers for enhanced lung cancer chemotherapy against multidrug resistance. Small. 2017 Aug;13(29):1700623. https://doi.org/10.1002/smll.201700623

[90] Hong, J., Murphy, A.B., Ashford, B. et al. Plasma-digital nexus: plasma nanotechnology for the digital manufacturing age. Rev. Mod. Plasma Phys. 4, 1 (2020). https://doi.org/10.1007/s41614-019-0039-8

[91] Kaushik NK, Kaushik N, Linh NN, Ghimire B, Pengkit A, Sornsakdanuphap J, Lee SJ, Choi EH. Plasma and nanomaterials: fabrication and biomedical applications. Nanomaterials. 2019 Jan;9(1):98. https://doi.org/10.3390/nano9010098

[92] Li W, Yu H, Ding D, Chen Z, Wang Y, Wang S, Li X, Keidar M, Zhang W. Cold atmospheric plasma and iron oxide-based magnetic nanoparticles for synergetic lung cancer therapy. Free Radical Biology and Medicine. 2019 Jan 1;130:71-81. https://doi.org/10.1016/j.freeradbiomed.2018.10.429